Embryos, Genes and Birth Defects

Embryos, Genes and Birth Defects

Edited by

PETER THOROGOOD

Institute of Child Health, London, UK

JOHN WILEY & SONS

Chichester · Weinheim · New York · Brisbane · Singapore · Toronto

Other Wiley Editorial Offices

John Wiley & Sons, Inc., 605 Third Avenue,
New York, NY 10158-0012, USA

VCH Verlagsgesellschaft mbH, Pappelallee 3,
D-69469 Weinheim, Germany

Jacaranda Wiley Ltd, 33 Park Road, Milton,
Queensland 4064, Australia

John Wiley & Sons (Asia) Pte Ltd, 2 Clementi Loop #02-01,
Jin Xing Distripark, Singapore 129809

John Wiley & Sons (Canada) Ltd, 22 Worcester Road,
Rexdale, Ontario M9W 1L1, Canada

Library of Congress Cataloging-in-Publication Data

Embryos, genes, and birth defects/edited by Peter Thorogood.
    p.   cm.
    Includes bibliographical references and index.
    ISBN 0-471-97196-0 (hbk : alk. paper). – ISBN 0-471-95565-5
(pbk.: alk paper)
    1. Abnormalities, Human. 2. Teratogenesis. 3. Embryology, Human.
I. Thorogood, Peter.
    [DNLM: 1. Embryo–abnormalities. 2. Gene Expression Regulation,
Developmental. QS 675 E535 1996]
QM691.E44 1996
616'.043–dc20
DNLM/DLC
for Library of Congress   96-46036
                                                            CIP

British Library Catologuing in Publication data

A catalogue record for this book is available from the British Library

ISBN   0-471-97196-0 (hardback)
       0-471-95565-5 (paperback)
Typeset in 10/12 Times from the author's disks by Mathematical Composition Setters, Salisbury, Wiltshire
Printed and bound in Great Britain by Bookcraft (Bath) Ltd, Midsomer Norton
This book is printed on acid-free paper responsibly manufactured from sustainable forestation, for
which at least two trees are planted for each one used for paper production.

Contents

continued

List of Contributors

Rudi Balling
Institut für Säugetiergenetik, GSF Forschungszentrum Neuherberg, Neuherberg, Germany

Michael Baraitser
Mothercare Unit of Molecular Genetics and Fetal Medicine, Institute of Child Health, 30 Guilford Street, London WC1N 1EH, UK

Nigel A. Brown
Department of Anatomy and Developmental Biology, St George's Hospital Medical School, Cranmer Terrace, London SW17 0RE, UK

Andrew J. Copp
Neural Development Unit, Institute of Child Health, 30 Guilford Street, London WC1N 1EH, UK

Susanne Dietrich
Department of Developmental Neurobiology, UMDS Guy's Hospital, London SE1 9RT, UK

Patrizia Ferretti
Developmental Biology Unit, Institute of Child Health, 30 Guilford Street, London WC1N 1EH, UK

Lowell A. Goldsmith
Department of Dermatology, University of Rochester School of Medicine and Dentistry, 601 Elmwood Avenue, Box 697, Rochester, New York 14642, USA

Michèle Kedinger
INSERM unité 381, 3 avenue Molière, 67200-Strasbourg, France

Michael Kessel
Max-Planck-Institut für biophysikalische Chemie, Abteilung Molekulare Zellbiologie, Am Fassberg, D-37077 Göttingen, Germany

Margaret L. Kirby
Developmental Biology Program & Heart Development Group, Institute of Molecular Medicine and Genetics, Medical College of Georgia, Augusta, GA 30912-2640, USA

Don Newgreen
The Murdoch Institute, Royal Children's Hospital, Flemington Road, Melbourne, Victoria, Australia 3052

Anne Reeves Haake
Department of Dermatology, University of Rochester School of Medicine and Dentistry, 601 Elmwood Avenue, Box 697, Rochester, New York 14642, USA

Peter J. Scambler
Molecular Medicine Unit, Institute of Child Health, 30 Guilford Street, London WC1N 1EH, UK

Irma Thesleff
Institute of Dentistry & Institute of Biotechnology, FIN-00014 University of Helsinki, Helsinki, Finland

Peter Thorogood
Developmental Biology Unit, Institute of Child Health, 30 Guilford Street, London WC1N 1EH, UK

Cheryll Tickle
Department of Anatomy and Developmental Biology, University College London, Medawar Building, Gower Street, London W1E 6BT, UK

Robin M. Winter
Mothercare Unit of Clinical Genetics and Fetal Medicine, Institute of Child Health, 30 Guilford Street, London WC1N 1EH, UK

Adrian S. Woolf
Developmental Biology Unit, Institute of Child Health, 30 Guilford Street, London WC1N 1EH, UK

Preface

This book has a single purpose. It is to provide, in an intellectually accessible and concise form, an overview of contemporary understanding of the mechanisms of embryonic development, as they pertain to dysmorphogenesis or the generation of birth defects. In order to do so we will explore a variety of systems and strategic approaches to analysis, and the layout of the book is designed to facilitate this. The first six chapters cover selected modern strategies of analysis and introduce some of the major themes. The subsequent nine chapters, all of which are structured according to a common pattern, review current knowledge of developmental mechanisms in those organ systems for which there has been particular progress in our understanding. Each of these 'systems' chapters presents an agenda for future research directions. It is perhaps necessary to point out that we do not attempt to cover the topics of inherited metabolic disease or those syndromes where the phenotype is exclusively behavioural; the emphasis in this volume is largely on physical birth defects.

Recognition of the need for a book of this type has had a gradual gestation. Vague thoughts on the form that such a book might take have been brought sharply into focus through discussion with my immediate colleagues at the Institute of Child Health: Andrew Copp, Patrizia Ferretti and Adrian Woolf. It is my pleasure to be able to acknowledge with gratitude their contributions not only as chapter authors but also through our various research interactions and the general support provided as we went about our everyday tasks of running busy research teams. The image of the human embryo on the front cover was provided by Rachel Moore and Simon Brown. Finally, my editor at John Wiley & Sons Ltd, Dr Sally Betteridge, and her assistant, Lisa Tickner, have guided the project to completion with wisdom, common sense, but most of all with patience! Thank you.

Peter Thorogood
Institute of Child Health

1 The Relationship Between Genotype and Phenotype: Some Basic Concepts

PETER THOROGOOD

Developmental Biology Unit, Institute of Child Health, London, UK

Up to 2% of live births display some kind of major abnormality. Actual incidences may vary according to locality, culture, ethnicity and the efficiency of recognition and reporting. If minor abnormalities are included, then the incidence is nearer to 5%. In the Western world, birth defects constitute the greatest single cause of infant mortality and have a major impact on national health care budgets (Sever et al, 1993). Most books published on birth defects, or **dysmorphology**, concentrate on developmental pathology, clinical genetics, syndromology or the consequences for health care of the affected newborn, but neglect to discuss, in anything other than superficial detail, the mechanisms whereby a particular abnormality might have come about. At the same time, there has been a tremendous increase in our understanding of the molecular, genetic and cellular mechanisms underlying normal development, emerging largely from work on animal model systems. Moreover, it is now apparent that many of the mechanisms of development, and indeed some of the critical regulatory genes involved, have been highly conserved. Thus, a significant proportion of this new knowledge is directly applicable and relevant to human development. However, to date, this increased understanding has not been communicated in any comprehensive way to the medical community involved in birth defects. The consequence is that there is a conceptual gulf between the average clinician's understanding of how particular defects come about and the developmental biologist's appreciation, now profoundly increased, of the actual or potential causal mechanism(s).This book is designed to bridge that gulf by providing the reader with a concise and 'accessible' overview of contemporary understanding of the mechanisms of embryonic development, as they pertain to **dysmorphogenesis**, or the generation of birth defects. The intention is to provide the reader with a basic understanding of how contemporary developmental biology is providing new paradigms for the study of dysmorphology.

In this introductory chapter some basic precepts and concepts are presented and explained. For a comprehensive introduction to embryonic development per se, the reader is referred to any one of several excellent publications that already exist (e.g. Alberts et al, 1989; Gilbert, 1991). What this chapter attempts to provide is the information that might be necessary for a clinician, or advanced

Embryos, Genes and Birth Defects. Edited by P. Thorogood.
© 1997 John Wiley & Sons Ltd.

student specializing in paediatric medicine, to understand and appreciate in context what follows. In that sense an element of unorthodoxy might be discerned by some readers. However, I hope that this rationale will be justified as the reader progresses through the book.

THE RELATIONSHIP BETWEEN GENOTYPE AND PHENOTYPE

The term **genotype** is generally used to refer to the genetic make-up or constitution of an individual organism, be it virus, fruit fly or human. In contrast, we use the word **phenotype** to cover the form and functioning of an individual, to the extent that it may encompass metabolism and behaviour (and thus we can refer to 'behavioural phenotypes'). The word genotype is subtly but distinctly different from the term **genome**, which refers not to the totality of genes in an individual cell but to the array of genes in a complete haploid set of genes characteristic for that species. In this sense, a genome is a species-specific concept whereas genotype is a concept applying to an individual of the species in question.

The complexity of the phenotype reflects largely but not entirely the complexity of the genotype. However, there is not necessarily a simple and direct relationship since genome size and genome complexity are rather different entities. Overall genome size, in terms of DNA, is to some extent determined by the relative proportion of non-coding sequences contained within it. Thus, some plant, insect and amphibian species contain far more total DNA in their genomes than does *Homo sapiens*, even though they are phenotypically simpler and contain fewer genes. (Indeed, some amphibian species contain up to 9×10^{11} nucleotide bases per haploid genome as opposed to the 3×10^9 characteristic of mammalian species, including humans; Alberts et al, 1989.) Much of this is thought to represent a greater than normal proportion of non-coding, repetitive sequences. If we consider genome complexity in terms of the number of genes present, then a more systematic relationship emerges. In simple organisms, such as viruses, the limited number of genes in the genome can be, and in some cases has been, calculated. However, for more complex multicellular organisms gene number is usually an estimate and the size of these estimates has changed as our understanding of genomic organization has evolved. Currently, *Drosophila melanogaster*, the fruit fly, is thought to contain some 15 000 genes in its genome whereas the genome of *Homo sapiens* is thought to comprise approximately 50 000–100 000. However, even this latter set of figures is a remarkably crude estimate and likely to be revised extensively over the coming years, as data accrue from the mapping of the human genome.

Whereas **gene mapping** refers to identification of the chromosomal location of an individual gene, **genome mapping** is a programme of research designed to identify the chromosomal location of all genes in the genome of a particular species. Although it is the international Human Genome Project that has received wide media attention, it should be noted that genome mapping projects for other species, particularly those of economically important food species such as cow, pig and chicken, are also currently under way (Burt et al, 1995). The mapping of individual genes, or of loci or of candidate gene loci, means that chromosomal 'maps' of congenital abnormality can be drawn up (Wilkie et al, 1994; and see Chapters 2 and 3) whereby the location of genes, in which mutation produces a particular dysmorphology or inherited metabolic disease, can be displayed (Figure 1.1).

At this point we should ask ourselves what kind of information is encoded within the genes. Are the genes really the 'blueprint' to which they are often analogized? A blueprint implies some kind of descriptive specification. Is that indeed how the genome is organized? In fact, the information content of genes is one-dimensionally complex, since it is specified by the nature of the linear sequence of nucleotide bases along the DNA molecule. In dramatic contrast, the phenotype is three-dimensionally complex (and four-dimensionally complex, if we include dynamic phenomena such as metabolism and homeostasis rather than just morphology); yet the linear nucleotide sequence itself conveys no sense of what the phenotype might look like. To appreciate just how phenotypic complexity might be generated we have to move away from the rather dated

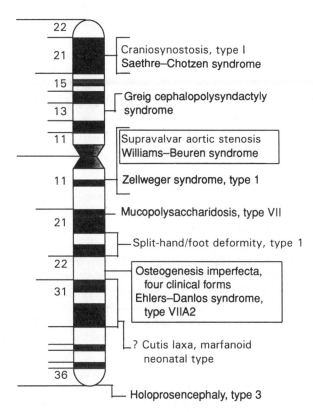

Figure 1.1 Congenital malformation loci for human chromosome 7. (After Wilkie et al, 1994; and see Chapter 2)

PRESUMED BY CLADISTS & ATOMIZERS

analogy of a descriptive specification and think of the genome and its implementation as a **generative programme**. The more appropriate and meaningful analogy of origami has been proposed to illustrate the characteristics of a generative programme (Wolpert, 1991). Here, the instructions for creating a topologically complex shape from a sheet of paper contain within them no description of the final outcome. The complexity is generated progressively by implementing those instructions, which may in themselves be very simple even though the outcome is complex. In this way, the genome, or at least the developmentally significant parts of it, can be seen as **assembly rules** for building an embryo.

In one sense, genes 'simply' encode proteins. Transcription of a gene produces a message that is translated from the 4-letter alphabet (nucleotides) of the nucleic acids to the approximately 20-letter alphabet (amino acids) of the proteins, by virtue of the genetic code. The primary structure of a protein, i.e. the linear sequence of amino acids, together with any post-translational modifications, determines its secondary and tertiary structure. Proteins endow cells with properties such as characteristic metabolisms, behaviour, polarity, adhesiveness and receptivity to signals (Figure 1.2) and it is this functional level that marks the implementation of those assembly rules. Within the increasingly multicellular embryo, cell interactions and inductions are initiated, cell lineages are established, and morphogenesis, growth and histogenesis proceed. Thus, interactions of proteins, of cells and of tissues during development generate progressively higher-order complexity (Figure 1.2), from the one-dimensional complexity of the genotype and primary protein structure to the three-dimensionally complex phenotype. Embryonic development is therefore a typical generative programme. From a limited range of fundamental cell properties, an almost infinite range of complex phenotypes can be built simply by deploying these cell properties in varying ways. The diverse range of phenotypic form across extant and extinct species bears witness to the morphogenetic power of these basic cell properties over an evolutionary time-scale.

Thus, it is the morphogenetic potential of cell properties and the mechanisms of embryonic development that causally link genotype and phenotype. And from this brief and perhaps simplistic rationalization, one can see that during development there will be significant, higher-order events taking place in the absence of direct genetic control but which are themselves the inevitable consequences of genetic specification (Figure 1.2, from the level of 'cell properties' upwards). This class of phenomena is sometimes described as epigenetic and, clearly, much morphological complexity is generated within this so-called **epigenetic domain** (Alberch, 1982; McLachlan, 1986).

Developmental biologists are interested in defining assembly rules and elucidating their operation at tissue, cellular and molecular/genetic levels. To understand dysmorphogenesis it is necessary to clarify what happens when certain assembly rules are either mis-specified or wrongly interpreted and a birth defect results. Clearly, understanding a particular birth defect involves much more than simply identifying a mutated gene or an environmental teratogen. It requires knowledge of the consequences of these on the mechanisms operating

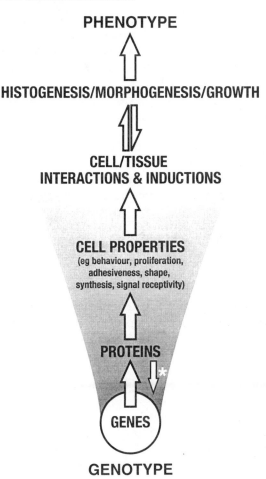

Figure 1.2 Causal relationship between genotype and phenotype. Higher-order complexity is generated progressively by the interaction of proteins, of cells and of tissues during development. The asterisked 'return' arrow between genes and proteins represents the controlling role on gene expression of transcription factors encoded by regulatory genes

within the embryo, an understanding of how the generative programme has been perturbed and how that produces an abnormal phenotype. Furthermore, just as an understanding of normal development can help clarify abnormal development, so analysis of abnormal development can sometimes throw light on hitherto unknown aspects of normal mechanisms.

Before leaving this topic, it should be noted that in Figure 1.2 there is feedback indicated from proteins to genes (see reverse arrow). This reflects the fact that the role of some proteins is to bind to DNA, typically in a highly sequence-specific manner. Genes that encode such proteins are referred to as **regulatory genes** and the proteins themselves known as **transcription factors** since they control (either up-regulate or down-regulate) transcriptional activity of the gene to which they have bound. In essence, genes work in hierarchies, with regulatory genes controlling the expression of 'downstream' genes and with elements of 'cross-talk' between regulatory genes themselves. The definition of such genetic cascades and signalling pathways is a very topical issue in contemporary developmental biology and this is reflected by the prominence given to it by many of the contributors to this volume. Such genes are, of course, pivotally important in the normal life of the cell, in its synthetic and metabolic activity, homeostasis and proliferation, but during embryonic development they have multiple and crucial roles in determining cell fate. Although many of the genes identified to date as being involved in birth defects encode enzymes or structural proteins, it is now emerging that some families of regulatory genes are also directly implicated in dysmorphogenesis (see later).

Having discussed some aspects of the genotype/phenotype relationship, it is now appropriate to point out that it can be simplistic to always interpret dysmorphogenesis on the basis of a 'one gene : one (dysmorphic) phenotype' model. It is now clear that, in some cases, a diversity of phenotypes can emerge from mutations in a single gene, each disease or dysmorphic phenotype reflecting a different mutation within that gene. Thus, different mutations in the receptor tyrosine kinase gene, RET, can result in familial medullary thyroid carcinoma, multiple endocrine neoplasia types 2A and 2B (all of which accords with its original recognition as an oncogene) and in Hirschsprung's disease, a developmental anomaly of the gut (reviewed by van Heyningen, 1994). This last disorder appears to be the consequence of a failure of RET-expressing neural crest cells to migrate normally and establish a parasympathetic innervation to the gut. The thyroid cancer-associated syndromes all result from mutations causing specific amino-acid substitutions that apparently alter the functionality of the receptor tyrosine kinase encoded by RET (i.e. gain-of-function mutations that may lead to hyperplasia of the RET-expressing tissues). In contrast, the Hirschsprung mutations comprise deletions and a loss of function. The phenotype can be explained as due to **haploinsufficiency**, whereby a threshold sensitivity to absence of 50% of the gene product (due to a mutated allele) is sufficient to perturb the development of the cells normally expressing that particular gene. In this case, it is the neural crest progenitors of the gut parasympathetic neurones that are affected, leaving other RET-expressing cell populations in the embryo apparently unscathed due to tissue-specific differences in the threshold sensitivity (van Heyningen, 1994; and see Chapter 9).

But, of course, not all birth defects are necessarily genetic in origin and various aetiological categories can be recognized:

- chromosomal anomalies (e.g. trisomies, translocations)
- polygenic disorders
- single gene mutations
- environmental/teratogenic factors
- multifactorial aetiology
- unknown aetiology

Each of these six categories presents its own set of problems in determining how a particular birth defect is generated (see Chapters 2, 3 and 6). It might be argued that events occurring within the epigenetic domain referred to earlier can be extended to **environmental influences** on development. The embryo does not occupy a completely protected and privileged environment and, in some respects, is as open to influences from its environment as the neonate, juvenile or adult. Indeed, the recent recognition that the intrauterine experience of the fetus, as determined by maternal nutritional or hormonal status, is pivotal in determining later susceptibility to a number of adult diseases such as diabetes and coronary heart disease (reviewed by Barker, 1995) is a prime example of this.

Clearly, the phenotype, be it adult or embryonic, is always the product of the combined effects of genetic and environmental influences (Sykes, 1993), but the relative contributions of each can differ for each aspect of the phenotype (Figure 1.3). Thus, Down syndrome, as a trisomy disorder, reflects a condition that is 100% genetic, whereas a neural tube defect such as spina bifida may have a strong environmental component in its aetiology, coupled with a possible genetic predisposition in some cases (reviewed by Marsh, 1994).

Even though the majority of birth defects have a genetic component, the extent of interaction between genotype and environment is typically ill understood and, in research studies, often neglected. Thus, the majority of animal studies assessing teratogenicity and reproductive toxicity of environmental factors have failed to take into account the different genotypes of the various strains of animal species used (discussed by Copp, 1994). Yet it appears that there exist genes which, in ways not yet understood, increase susceptibility to environmental teratogens. We may conclude that, in elucidating the complex relationship between genotype and embryonic phenotype, whether it be in the context of normal development or dysmorphogenesis, environmental factors may sometimes be critical (see Chapter 5).

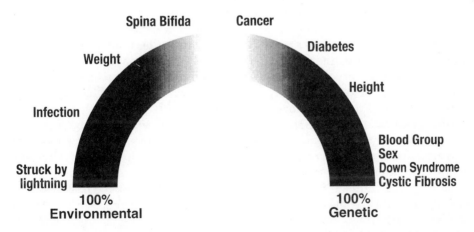

Figure 1.3 Interplay between environmental and genetic factors in the determination of phenotype. The relative importance of each will vary according to the particular phenotype, or aspect of phenotype, under consideration. (After Sykes, 1993)

THE ROLE OF 'MODEL SYSTEMS'

To understand the mechanisms of development inevitably means dismantling and/or perturbing the embryo in some way. Very little has ever been learnt of mechanisms by simply observing embryonic development. Traditionally, developmental biologists dismantle and reassemble embryos, or parts of embryos, at the level of gene, cell, tissue or organ. In this way we learn how the system responds to perturbation, and through that we can elucidate the functional role of the component parts, sometimes down to the level of an individual nucleotide base within a DNA codon. For example, a change in a single nucleotide in the *bicoid* gene of *Drosophila* will actually reverse the anteroposterior axis of the embryo (Fronhöfer and Nüsslein-Volhard, 1986; Struhl et al, 1989).

Recombinant DNA technology has now brought an unparalleled precision and finesse to developmental analysis and perturbation strategies. Thus, **transgenic technology** (see Chapter 4) can be considered as the latest and most sophisticated of perturbation strategies, following in the great tradition of experimental perturbation started in the nineteenth century with the emergence of Experimental Embryology, epitomized by the German *Entwicklungsmechanik* ('developmental mechanics') school established by Wilhelm Roux and colleagues. However, it is important to comment that molecular biology as it exists now has not rendered traditional experimental embryology redundant. The molecular biology mono-culture that some feared 10 to 15 years ago has not prevailed and what we see emerging today, and which is well reflected in the following chapters, is a pragmatism in which molecular approaches are creatively integrated with cellular and tissular approaches. For instance, a well-designed 'cut 'n paste' tissue grafting experiment can generate results with profound implications at the molecular level (see, for example, some of the grafting experiments described in Chapter 7), and can itself direct further analysis at the molecular level.

This theme of perturbational analysis to reveal mechanisms means that the human embryo is generally not a system of choice, at least not after the 14-day limit set by the regulating authorities in Britain, and manifest in the Human Fertilization and Embryology Act, 1990 (and see Burn and Strachan, 1995: Table 1). Most dysmorphogenesis is likely to have its inception during the major stages of morphogenesis and organogenesis, starting with neurulation during the fourth week in the human embryo (Larsen, 1993). Disruptions earlier than that are likely to result in spontaneous abortion and be lost; indeed, it has been estimated that about 15% of all human pregnancies end as spontaneous abortions after implantation (Warburton and Fraser, 1964).

Nevertheless, human fetal tissues are being used in biomedical research, particularly in the context of somatic gene therapy, fetal cell transplantation, haematopoietic stem cell transplantation and fetal organ transplantation (reviewed by Reed et al, 1995). However, such research programmes almost always use developmentally late fetal material, which is of little if any use in studying embryonic expression of genes implicated in birth defects. For this specific purpose, **human embryo banks** are currently being established (reviewed by Burn and Strachan, 1995), using material obtained from terminations and collected with full ethical approval. The first reports on expression of genes causally involved in dysmorphogenesis are now beginning to appear (e.g. Duke et al, 1995; and see Chapter 10) and the use of such data in the long-term development of preventive and therapeutic clinical strategies is likely to escalate over the next few years.

However, in order to study developmental mechanisms during the crucial stages of morphogenesis and organogenesis we are, of necessity, obliged to use **animal model systems**. In Chapters 7 to 15 you will find reference to work using embryonic systems as diverse as zebrafish, *Xenopus*, chick and mouse. Are we to view these simply as models or research surrogates for the human embryo (see discussion by Monk, 1994)? In fact, most developmental research is driven by reasons of scholarship, and animal models are more typically studied for their own intrinsic interest, in the context of comparative biology and evolution (Bard, 1993). Nevertheless, several essential concepts that have significantly enhanced our understanding of human dysmorphology have emerged from analysis of animal model systems; the Developmental Field Concept, as applied to dysmorphogenesis (Opitz, 1985), and chromosomal imprinting (Monk, 1994; see Chapter 2) are two obvious examples. However, when animal model systems are seen as 'research surrogates' for the human embryo and fetus in the sense that extrapolations are made, we must ask ourselves to what extent is this justified?

THE CHANGING CONCEPT OF HOMOLOGY

For many years, developmental biologists, if challenged, have sought to justify the use of animal model systems by virtue of homology of form. This is likely to have been based loosely upon the a-priori argument that, at least in early development, phenotypic similarities between human and non-human vertebrate species must reflect equivalence of the underlying generative mechanism. However, only slowly has evidence for such assumptions about homology of mechanism begun to accumulate. Perhaps one of the clearest early demonstrations of this related to the zone of polarizing activity (ZPA): the region of a limb bud which, by release of a diffusible morphogen, polarizes the distal part of the growing limb and controls the anteroposterior pattern of digits (see Chapter 7). It has been found that the ZPA taken from a human limb bud will, when assayed by grafting ectopically into a chick embryo wing bud, display the same activity as the equivalent region of a chick bud. Extra digits are formed in a predictable and organized fashion by the host, demonstrating that irrespective of the graft species, chick host cells recognize the ZPA signal and respond accordingly (Fallon and Crosby, 1977). In other words, there is an equivalence of mechanism in the building of this particular bit of anatomy. Although this example deals with just a small part of the body plan (digit specification), it can be seen as exemplifying a widely held belief that similar equivalences exist at the mechanistic level in the building of much of the anatomy or, at least, that portion of it which is characteristically and uniquely 'vertebrate' in character.

This type of assumption has been cautiously held for a number of years and, in a rather piecemeal and limited fashion, evidence gradually accumulated to give it some justification. However, it has become clear in the last few years that the concept of homology is underpinned by an amazing degree of conservation of both gene sequence and function (reviewed by Scott, 1994). So fundamental is this to our understanding of the genotype/phenotype relationship and to our interpretation of data from model systems, that it is necessary to deal with the topic at some length.

The existence of *Drosophila* mutants in which body parts are transformed into recognizable structures but develop at an inappropriate site, the so-called **homeotic mutants**, has been known since the nineteenth century when the phenomenon of **homeosis** was first discovered. Certain unidentified genes were thought to be involved in the specification of the segmented body plan of *Drosophila*, with mutation resulting in mis-specification of particular body parts. Cloning and sequencing revealed that the homeotic genes are in fact regulatory genes and contain a highly conserved motif, the **homeobox** (McGinnis et al, 1984), encoding a DNA-binding domain that subsequently became known as the **homeodomain**. Further analysis of homeobox-containing genes confirmed their role in morphogenetic specification and revealed a complex and hierarchical genetic control of the body plan in this arthropod (reviewed by Akam et al, 1994). The cloning of these genes provided probes with which to screen the genomes of other species, and screening revealed a surprising degree of conservation, with homologous genes being found in a very wide and diverse range of species examined. The largest and best known of these homeobox-containing gene families are the **Hox genes** of which there are 38, organized in four clusters on different chromosomes in all vertebrates including humans. Sequence homology and position within each cluster is such that derivation of each gene can be traced from a single ancestral cluster similar to the **HOM-C complex** in *Drosophila*. Excellent reviews of the organization, evolution and functional roles of Hox genes have been published elsewhere (McGinnis and Krumlauf, 1992; Krumlauf, 1994) and accounts of their role in specification of major features of the vertebrate body plan are given here in Chapters 7, 10 and 13.

Although these genes and others like them have only been identified in vertebrate genomes by virtue of their sequence homology with their *Drosophila* counterparts (remember that *Drosophila* probes were used in the screening), conservation of gene sequence is only one aspect of this remarkable evolutionary story. If there is truly homology of function, then we might expect conservation of expression domains of the gene(s) in question across a range of species, and this is indeed often found. The most rigorous test, however, has to be an operational one in which genes are moved into the genome of another and distant species, preferably into individuals in which the homologue has been inactivated. Will the introduced 'foreign' gene be switched on in the correct spatiotemporal pattern and will it function to produce a normal embryo?

Homeobox-containing genes provide a number of examples in which these three criteria of sequence homology, equivalence of expression domain and **functional homology** are satisfied (reviewed by Krumlauf, 1994; Scott, 1994). Thus, the regulatory element of the *Drosophila* homeotic gene, *Deformed*, can be substituted for the equivalent region of its mouse homologue and support normal embryonic development (Awgulewitsch and Jacobs, 1992). The mouse gene, *Hoxb-6*, can be moved into the *Drosophila* embryo and specify normal thoracic segments (Malicki et al, 1990) and even the regulatory element of a human Hox gene, *HOXB4*, is expressed rostrally and supports head development when introduced into *Drosophila* (Malicki et al, 1992). Finally, we should not assume that such exchanges only operate between species with segmented body plans, no matter how divergent they may be; recently it has been shown that equivalent functional homology even exists between the Hox genes of *Drosophila* and those of the unsegmented nematode worm, *Caenorhabditis elegans* (Hunter and Kenyon, 1995).

The existence of such amazing functional homology might suggest that there has been some conservation of downstream target genes for the homeoproteins. But how would this degree of conservation of homeobox gene function across a wide range of species correlate with the diverse range of phenotypic form displayed by these species? In other words, how do we reconcile functional homology, and all that that entails, with the evolution of the disparate body plans displayed by mammals and insects, for example? Such questions are currently unresolved but various possibilities such as homeoproteins acquiring new targets, homeobox genes changing expression domains, changes in the function of downstream target genes and the emergence of new modes of regulation, are all under consideration (Kenyon, 1994; Manak and Scott, 1994). Meanwhile, similar levels of conservation for genes involved in major morphogenetic events are being discovered, with functional homology apparently being retained by other key regulatory genes, such as *goosecoid* and *Brachyury*, controlling the very different modes of gastrulation across species as diverse as zebrafish, *Xenopus*, chick and mouse (Beddington and Smith, 1993; De Robertis et al, 1994).

However, it is not just regulatory genes that display such conservation of sequence, expression domain and function. It is rapidly emerging that genes encoding a number of secreted molecules involved in signalling between cells have been similarly conserved. Genes homologous to the *Drosophila hedgehog* gene family (so named because of the 'spiny' appearance of the mutant larvae) encode secreted proteins that appear to have a pivotal role in patterning a number of structures in vertebrates (reviewed by Fietz et al, 1994). The product of *sonic hedgehog* (*shh*) has a major role in notochord induction of the ventral floor plate of the neural tube (e.g. Roelink et al, 1994; and see Chapter 8). A parallel signalling role for this secreted protein is seen in limb development. Thus, *shh* is expressed in the posterior region of both fin (zebrafish) and limb buds (chick and mouse) where it is thought to be active in establishing pattern across the anteroposterior axis of the bud and an active component of the ZPA (see earlier). Ectopic expression of this gene in the anterior part of the chick limb bud produces duplication of anterior structures paralleling the mirror-image duplication of the anterior wing compartment in *Drosophila* resulting from ectopic *hedgehog* expression (Fietz et al, 1994). Functional homology is even maintained amongst some of the other signalling molecules thought to be downstream from the hedgehog proteins, such as *decapentaplegic* (*dpp*) in *Drosophila*, and the related *transforming growth factor-β* (*TGF-β*) gene family in vertebrates (reviewed by Hogan et al, 1994), and the proteins with which they interact during specification of dorsoventral pattern in the neural primordium (Holley et al, 1995).

The full extent of regulatory gene involvement in birth defects is unclear at present (Redline et al, 1992) but one particular regulatory gene family not only displays functional homology but also has been directly implicated in dysmorphogenesis and neoplasia (reviewed by Read, 1995). Most members of the **Pax gene** family appear to be expressed early on in the development of the nervous system but their function and downstream target genes remain unknown. Table 1.1 lists the human syndromes and mouse mutant phenotypes associated with each member of the family (from Read, 1995). Thus, loss-of-function mutations in *PAX3* and *PAX6* are responsible for Waardenburg syndrome type I and aniridia respectively; haploinsufficiency is assumed to be responsible. Not

Table 1.1 Classification of the nine humans *PAX* genes into families of paralogous genes (after Read, 1995)

Gene	Location	PB	OP	HB	Loss-of-function phenotype	Gain-of-function phenotype
PAX1	20p11	+	+	–	Mouse: *undulated* Human: ?	?
PAX9	14q12	+	+	–	?	?
PAX2	1–q25	+	+	(–)	Mouse[a]: *Krd* Human: kidney and retinal problems	Mouse: abnormal kidney development Human: role in Wilms' tumour?
PAX5 (*BSAP*)	9p13	+	+	(–)	Mouse[a]: B-cell and brain abnormalities	Human: role in astrocytoma?
PAX8	2q12–q14	+	+	(–)	?	Human: role in Wilms' tumour?
PAX3	2q35	+	+	+	Mouse: *Splotch* Human: WS1, WS3, craniofacial– deafness–hand syndrome	Human: rhabdomyosarcoma
PAX7	1p36	+	+	+	?	?
PAX4	7q22–qter	+	–	+	?	?
PAX6	11p13	+	–	+	Mouse: *Small eye* Human: aniridia, Peter's anomaly, cataract	?

Genes within a family contain similar structural elements (PB, paired box; OP, octapeptide; HB, homeobox), show strong sequence homology and have similar though not identical patterns of expression in the embryo.
[a] Phenotypes of transgenic mice.

all sites of gene expression are necessarily affected in each syndrome and this is thought to reflect, at least in part, differential sensitivity by different tissues to the amount of Pax gene product present.

From Table 1.1 it can also be seen that the mouse homologue for the *Aniridia/PAX6* gene has been cloned and turns out to be a gene formerly known as *Small eye*, since a loss-of-function mutation produced a microphthalmic phenotype. Recent sequencing revealed that these two genes both show a high sequence homology with the *eyeless (ey)* gene of *Drosophila* (Quiring et al, 1994); *ey* also is involved in eye development, and a loss-of-function mutation eliminates the compound eye. As a result, *Aniridia*, *Small eye* and *eyeless* are collectively regarded as *Pax-6* homologues with pivotal roles in eye development, whether it be the compound eye of an arthropod or the vertebrate eye (Quiring et al, 1994). This has been assessed by ectopic expression of the *ey* gene, which results in ectopic compound eyes with relatively normal facet organization and arrays of photoreceptor cells (Figure 1.4a). More relevant to this discussion is the finding that ectopic expression of the mouse *Pax-6/Small eye* gene introduced into *Drosophila* will also generate ectopic compound eyes that are morphologically equivalent to the normal compound eye (Figure 1.4b; Halder et al, 1995). In other words, the generative programme for assembling an arthropod compound eye can be activated and controlled by a mouse *Pax-6* gene. It is concluded that these various *Pax-6* homologues constitute **master genes**, arising from a common ancestral gene and with conserved function in controlling eye morphogenesis.

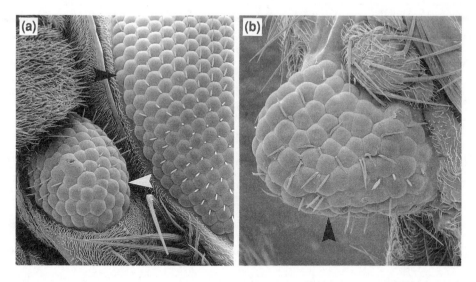

Figure 1.4 (a) Ectopic compound eye (white arrowhead) formed adjacent to the normally located compound eye (on the right) in the head of a *Drosophila* fly; this is the result of the ectopic expression of the *eyeless* gene. (b) Ectopic compound eye formed, in this case, on the leg of a fly, under the control of an ectopically expressed mouse *Pax-6* gene introduced experimentally. In both (a) and (b), note the similarity of the ommatidial organization and interommatidial bristles, in the ectopic eyes and in their normal counterpart in (a). (Photographs supplied by Professor Walter Gehring)

The existence of such homology of function in the development of structures that have traditionally been regarded as anatomical analogues (arising by convergent evolution), rather than anatomical homologues, suggests that long-held views on the evolution of phenotypic form are about to be fundamentally revised. At the very least, it demonstrates that there is a basic, genetic 'tool-kit' of development (Akam et al, 1994) which has been retained over many millions of years and that the different generative programmes of development have deployed this in a multitude of ways to build different phenotypes. Not surprisingly, those phenotypes are sometimes dysmorphic as in the case of *Pax-6* mutations. Earlier assumptions about the extent of homology of developmental mechanism, between human and various animal model systems, have been vindicated more powerfully than could have been anticipated even a few years ago.

ACKNOWLEDGEMENT

I am most grateful to Professor Walter Gehring, who generously provided the photographs used in Figure 1.4.

REFERENCES

Akam, M., Holland, P., Ingham, P. and Wray, G. (Eds) (1994) Preface. In *The Evolution of Developmental Mechanisms. Development* Suppl.

Alberch, P. (1982) Developmental constraints in evolutionary processes. In *Evolution and Development* (Ed.: J.T. Bonner), pp. 313–332. Springer-Verlag: Berlin.

Alberts, B., Bray, D., Lewis, J. et al. (1989) *Molecular Biology of the Cell*, 2nd edn. Garland: New York.

Awgulewitsch, A. and Jacobs, D. (1992) *Deformed* autoregulatory element from *Drosophila* functions in a conserved manner in transgenic mice. *Nature* 358, 341–344.

Bard, J. (1993) *Embryos: Color Atlas of Development*. Wolfe: London.

Barker, D.J.P. (1995) Intrauterine programming of adult disease. *Molec. Med. Today*, 418–423.

Beddington, R.S.P. and Smith, J.C. (1993) Control of vertebrate gastrulation: inducing signals and responding genes. *Curr. Opin. Genet. Dev.* 3, 655–661.

Bolker, J.A. (1995) Model systems in developmental biology. *BioEssays* 17, 451–455.

Burn, J. and Strachan, T. (1995) Human embryo research in developmental research. *Nature Genetics* 11, 3–6.

Burt, D.W., Bumstead, N., Bitgood, J., Ponce de Lyon, F.A. and Crittenden, L.B. (1995) Chicken genome mapping: a new era in avian genetics. *Trends Genet.* 11, 190–194.

Copp, A.J. (1994) Birth defects: from molecules to mechanisms. *J. Roy. Coll. Phys. London* 28, 294–300.

De Robertis, E.M., Fainsod, A., Gont, L.K. and Steinbesser, H. (1994) The evolution of gastrulation. *Development* Suppl., 117–124.

Duke, V., Winyard, P., Thorogood, P. et al (1995) *KAL*, a gene mutated in Kallmann's syndrome, is expressed in the first trimester of human development. *Molec. Cell. Endocrinol.* 110, 73–79.

Fallon, J.F. and Crosby, G.M. (1977) Polarizing zone activity in limb buds of amniotes. In *Vertebrate Limb and Somite Morphogenesis* (Eds: D.A. Ede, J.R. Hinchliffe and M. Balls), pp. 55–69. Cambridge University Press: Cambridge.

Fietz, M.J., Concordet, J.-P., Barbosa, R. et al (1994) The *hedgehog* gene family in *Drosophila* and vertebrate development. *Development* Suppl., 43–51.

Fronhöfer, H.G. and Nüsslein-Volhard, C. (1986) Organisation of anterior pattern in the *Drosophila* embryo by the maternal gene *bicoid*. *Nature* 324, 120–125.

Gilbert, S.F. (1991) *Developmental Biology*, 3rd edn. Sinauer: Sunderland, MA.

Halder, G., Callaerts, P. and Gehring, W.J. (1995) Induction of ectopic eyes by targeted expression of the *eyeless* gene in *Drosophila*. *Science* 267, 1788–1792.

Hogan, B.L.M., Blessing, M., Winnier, G.E., Suzuki, N. and Jones, C.M. (1994) Growth factors in development: the role of TGF-β related polypeptide signalling molecules in embryogenesis. *Development* Suppl., 53–61.

Holley, S.A., Jackson, P.D., Sasai, Y. et al (1995) A conserved system for dorsal-ventral patterning in insects and vertebrates involving *sog* and *chordin*. *Nature* 376, 249–253.

Hunter, C.P. and Kenyon, C. (1995) Specification of anterioposterior cell fates in *Caenorhabditis elegans* by *Drosophila Hox* proteins. *Nature* 377, 229–232.

Kenyon, C. (1994) If birds can fly, why can't we? Homeotic genes and evolution. *Cell* 78, 175–180.

Krumlauf, R. (1994) *Hox* genes in vertebrate development. *Cell* 78, 191–201.

Larsen, W.J. (1993) *Human Embryology*. Churchill Livingstone: Edinburgh.

Malicki, J., Schughart, K. and McGinnis, W. (1990) Mouse *Hox-2.2* specifies thoracic segmental identity in Drosophila embryos and larvae. *Cell* 63, 961–967.

Malicki, J.L.C., Cianetti, C., Peschle, C. and McGinnis, W. (1992) A human HOX4B regulatory element provides head-specific expression in *Drosophila* embryos. *Nature* 358, 345–347.

Manak, J.R. and Scott, M.P. (1994) A class act: conservation of homeodomain protein functions. *Development* Suppl., 61–71.

Marsh, J. (Ed.) (1994) *Neural Tube Defects*. Ciba Foundation Symposium, vol. 181. Wiley: Chichester.

McGinnis, W. and Krumlauf, R. (1992) Homeobox genes and axial patterning. *Cell* 68, 283–302.

McGinnis, W., Garber, R.L., Wirz, J., Kuriowa, A. and Gehring, W. (1984) A homologous protein-coding sequence in *Drosophila* and its conservation in other metazoans. *Cell* 37, 403–409.

McLachlan, J.C. (1986) Self-assembly of structures resembling functional organs by pure populations of cells. *Tissue Cell* 18, 313–320.

Monk, M. (1994) The value of man–mouse homology in human embryology. In *Early Fetal Growth and Development* (Eds: R.H.T. Ward, S.K. Smith and D. Donnai), pp. 63–74. Royal College of Obstetricians and Gynaecologists: London.

Opitz, J. (1985) The Developmental Field Concept. *Am. J. Med. Genet.* 21, 1–11.

Quiring, R., Walldorf, U., Kloter, U. and Gehring, W.J. (1994) Homology of the *eyeless* gene of *Drosophila* to the *Small eye* gene in mice and *Aniridia* in humans. *Science* 265, 785–789.

Read, A.P. (1995) Pax genes – *Paired* feet in three camps. *Nature Genetics* 9, 333–334.

Redline, R.W., Neish, A., Holmes, L.B. and Collins, T. (1992) Biology of disease: homeobox genes and congenital malformation. *Lab. Invest.* 66, 659–670.

Reed, G.B., Rajan, K.T., Ballard, P.L., Shephard, T.H. and Wong, L. (1995) The uses of human embryonic and fetal tissues in treatment and research. In *Diseases of the Fetus and Newborn* (Eds: G.B. Reed, A.E. Claireaux and F. Cockburn), 2nd edn, pp. 389–397. Chapman & Hall: London.

Roelink, H., Augsburger, A., Heemskerk, J., et al., (1994) Floor plate and motor neuron induction by vhh-1, a vertebrate homologue of hedgehog expressed by the notochord. *Cell* 76, 761–775

Scott, M.P. (1994) Intimations of a creature. *Cell* 79, 1121–1124.

Sever, L., Lynberg, M.C. and Edmonds, L.D. (1993) The impact of congenital malformations on public health. *Teratology* 48, 547–549.

Struhl, G., Struhl, K. and Macdonald, P.M. (1989) The gradient morphogen bicoid is a concentration dependent transcriptional activator. *Cell* **57**, 1259–1273.

Sykes, B. (1993) Introduction to medical genetics. In *Connective Tissue and its Heritable Disorders*, pp. 7–50. Wiley-Liss: New York.

van Heyningen, V. (1994) One gene – four syndromes. *Nature* **367**, 319–320.

Warburton, D. and Fraser, C. (1964) Spontaneous abortion risks in man: data from reproductive histories collected in a medical genetics unit. *Am. J. Hum. Genet.* **16**, 1–15.

Wilkie, A.O.M., Amberger, J.S. and McKusick, V.A. (1994) A gene map of congenital malformations. *J. Med. Genet.* **31**, 507–517.

Wolpert, L. (1991) *The Triumph of the Embryo*. Oxford University Press: Oxford.

2 Mapping Syndromes to Genes

ROBIN M. WINTER

Mothercare Unit of Clinical Genetics and Fetal Medicine, Institute of Child Health, London, UK

Genetic malformation syndromes are associated with considerable morbidity in childhood. About 1 in 50 children is born with significant congenital abnormalities and in many cases these malformations have a strong genetic component. Most genetic conditions leading to abnormal physical development have not been mapped and the genes responsible have not been identified. All of these genes would be expected to play an important role in normal development. Thus, the elucidation of the genetic malformation syndromes will lead to greater understanding of normal embryological development, as well as providing a means of explaining and preventing congenital abnormalities.

Genetic mapping is often the first step in the isolation of genes causing clinical syndromes. Examination of 'candidate genes' for mutations is also becoming an important strategy (Ballabio, 1993). These methods are greatly accelerated if there is information about where in the genome a particular locus might be situated. Such clues can come from homology to mouse mutants that have been mapped and from knowledge of homology between mouse and human chromosomal segments. Further clues come from chromosome aberrations (i.e. from balanced translocations, deletions or duplications) giving a similar phenotype, or from knowledge of the function, expression and map location of possible candidate genes.

This chapter will review the approach to mapping genes responsible for malformation syndromes and outline the groups of disorders where genes have been isolated or mapped. Appendix 2.1 provides a list of single gene disorders giving rise to malformations; an indication is given of the method by which each gene was mapped or isolated. The appendix has been assembled from a variety of sources (McKusick, 1994; Wilkie et al, 1994; Winter and Baraitser, 1996; and see Chapter 6). Where a condition appears in McKusick's catalogue (McKusick, 1994), a McKusick number is given. Other conditions are referenced by Winter and Baraitser (1996).

LINKAGE AND MAPPING

If two loci are close together on the same chromosome, they are said to be **linked**. This implies that alleles at the two loci tend to co-segregate (in other

Embryos, Genes and Birth Defects. Edited by P. Thorogood.
© 1997 John Wiley & Sons Ltd.

words they are passed on together at a greater frequency than would be expected by chance). It is possible for two loci to be situated on the same chromosome, but not to be linked. This would occur if they were so far apart that at least one crossover was almost certain to occur between them at meiosis. Loci on the same chromosome are said to be **syntenic**. Linked loci are therefore, by definition, syntenic but not all syntenic loci are linked.

One statistic that is used to indicate how close two loci are situated on a chromosome is the **recombination fraction**. This is the chance of alleles at the two loci being separated by crossing over at meiosis. If the recombination fraction is less than 0.5, then the two loci are by definition linked. The recombination fraction between two unlinked loci is 0.5. Genetic distance is also expressed in terms of **morgans**. One morgan corresponds to the average distance between which one crossover occurs. For short genetic distances of less than a recombination fraction of 0.2, the distance expressed in morgans (or centimorgans; cM) has roughly a linear relationship to the recombination fraction. Thus, a recombination fraction of 0.05 is equivalent to a distance of 5 cM. However, for greater distances, the relationship between recombination fraction and distance in centimorgans becomes non-linear, because of the chance of two or more crossovers occurring. The mathematical conversion of recombination fraction to centimorgans then depends upon assumptions about interference (the chance of one crossover inhibiting another close by). As a result, various mapping functions have been derived depending on different assumptions (White and Lalouel, 1987).

When investigating the possibility of linkage, families must be found where a genetic condition is segregating – the **trait locus**. Alleles at **marker loci** can then be investigated to see whether co-segregation occurs. Over the past few years microsatellite markers that can be detected by polymerase chain reaction (PCR) technology have been developed. These span the whole genome and the latest map contains 5264 such markers (Dib et al, 1996).

Because human families are often small, and key individuals in the family may be deceased or unavailable for study, simple counting techniques to look for co-segregation of trait and marker alleles cannot easily be used. Probability methods and computer programs have therefore been developed to combine data from different families and to allow for the irregular nature of human pedigrees (Ott, 1976, 1987, 1991; Lathrop et al, 1984). A universal statistic to express the likelihood of linkage is the **LOD score**. This is the logarithm to the base 10 of the ratio of the chance of observing the segregation of the phenotypes at the trait and marker loci assuming a given recombination fraction to the chance given no linkage (i.e. a recombination fraction of 0.5).

A LOD score is taken as significant at a given recombination fraction if it is greater than 3. Thus a LOD score of 3 at a recombination fraction of 0.1 means that the two loci have a 1000:1 chance of being linked at a recombination fraction of 0.1 or less. Because there are 22 autosomes there is a 50:1 prior chance that two loci are **not** linked and this must be taken into account when interpreting a LOD score of 3. Combining the prior and posterior odds gives final odds of 20:1 on linkage when a LOD score of 3 is observed.

LOD scores can be summed for different recombination fractions over different families to give a final LOD score. An example taken from a linkage study on Crouzon syndrome, a form of craniosynostosis (early fusion of the cranial sutures), is shown in Table 2.1. This demonstrates that the maximum LOD score is 9.02 at a recombination fraction of 0.0, indicating that the Crouzon locus and the marker are closely linked.

Where several markers on a chromosome are tested, a multipoint map can be obtained. Figure 2.1 shows the LOD scores for the Saethre–Chotzen locus (another dominant form of craniosynostosis) mapped against three marker loci on the short arm of chromosome 7 (D7S488, D7S493, D7S516) (van Herwerden et al, 1994). The order and distance between these marker loci is known and the

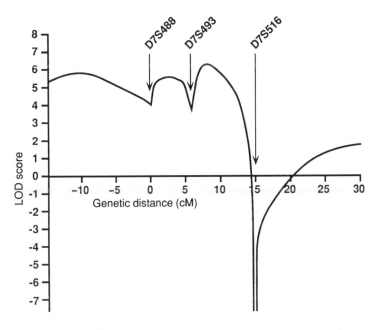

Figure 2.1 LOD scores for the Saethre–Chotzen locus mapped against three marker loci (D7S488, D7S493 and D7S516) on the short arm of chromosome 7

Table 2.1 Two-point LOD scores for Crouzon syndrome with a fibroblast growth factor receptor 2 (FGFR2) polymorphism

	Recombination fraction					
	0.0	0.05	0.1	0.2	0.3	0.4
Family 1	5.11	4.68	4.24	3.27	2.17	0.94
Family 2	3.01	2.77	2.51	1.94	1.31	0.62
Family 3	0.9	0.82	0.73	0.54	0.36	0.18
Total	9.02	8.27	7.48	5.75	3.84	1.74

From Reardon et al, 1994.

graph shows the relative likelihood of different positions of the Saethre–Chotzen locus. Although the trait locus is linked to marker loci, it is not possible to say that it is definitely situated between two particular marker loci.

GENETIC HETEROGENEITY

The ability to map and isolate developmental genes has revealed that some disorders are genetically heterogeneous, with abnormal alleles at different loci giving similar clinical pictures (**non-allelic** or **locus heterogeneity**). A number of well-established examples are given in Table 2.2. In some instances, for example Bardet–Biedl syndrome and multiple exostoses, alleles at three or more separate loci appear to give the same phenotype. In other cases, the locus for one form of a disorder has been found, but not the other locus or loci. For example, a locus for Holt–Oram syndrome has been found at 12q, but other families can be shown not to map to 12q, and the locus or loci for these cases remain undiscovered.

CHROMOSOME ABERRATIONS, MOUSE/HUMAN HOMOLOGY AND IDENTIFICATION OF DEVELOPMENTAL GENES

Clues to the mapping and identification of genes responsible for human malformation syndromes can be gained from studies of the phenotypic effects of human chromosome aberrations and of mouse mutants.

Table 2.2 Examples of locus heterogeneity

Disorder	Map locations
Alport syndrome (deafness; nephropathy)	2qter; Xq21–22
Bardet–Biedl (Laurence–Moon–Bardet–Biedl) syndrome	3p11–13; 11q13; 15q22; 16q13–22
Cockayne syndrome	2q21; 10q11; 13q32–33
Fanconi anaemia	9q22; 20q13
Glutaric aciduria type 2	15q23–25; 19q13
Hirschsprung's disease (familial)	10q11–21; 13q22; 20q13
Holoprosencephaly	2p21; 3p24; 7q36; 13q; 18p
Holt–Oram syndrome	12q21–ter; 14q23–24
Multiple exostoses (diaphyseal aclasis)	8q24; 11p11–12; 19p11–13
Stickler syndrome (hereditary arthro-ophthalmopathy)	6p21–22; 12q13–14
Tuberous sclerosis	9q34; 16p13
Usher syndrome (retinitis pigmentosa; deafness)	1q41; 3q21–25; 11p15; 11q13; 14q32
Waardenburg syndrome	2q37 (type I); 3p12–14 (type II)

HUMAN CYTOGENETIC ABERRATIONS

Human chromosome deletions and duplications can give rise to a malformation phenotype that resembles that seen in a single gene disorder and in this case there is a possibility that the gene resides in that chromosomal segment, and that haploinsufficiency or excess has caused the clinical picture. In other cases an apparently balanced chromosome translocation may be associated with a specific phenotype and, if the translocation is de novo, it is possible that an important developmental gene has been disrupted. Tommerup (1993) summarizes cases where genes have been mapped by finding chromosome aberrations that give rise to specific phenotypes. Schinzel (1994) has compiled a computerized database of the clinical effects of human chromosomal aberrations that can be used to generate clues to the possible location of human malformation genes. Appendix 2.1 shows genes that have been mapped or isolated by reference to cytogenetic clues. To date, over 50 examples have been reported, indicating the importance of this approach.

MOUSE MUTANTS

Mouse malformation mutants have been classified in detail and most have been mapped (Winter 1988b; Lyon and Searle, 1989). Analysis of the map locations of specific genes in mouse and man has shown that there is conservation of chromosome segments, so that, for example, part of mouse chromosome 13 is homologous to part of the short arm of human chromosome 7 (Edwards, 1991). If there is phenotypic homology between a specific mouse mutant and a (non-mapped) human syndrome and the mouse mutant is mapped, then tables of mouse/human homology can be used to suggest the possible map location in the human. Further evidence that the gene might be located in that region could be gained from human chromosome deletions or duplications that may give similar clinical features (Schinzel, 1994). Finally a search can be made for candidate genes using the criteria of expression pattern and map location. Direct mutation and linkage analysis can then be carried out using the candidate genes or random markers mapping to the appropriate chromosomal region.

There are several examples of the fruitfulness of the approach of combining human cytogenetic and mouse homology clues:

(1) Genetic studies of **Waardenburg syndrome**, where there is the association between sensorineural deafness and pigmentary abnormalities of the hair, skin and irises, have benefited greatly from this approach. There are two main types, distinguished by facial features. **Type I** was localized to 2q37 after a case with features of the condition, associated with a chromosome rearrangement of that region, was reported (Foy et al, 1990). In the mouse both the *Splotch (Sp)* mutant (which had been suggested as a homologue) and paired-box gene *Pax-3*, had been shown to map to a homologous region on mouse chromosome 1. Baldwin et al (1992) and Tassabehji et al (1992) demonstrated mutations in the *HuP2* gene (the human homologue of mouse *Pax-3*) in type I cases. This confirmed the homology to the *Splotch* mutant in the mouse. Tassabehji et al

(1994a) point out that *PAX3* mutations in human Waardenburg cases, and the *Splotch* mouse, have close analogies including deletions, splice-site mutations and similar amino-acid substitutions. Meanwhile, Hughes et al (1994) mapped the gene for **type II** Waardenburg syndrome to 3p12–p14 close to the human homologue of the mouse *microphthalmia* (*mi*) gene. Subsequently, Tassabehji et al (1994b) showed that mutations in the human homologue (*MITF*) of the mouse *mi* gene caused Waardenburg syndrome type II; this gene codes for a basic helix-loop-helix leucine zipper (bHLH-ZIP) protein. It was found that two Waardenburg syndrome type II families had mutations affecting splice sites in the *MITF* gene.

(2) **Greig syndrome** is an autosomal dominant form of polydactyly in humans causing the combination of pre-axial polysyndactyly and post-axial polydactyly. The gene was shown to map to 7p13 (Brueton et al, 1988) after cases with balanced translocations involving 7p13 had been reported (Tommerup and Nielsen, 1983; Kruger et al 1989). Winter and Huson (1988) suggested, from chromosome homology and morphological clues, that the mouse mutant *Extra toes* (*Xt*) was homologous. Vortkamp et al (1991) reported that the *GLI3* zinc-finger gene was interrupted by translocations in Greig syndrome families. Subsequently, Schimmang et al (1992) and Hui and Joyner (1993) demonstrated that the mouse *Gli-3* gene was disrupted in the *Extra toes* mouse.

(3) Deletions of human 11p13 are known to cause the association of **Wilms' tumour** of the kidney, aniridia, genital anomalies and mental retardation (WAGR syndrome; Riccardi et al, 1980; Friedman, 1986). Ton et al (1991) isolated a paired box-like gene (*PAX6*) from the 11p13 region and showed that it was deleted in two patients with aniridia. *Small eye* (*Sey*) in the mouse was postulated to be the human aniridia homologue and the mouse *Pax-6* gene was shown to contain mutations (Hill et al, 1991). Point mutations in the human *PAX6* gene have been shown to cause isolated aniridia (Davis and Cowell, 1993).

(4) The c-*kit* proto-oncogene encodes the cellular tyrosine kinase receptor for mast/stem cell growth factor and has been found to be mutated in the mouse mutant dominant *White spotting* (*W*). In human families with **piebaldism** linkage was demonstrated to the c-*kit* gene on 4q and mutations in this gene have been found (Spritz, 1992).

(5) **Type II oculocutaneous albinism** maps to 15q11–12. Lee et al (1994) demonstrated mutations in the *P* gene (the homologue of the mouse *pink-eye dilution*, *p*, gene) in three patients with type II oculocutaneous albinism, one of whom also had **Prader–Willi syndrome**. The presence of skin and hair hypopigmentation in some cases of Prader–Willi syndrome has long been recognized and the finding of *P* gene mutations provides a molecular explanation.

Reviews of mouse/human homology, both confirmed and speculative, are available and constantly updated (Winter, 1988a,b; Erickson, 1990; Jacenko et al, 1994; Searle et al 1994). Clearly, researchers interested in human malformations need to be aware of this literature and of the relevant databases (see Chapter 6) and of the potential in identifying homologies emerging from the analysis of developmental mutants in other species.

Appendix 2.1 Mapped or isolated genes causing human malformations

Map position	Condition	Gene	Method[a]	McKusick number
1p36	Ehlers–Danlos syndrome type VI	*Lysyl oxidase*	B	225400
1p34–36	Hypophosphatasia	*Alkaline phosphatase (liver/bone/kidney)*	B	241500
1p34–36	Schwartz–Jampel syndrome		M	255800
1p32–33	Multiple epiphyseal dysplasia type 2		M	600204
1p21–22	Zellweger (cerebro-hepato-renal) syndrome	*Peroxisomal membrane protein-1 (70 kD)*	B	214100
1q21	Pyknodysostosis		M	265800
1q41	Usher syndrome (retinitis pigmentosa; deafness)		M	276900
1q32–41	Van der Woude syndrome (cleft lip and palate; lip pits)		CM	119300
2p	Torre syndrome (sebaceous gland tumours; internal carcinomas)	*MSH2*	MG	158320
2p12/2q14	Baraitser–Winter syndrome (iris coloboma; ptosis; hypertelorism; mental retardation)		C	243310
2p21	Holoprosencephaly		C	157170
2p16	Carney complex		M	160980
2q21	Cockayne syndrome	*ERCC3*	M	216400
2q31	Ehlers–Danlos syndrome type IV	*Collagen α3(I)*	B	130050
2q31	Syndactyly type II	*HOXD13*	MG	186000
2q31–ter	Osteopoikilosis		M	166700
2q37	Klein–Waardenburg syndrome	*Pax3*	G	148820
2q37	Waardenburg syndrome type I	*Pax3*	ACM	193500
3p26–25	von Hippel–Lindau disease	*VHL tumour suppressor*	M	193300
3p24–25	Marfan syndrome type 2		M	154700
3p24	Holoprosencephaly		C	
3p22–23	Pseudo-Zellweger syndrome	*Peroxisomal bifunctional enzyme*	B	261510
3p14–21	Larsen syndrome		M	150250
3p12–14	Waardenburg syndrome type II	*MITF*	AGM	193510
3p11–13	Bardet–Biedl syndrome		M	209900
3q22–23	Blepharophimosis–ptosis–epicanthus inversus		C	110100
3q26	De Lange syndrome		C	122470
3q2	Hyperparathyroidism (neonatal familial)	*Parathyroid sensing receptor*	G	239200
4p	Diabetes insipidus–diabetes mellitus–optic atrophy–deafness (DIDMOAD)		M	222300

(*continued*)

Appendix 2.1 *Continued*

Map position	Condition	Gene	Method[a]	McKusick number
4p16	Hypochondroplasia	*Fibroblast growth factor receptor 3 (FGFR3)*	MG	146000
4p16	Achondroplasia	*Fibroblast growth factor receptor 3 (FGFR3)*	GM	100800
4p16	Thanatophoric dysplasia	*Fibroblast growth factor receptor 3 (FGFR3)*	G	187600
4p16	Craniosynostosis (Adelaide type)		M	600593
4p16	Ellis–van Greveld syndrome		M	225500
4q12–13	Piebaldism	*KIT*	AM	172800
4q25–27	Rieger syndrome		CM	180500
4q33–35	Aspartylglucosaminuria	*Aspartylglucosaminidase*	B	208400
5q21–34	Diastrophic dysplasia	*DTDST*	M	222600
5q22–23	Gardner syndrome		C	175300
5q23–31	Beal contractural arachnodactyly	*Fibrillin-2*	G	121050
5q32–33	Treacher Collins syndrome	*Treacle*	M	154500
5q34–ter	Boston craniosynostosis	*MSX2*	GM	123101
6	Cleidocranial dysplasia		ACM	119600
6pter–p24	Agnathia-holoprosencephaly		C	202650
6p23	Cleft lip and palate; ectodermal dysplasia		C	
6p21–22	Stickler syndrome (hereditary arthro-ophthalmopathy)	*COL11A2*	GM	108300
6q21–22	Schmid metaphyseal dysplasia	*COL10A1*	M	156500
6q	Volar nails		C	
7p21	Saethre–Chotzen syndrome (acrocephalo-syndactyly)		CM	101400
7p13	Greig syndrome (digital anomalies; macrocephaly)	*GLI3*	ACM	175700
7q11	Aortic stenosis (autosomal dominant)	*Elastin*	GM	185500
7q11	Argininosuccinic aciduria	*Argininosuccinate lyase*	B	207900
7q11	Williams syndrome	*Elastin*	GM	194050
7q21–22	Ectrodactyly (autosomal dominant)		C	183600
7q21–22	Ectrodactyly–ectodermal dysplasia-clefting		C	129900
7q21–22	Osteogenesis imperfecta type I	*COL1A2*	GM	166200
7q21–22	Osteogenesis imperfecta type II	*COL1A2*	G	166210
7q21–22	Osteogenesis imperfecta type III	*COL1A2*	G	259420
7q21–22	Ehlers–Danlos syndrome type VIIA2	*COL1A2*	B	130060

Appendix 2.1 *Continued*

Map position	Condition	Gene	Method[a]	McKusick number
7q31	Pendred syndrome		M	274600
7q32	Smith–Lemli–Opitz syndrome	*7-Dehydrocholesterol reductase*	B	268670
7q35–ter	Triphalangeal thumb		M	174500
7q36	Nicolai–Hamel polysyndactyly		M	190605
7q36	Holoprosencephaly	*SHH*	CM	142945
7q36	Currarino triad		CM	176450
8p12	Werner syndrome	*WRN*	M	277700
8p11	Pfeiffer syndrome	*Fibroblast growth factor receptor 1 (FGFR1)*	GM	101600
8q11–13	Branchio-oto-renal (BOR) syndrome		C	113650
8q22	Carbonic anhydrase II deficiency (marble brain disease)	*Carbonic anhydrase II*	B	259730
8q22–23	Cohen syndrome		M	216550
8q24	Langer–Giedion syndrome		C	150230
8q24	Tricho-rhino-phalangeal (TRP) syndrome		C	190350
8q24	Multiple exostoses (diaphyseal aclasis)	*EXT1*	CM	133700
9p13–22	Venous malformations (familial)		M	600195
9cen	McKusick syndrome (cartilage–hair hypoplasia)	*FAC*	M	250250
9q22	Fanconi anaemia		M	227645
9q22–31	Naevoid basal cell carcinoma syndrome	*PTC*	MG	109400
9q31–33	Riley–Day syndrome (familial dysautonomia)		M	223900
9q33–34	Rendu–Osler–Weber hereditary telangiectasia	*Endoglin*	M	187300
9q34	Citrullinemia-pili torti	*Argininosuccinate synthetase*	B	215700
9q34	Nail–patella syndrome (osteo-onychodysplasia)		M	161200
9q34	Tuberous sclerosis	*Tuberin*	M	191100
9q34	Ehlers–Danlos syndrome I	*COL5A1*	CG	130000
10q11	Multiple endocrine adenomatosis type 2B	*RET*	GM	162300
10q11–21	Hirschsprung's disease (familial)	*RET*	GM	142623
10q24–25	Renal–coloboma syndrome	*PAX2*	G	120330
10q24–24	Ectrodactyly		M	183600
10q25–26	Crouzon syndrome (craniofacial dysostosis)	*Fibroblast growth factor receptor 2 (FGFR2)*	GM	123500
10q25–26	Apert syndrome	*Fibroblast growth factor receptor 2 (FGFR2)*	G	101200

(*continued*)

Appendix 2.1   *Continued*

Map position	Condition	Gene	Method[a]	McKusick number
10q25–26	Pfeiffer syndrome type 2	*Fibroblast growth factor receptor 2 (FGFR2)*	G	101200
10q25–26	Jackson–Weiss syndrome	*Fibroblast growth factor receptor 2 (FGFR2)*	GM	123150
10q26	Gyrate atrophy of choroid and retina	*Ornithine aminotransferase*	B	258870
10q26	Schizencephaly	EMX2	G	269160
11p15	Beckwith–Wiedemann (EMG) syndrome		CM	130650
11p15	Drash syndrome (nephritis; pseudohermaphroditism; Wilms' tumour)	WT1	G	194080
11p13	Aniridia–Wilms' tumour/ WAGR syndrome	*PAX6* (aniridia) WT1 (Wilms' tumour)	AC	194070
11p13	Aniridia; microphthalmia microcephaly	*PAX6*	G	
11p11–12	Multiple exostoses (diaphyseal aclasis)	EXT2	CM	133700
11q13	Usher syndrome (retinitis pigmentosa; deafness)	*Myosin VIIA*	M	276900
11q13	Bardet–Biedl syndrome		M	209900
11q22–23	Louis–Bar syndrome (ataxia–telangiectasia)	ATM	M	208900
12p11–13	Jansen metaphyseal dysplasia	PTHR	G	156400
12p11–13?	Acrocallosal syndrome		C	200990
12p11–13	Fibrosis of extraocular muscles		M	135700
12q	Rendu–Osler–Weber type 2	ACVRLK1	MG	187300
12q13	Namaqualand hip dysplasia		G	142670
12q13	Ivemark syndrome	Connexin43	G	208530
12q13–14	Kniest syndrome	COL2A1	G	156550
12q13–14	Spondyloepiphyseal dysplasia congenita	COL2A1	GM	183900
12q13–14	Hypochondrogenesis	COL2A1	G	200600
12q13–14	Achondrogenesis type 2	COL2A1	G	200610
12q13–14	Stickler syndrome (hereditary arthro-ophthalmopathy)	COL2A1	GM	108300
12q13–14	Lipomatosis (multiple)		C	151900
12q21–ter	Holt–Oram syndrome		M	142900
12q22	Noonan syndrome		M	163950
13q22	Hirschsprung's disease	EDNRB	GM	131244
13q32–33	Cockayne syndrome	XPGC	M	216400
13q	Holoprosencephaly		C	
13q	Clouston ectodermal dysplasia		M	126500
14q32	Usher syndrome (retinitis pigmentosa; deafness)		M	276900

Appendix 2.1 *Continued*

Map position	Condition	Gene	Method[a]	McKusick number
15q11	Angelman ('happy puppet') syndrome		C	234400
15q11	Prader–Willi syndrome		C	176270
15q15–21	Ectopia lentis (isolated)	*Fibrillin-1*	G	129600
15q15–21	Marfan syndrome (severe neonatal)	*Fibrillin-1*	G	154700
15q15–21	Marfan syndrome	*Fibrillin-1*	GM	154700
15q23–25	Glutaric aciduria type 2	*Electron transfer flavoprotein*	B	231680
15q26	Bloom syndrome	*RecQ helicase-like* gene	M	210900
16p13	Rubinstein–Taybi syndrome	*CBP*	CG	268600
16p13	Alpha thalassaemia–mental retardation		C	141750
16p13	Tuberous sclerosis	*Tuberin*	M	191100
16p13	Carbohydrate-deficient glycoprotein syndrome		BM	212065
16q13–22	Bardet–Biedl syndrome		M	209900
16q22	Richner–Hanhart tyrosinaemia type II	*Tyrosine aminotransferase*	B	276600
16q24	Fanconi anaemia		M	227650
17p13	Miller–Dieker lissencephaly		C	247200
17q11	Neurofibromatosis type 1	*Neurofibromin*	M	162200
17q11	Watson syndrome (*café au lait* patches; pulmonary stenosis)	*Neurofibromin*	M	193520
17q12–21	Pachyonychia congenita	*Keratin 17/16*	M	167210
17q21–22	Osteogenesis imperfecta type I	*COL1A1*	GM	166200
17q21–22	Osteogenesis imperfecta type II	*COL1A1*	G	166210
17q21–22	Osteogenesis imperfecta type III	*COL1A1*	G	259420
17q21	Proximal symphalangism		M	185800
17q21–22	Ehlers–Danlos syndrome type VIIA1	*COL1A1*	G	130060
17q21–22	Meckel–Gruber syndrome		M	249000
17q24–25	Camptomelic dysplasia	*SOX9*	CG	211970
18p	Holoprosencephaly		C	236100
18q21–22	Osterberg familial expansile osteolysis		M	174810
19p13	Persistent Müllerian duct syndrome	*Müllerian inhibition factor*	G	261550
19p13.1	Pseudoachondroplasia	*COMP*	MG	177170
19p11–13	Multiple exostoses (diaphyseal aclasis)		CM	133700
19q13	Pollitt syndrome	*DNA helicase*	G	275550
19q13	Multiple epiphyseal dysplasia	*COL9A2*	MG	132400

(continued)

Appendix 2.1 *Continued*

Map position	Condition	Gene	Method[a]	McKusick number
19q13	Glutaric aciduria type 2	*Electron transfer flavoprotein*	B	231680
20p11	Alagille syndrome (arterio-hepatic dysplasia)		C	118450
20q13	Albright syndrome (pseudo, and pseudo-pseudohypoparathyroidism)	*G protein α subunit*	BG	103580
20q13	McCune–Albright syndrome (polyostotic fibrous dysplasia)	*G protein α subunit*	G	174800
20q13	Dwarfism–immunodeficiency type 1	*Adenosine deaminase deficiency*	B	200900
20q13	Acromesomelia type Hunter–Thompson	*CDMP1*	AG	228900
20q13	Fanconi anaemia	*Fanconi anaemia-1*	GM	227650
20q13	Hirschsprung's disease	*EDN3*	G	131242
21q22	Autoimmune polyendocrinopathy–candidosis–ectodermal dysplasia (APECED)		M	240300
21q22	Homocystinuria	*Cystathione β-synthase*	B	236200
21q22	Multiple carboxylase deficiency	*Biotinidase*	B	253270
21q22	Knoblock–Layer syndrome		M	267750
22q11	Velo-cardio-facial syndrome		C	192430
22q11	DiGeorge syndrome		C	188400
22q11	Optiz–G syndrome		M	145410
Xpter–22	X-linked ichthyosis	*Steroid sulphatase*	B	308100
Xp22	Aicardi syndrome		C	304050
Xp22	Optiz–G syndrome		G	145410
Xp22	Coffin–Lowry syndrome		M	303600
Xp22	Goltz focal dermal hypoplasia		C	305600
Xp22	Ichthyosis–hypogonadism–mental retardation		C	308200
Xp22	Kallmann syndrome	*Kalig-1*	C	308700
Xp22	Microphthalmia–dermal aplasia–sclerocornea		C	309801
Xp22	Nance–Horan syndrome (mesiodens; cataract)		M	302350
Xp22	Spondyloepiphyseal dysplasia tarda		M	313400
Xp22	Chondrodysplasia punctata	*ARSE*	C	302950
Xp22	Pyruvate dehydrogenase complex deficiency	*E1 α subunit*	B	208800
Xp21–22	X-linked reticular pigmentary disorder		M	301220
Xp21–22	Keratosis follicularis; spinulosa decalvans		M	308800

Appendix 2.1 *Continued*

Map position	Condition	Gene	Method[a]	McKusick number
Xp11	Åarskog syndrome	*FGDY*	CM	305400
Xp11	Norrie disease	*NDP*	M	310600
Xp11–cen	Wilson syndrome (mental retardation; gynaecomastia; obesity)		M	309585
Xp11–21	Prieto syndrome (dysmorphic features; mental retardation)		M	309610
Xp11–21	Proud syndrome (mental retardation; seizures; microcephaly; corpus callosum agenesis)		M	
Xp11	Incontinentia pigmenti		CM	308300
Xp21–q21	Hamel syndrome (mental retardation; congenital heart defects)		M	
Xq11–12	Kennedy's syndrome (X-linked spinal and bulbar muscular atrophy)	*Androgen receptor*	GM	313200
Xq11–21	Sutherland syndrome (mental retardation; microcephaly; spastic diplegia)		M	
Xq12–13	Ectodermal dysplasia (hypohidrotic type)		CM	305100
Xq12–21	Mental retardation–deafness–hypogenitalism		M	309590
Xq12–21	Alpha thalassaemia–mental retardation	*XNP(XH2)*	M	301040
Xq12–26	X-linked megalocornea		M	309300
Xq13	Menkes (kinky hair) syndrome	*Copper-transporting ATPase*	ACM	309400
Xq13–21	Wieacker–Wolff syndrome		M	314580
Xq21	Cleft palate (X-linked)		M	303400
Xq21	Nance syndrome (stapes fixation with perilymphatic gusher)	*POU3F4*	M	304400
Xq21	Miles–Carpenter syndrome (mental retardation; fingertip arches; contractures)		M	309605
Xq21	Allan–Herndon syndrome		M	309600
Xq21–22	Goldblatt syndrome (spastic paraplegia; mental retardation; optic atrophy)		GM	312920
Xq21–22	Alport syndrome (deafness; nephropathy)	*COL4A5*	GM	104200
Xq24–27	Mathias syndrome (X-linked laterality sequence)		M	304750

(continued)

Appendix 2.1 *Continued*

Map position	Condition	Gene	Method[a]	McKusick number
Xq25	Lowe (oculo-cerebro-renal) syndrome	*Inisotol polyphosphate-5-phosphatase*	M	309000
Xq25–26	Thoracoabdominal syndrome		M	313850
Xq25–27	Simpson–Golabi–Behmel syndrome	*GPC3*	M	312870
Xq26	Ectrodactyly (X-linked recessive)		M	313350
Xq26	Pettigrew syndrome (mental retardation; Dandy–Walker; basal ganglia disease)		M	304340
Xq26	Gustavson syndrome (mental retardation; blindness; deafness; seizures; spasticity)		M	309555
Xq26–27	Borjeson–Forssman–Lehmann syndrome		M	301900
Xq26–27	Rosenberg–Chutorian syndrome (optic atrophy; peroneal muscular atrophy; deafness)		M	311070
Xq26–27	Ziprkowski syndrome (partial albinism; deafness)		M	300700
Xq27–28	Fragile X-linked mental retardation	*FMR1*	M	309550
Xq27–28	X-linked anophthalmos		M	301590
Xq27–ter	Christian syndrome (skeletal dysplasia; mental retardation)		M	309620
Xq28	Adrenoleukodystrophy	*Peroxisomal membrane protein 70-like* gene	B	300100
Xq28	Conradi chondrodysplasia punctata (X-linked dominant)		AM	118650
Xq28	Dyskeratosis congenita		M	305000
Xq28	Taybi (oto-palato-digital) syndrome		M	311300
Xq28	Mental retardation–Aphasia–shuffling gait–adducted thumbs (MASA)	*L1CAM*	GM	309250
Xq28	X-linked hydrocephalus	*L1CAM*	GM	307000
Xq28	Incontinentia pigmenti		M	308300
Xq28–ter	Goeminne syndrome (torticollis; keloids; cryptorchidism)		C	314300

[a] A, animal model (mouse); B, biochemical evidence; C, chromosomal evidence; G, candidate gene; M, genome mapping

REFERENCES

Baldwin, C.T., Hoth, C.F., Amos, J.A. et al (1992) An exonic mutation in the *HuP2* paired domain gene causes Waardenburg's syndrome. *Nature* **355**, 637–638.

Ballabio, A. (1993) The rise and fall of positional cloning? *Nature Genetics*, **3**, 277–279.

Brueton, L., Huson, S.M., Winter, R.M. and Williamson, R. (1988) Chromosomal localisation of a developmental gene in man: direct DNA analysis demonstrates that Greig cephalopolysyndactyly maps to 7p13. *Am. J. Med. Genet.* **31**, 799–804.

Davis, A. and Cowell, J.K. (1993) Mutations in the *PAX6* gene in patients with hereditary aniridia. *Hum. Molec. Genet.* **2**, 2093–2098.

Dib, C., Faure, S., Fizames, C. et al. (1996) A comprehensive genetic map of the human genome based on 5264 microsatellites. *Nature* **380**, 152–154.

Edwards, J.H. (1991) The Oxford Grid. *Ann. Hum. Genet.* **55**, 17–31.

Erickson, R.P. (1990) Mapping dysmorphic syndromes with the aid of the mouse/human homology map. *Am. J. Hum. Genet.* **46**, 1013–1016.

Foy, C., Newton, V., Wellesley, D. et al. (1990) Assignment of the locus for Waardenburg syndrome type I to human chromosome 2q37 and possible homology to the *splotch* mouse. *Am. J. Hum. Genet.* **46**, 1017–1023.

Friedman, A.L. (1986) Wilms' tumor detection in patients with sporadic aniridia. *Am. J. Dis. Child.* **140**, 173–174.

Hill, R.E., Favor, J., Hogan, B.L.M. et al. (1991) Mouse *Small eye* results from mutations in a paired-like homeobox-containing gene. *Nature* **354**, 522–525.

Hughes, A.E., Newton, V.E., Liu, X.Z. and Read, A.P. (1994) A gene for Waardenburg syndrome type 2 maps close to the human homologue of the *microphthalmia* gene at chromosome 3p12–p14.1. *Nature Genetics* **7**, 509–512.

Hui, C-C. and Joyner, A.L. (1993) A mouse model of Greig cephalopolysyndactyly syndrome: the *extra-toes**J mutation contains an intragenic deletion of the Gli3 gene. *Nature Genetics* **3**, 241–246.

Jacenko, O., Olsen, B.R. and Warman, M.L. (1994) Of mice and men: heritable skeletal disorders. *Am. J. Hum. Genet.* **54**, 163–168.

Kruger, G., Gotz, J., Kvist, U. et al. (1989) Greig syndrome in a large kindred due to reciprocal chromosome translocation t(6;7)(q27;p13). *Am. J. Med. Genet.* **32**, 411–416.

Lathrop, G.M., Lalouel, J.M., Julier, C. and Ott, J. (1984) Strategies for multilocus linkage analysis in humans. *Proc. Natl. Acad. Sci. USA* **81**, 3443–3446.

Lee, S.-T., Nicholls, R.D., Bundey, S. et al. (1994) Mutations of the *P* gene in oculocutaneous albinism, ocular albinism, and Prader–Willi syndrome plus albinism. *New Engl. J. Med.* **30**, 529–534.

Lyon, M. and Searle, A.G. (Eds) (1989) *Genetic Variants and Strains of the Laboratory Mouse*. Oxford University Press: Oxford.

McKusick, V.A. (1994) *Mendelian Inheritance in Man*, 11th edn. Johns Hopkins University Press: Baltimore, MD.

Ott, J. (1976) A computer program for linkage analysis of general human pedigrees. *Am. J. Hum. Genet.* **28**, 528–529.

Ott, J. (1987) A short guide to linkage analysis. In *Genome Analysis – A Practical Approach* (Ed.: K.E. Davies), pp. 19–32. IRL Press: Oxford.

Ott, J. (1991) *Analysis of Human Genetic Linkage*. Johns Hopkins University Press: Baltimore, MD.

Reardon, W., Winter, R.M., Rutland, P. et al. (1994) Mutations in the fibroblast growth factor receptor 2 gene cause Crouzon syndrome. *Nature Genetics* **8**, 98–103.

Riccardi, V.M., Hittner, H.M., Francke, U. et al. (1980) The aniridia–Wilms tumor association: the critical role of chromosome band 11p13. *Cancer Genet. Cytogen.* **2**, 131–135.

Schimmang, T., Lemaistre, M., Vortkamp, A. and Ruther, U. (1992) Expression of the zinc finger gene *Gli3* is affected in the morphogenetic mouse mutant extra-toes (Xt). *Development* **116**, 799–804.

Schinzel, A. (1994) *Cytogenetics Database: Oxford Medical Databases*. (Eds: R.M. Winter and M. Baraitser). Oxford University Press: Oxford.

Searle, A.G., Edwards, J.H. and Hall, J.G. (1994) Mouse homologues of human hereditary disease. *J. Med. Genet.* **31**, 1–19.

Spritz, R.A. (1992) The molecular basis of human piebaldism. *Pigment Cell Res.* **5**, 340–343.

Tassabehji, M., Read, A.P., Newton, V.E. et al. (1992) Waardenburg's syndrome patients have mutations in the human homologue of the *Pax-3* paired box gene. *Nature* **355**, 635–636.

Tassabehji, M., Newton, V.E., Leverton, K. et al. (1994a) *PAX3* gene structure and mutations: close analogies between Waardenburg syndrome and the *Splotch* mouse. *Hum. Molec. Genet.* **3**, 1069–1074.

Tassabehji, M., Newton, V.E. and Read, A.P. (1994b) Waardenburg syndrome type 2 caused by mutations in the human *microphthalmia* (*MITF*) gene. *Nature Genetics* **8**, 251–255.

Tommerup, N. (1993) Mendelian cytogenetics: chromosome rearrangements associated with Mendelian disorders. *J. Med. Genet.* **30**, 713–727.

Tommerup, N. and Nielsen, F. (1983) A familial reciprocal translocation t(3;7)(p21.1;p13) associated with the Greig polysyndactyly–craniofacial anomalies syndrome. *Am. J. Med. Genet.* **16**, 313–321.

Ton, C.C.T., Hirvonen, H., Miwa, H. et al. (1991) Positional cloning and characterization of a paired box- and homeobox-containing gene from the aniridia region. *Cell* **67**, 1059–1074.

van Herwerden, L., Rose, C.S.P., Reardon, W. et al (1994) Evidence for locus heterogeneity in acrocephalosyndactyly: a refined localization for the Saethre–Chotzen syndrome locus on distal chromosome 7p. *Am. J. Hum. Genet.* **54**, 669–674.

Vortkamp, A., Gessler, M. and Grzeschik, K.-H. (1991) *GLI3* zinc-finger gene interrupted by translocations in Greig syndrome families. *Nature* **352**, 539–540.

White, R. and Lalouel, J.M. (1987) Investigation of genetic linkage in human families. *Adv. Hum. Genet.* **16**, 121–228.

Wilkie, A.O.M., Amberger, J.S. and McKusick, V.A. (1994) A gene map of congenital malformations. *J. Med. Genet.* **31**, 507–517.

Winter, R.M. (1988a) A mouse malformation mutant supplement to the London Dysmorphology Database. *Am. J. Med. Genet.* **30**, 819–820.

Winter, R.M. (1988b) Malformation syndromes: a review of mouse/human homology. *J. Med. Genet.* **25**, 480–487.

Winter, R.M. and Baraitser, M. (1996) *The London Dysmorphology Database*. Oxford University Press: Oxford.

Winter, R.M. and Huson, S.M. (1988) Greig cephalopolysyndactyly syndrome: a possible mouse homologue (*Xt–extra toes*). *Am. J. Med. Genet.* **31**, 793–798.

3 Positional Cloning and Analysis of Loci Implicated in Human Birth Defects

PETER J. SCAMBLER

Molecular Medicine Unit, Institute of Child Health, London, UK

Positional cloning (Collins, 1992) (or 'reverse genetics' in an earlier incarnation) has been used extensively in the search for genes that when mutated cause or predispose to human disease. The advances and achievements of the positional cloning approach have gone hand-in-hand with the development of the human (and murine) genome mapping projects. There have already been notable successes in the identification of genes at fault in several disorders involving abnormal development, including Wilms' tumour, aniridia, Hirschsprung's disease, Greig syndrome and fragile-X mental retardation (Ballabio, 1993). The purpose of this chapter is to outline the various methodologies that can now be applied to positional cloning. It is hoped that it will become apparent that the cloning of genes responsible for very rare disorders, or even single cases, is now a realistic possibility given the resources and technology arising out of genome projects. While the clinical load presented by these individual congenital defects is not great, genetic problems as a whole constitute a major burden on health care resources. In addition, elucidation of the genetic causes of human birth defects can be of importance in providing new avenues of research in the investigation of biological mechanisms underlying development. The major steps involved in the identification of such loci are presented in Figure 3.1, and described in more detail below.

MAPPING OF DISEASE LOCI

Many disease loci have been mapped by detecting the disease phenotype in individuals carrying various chromosomal abnormalities. These can be in the form of large cytogenetically visible aberrations including duplications, deletions, inversions, balanced translocations and fragile sites. Large duplications are very rare, but they have been used in phenotype/genotype correlations in Down syndrome (Korenberg et al, 1992), although the critical regions suggested are somewhat controversial. Smaller duplications such as

Embryos, Genes and Birth Defects. Edited by P. Thorogood.
© 1997 John Wiley & Sons Ltd.

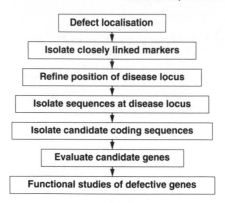

Figure 3.1 Steps in the positional cloning of disease genes

cat-eye syndrome (trisomy or tetrasomy of 22pter–q11) (Mears et al, 1994) and the marker chromosome 15 inv dup 15 (Robinson et al, 1993) may be due to the action of single genes.

Deletions are more common, and have been used extensively to map disease loci. A commonly used approach is to create a shortest region of deletion overlap (SRO) map in which deletions in several individuals with the same phenotype are compared, the gene(s) of interest being in the deleted region common to all patients. Occasionally, non-overlapping deletions allow a single gene to be incriminated, as exemplified by the identification of the *LIS1* gene at the Miller–Dieker lissencephaly locus (Reiner et al, 1993).

Inversions and balanced translocations can cause defects as a consequence of gene disruption by the chromosomal breakpoints, or position effects mediated by control elements brought into juxtaposition with a novel gene. Fragile sites are also visible cytogenetically. Two such sites on the X chromosome are associated with mental retardation and the presence of an expanded number of trinucleotide repeat elements (Verkerk et al, 1991; Knight et al, 1993). It is now possible to search for expanding trinucleotide repeats directly, using a variation of the ligase chain reaction (Schalling et al, 1993).

In addition to standard karyotyping and fragile site analysis, **fluorescence in-situ hybridization** (FISH; see later) has now become an indispensable tool for the analysis of chromosome structure. **Cosmid** and **yeast artificial chromosome** (YAC; see later) probes are available for most areas of the human genome, including centromeres and telomeres, and the **polymerase chain reaction** (PCR) has been used to provide 'paints' for whole chromosomes (Telenius et al, 1992). Region-specific paints can be produced by amplifying probe from template provided by the human component of somatic cell hybrids, or contiguous arrays of YAC clones. A particularly useful method for the initial characterization of a chromosome abnormality is the 'reverse paint' (Rack et al, 1993). Here, the abnormal chromosome is flow-sorted and degenerate primers are used to amplify probe which gives an even paint on a normal metaphase. This procedure allows the identification of the various chromosomes involved in a rearrangement, for instance where small marker chromosomes or complex rearrangements and/or deletions are involved.

However, many chromosomal abnormalities are not visible even using high-resolution (>800) band karyotype (Carey et al, 1992; Wilson et al, 1992). Mapping these aberrations therefore comes under the heading of refining disease locus position, but it is possible that genome scanning procedures will be developed in the near future that will allow such abnormalities to be detected earlier. The main contender in the race to provide such a method is **comparative genome hybridization** (CGH) (du Manoir et al, 1993), shown in Figure 3.2. In essence, total genomic DNA from the test individual or cell line is labelled with one fluorescent tag and hybridized to normal chromosomes in competition with similarly prepared, but differently tagged, probe from normal genomic DNA. The relative fluorescent intensities of the two probes are then compared along the length of the chromosome, duplications detected as gain of relative intensity and deletions as loss of intensity within the region concerned. At present the utility of this procedure is in the detection of several-fold amplification in tumours, or homozygous deletions. It is not yet clear what the practical limits of the technique will be, but it may yet find a place in the armamentarium of the positional cloner.

In a similar vein, it has been postulated that some cases of mental retardation are due to terminal deletions of chromosomes. Early studies to test this

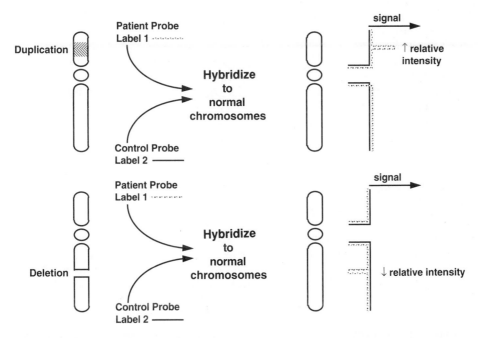

Figure 3.2 Comparative genome hybridization (CGH). A fluorescent probe from patient chromosomes is hybridized to normal chromosomes along with differentially labelled probe from control chromosomes. In the case of a duplication the relative signal strength of the test probe is greater over the duplicated sequences, whereas relative signal strength is lower over any deleted region

hypothesis are utilizing highly polymorphic markers to look for loss of obligate heterozygosity in these chromosomal regions. Such work may be replicated with other syndromes or, with multiplexing, be used to scan whole chromosomes.

Occasionally, a chromosomal or subchromosomal isodisomy can result in homozygosity for a recessive mutation. Detection of such isodisomy can be useful in the regional localization of disease genes, as was shown recently for Bloom syndrome (Woodage et al, 1994).

As linkage studies are described in more detail in Chapter 2, they are described only briefly here, for the sake of completeness. Disease genes are often localized by linkage analysis, using polymorphic markers and families segregating the disease phenotype. These studies are facilitated by the availability of a high density of very informative polymorphisms across the whole human genome (Dib et al, 1996), existing genetic maps and sophisticated statistical analyses. These advances mean that it is now possible to detect linkage in very rare disorders, for instance in single large families. It is also possible to contemplate the positional cloning of genes for more complex disorders with a genetic susceptibility such as diabetes (Davies et al, 1994), schizophrenia and hypertension. The application of homozygosity mapping has proved extremely useful in situations where standard linkage analysis is not applicable (small samples with consanguineous matings; Farrall, 1993). The position of disease loci may, in certain circumstances, be refined by allelic association studies (Ramsay et al, 1993; Jorde et al, 1994).

Occasionally there may be biochemical or physiological clues as to which gene might be mutated in certain diseases. Investigators may then choose to examine such **candidate genes** for linkage to, or association with, the disease phenotype, or even screen the candidate for mutations. There are now many successful applications of this strategy; however, negative data are less useful than global approaches in creating an exclusion map of the genome.

Two recent innovations for the localization of disease genes are **representational difference analysis** (RDA) and **genomic mismatch scanning** (GMS) (Lisitsyn et al, 1993; Nelson et al, 1994). Essentially, these techniques offer a short cut to genetic localization and both are still in the development phase, as far as human disorders are concerned. The reader is referred to Brown (1994) for a more detailed review of these procedures and their applications.

The basic approach is to isolate and map regions of identity (GMS) or difference (RDA) between genomes. RDA is a powerful application of subtractive hybridization. PCR amplicons are generated from 'Tester' and 'Driver' genomes in order to create a simplified representation of both samples. An adapter is ligated to the 5' end of the Tester amplicons which are melted and reannealed in the presence of a large molar excess of Driver. If a particular Tester amplicon is not represented or under-represented in the Driver, it may reanneal, allowing the ligation of an adapter to the 3' end and subsequent amplification. The procedure is iterated to achieve a good enrichment. One recent paper described the direct isolation of polymorphic markers linked to the *nude* locus using DNA from congenic mouse strains to minimize individual variation (restriction fragment length polymorphisms, RFLPs, may result in restriction fragments too large to be amplified in the Driver, allowing amplification of the Tester fragments) (Lisitsyn et al, 1994). Several other potential applications have been mooted for this elegant and powerful technique (Lander, 1993).

PHYSICAL MAPPING

Once the approximate map position of a disease locus has been ascertained there are several techniques that allow a refined map to be constructed. This will give probe order and often an estimate of the distance between the markers being examined. Somatic cell hybrids, which contain various human chromosomes and derivative chromosomes on a rodent background, are usually the first resource employed. Hybrids containing single chromosomes as their only human component are available from cell bank repositories for each of the human chromosomes. Where chromosomal rearrangements are associated with the disorder being studied, investigators can create hybrids from patients in order to segregate the abnormal chromosome from its normal homologue. This is particularly useful in birth defects associated with autosomal deletions as the resulting hybrids offer a plus/minus assay for the deletion instead of the vagaries of dosage analysis.

Radiation-reduced hybrids and telomere insertion hybrids may also be used for mapping. In the former, single chromosome hybrids are irradiated and then fused with a host cell line. The resulting hybrids then usually contain a few subchromosomal fragments whose size depends on the radiation dose. The presence or absence of markers in the hybrids and their co-segregation within the hybrid set allow a physical map to be constructed in a manner analogous to linkage mapping. Radiation hybrid maps of the entire genome are available, integrated with the physical map, and any sequence can be placed on this map easily (Hudson et al, 1996). Telomere-associated chromosome fragmentation is an approach based on the non-targeted (Farr et al, 1992) or targeted (Itzhaki et al, 1992) breakage of mammalian chromosomes with cloned telomeric DNA being introduced into hybrid cell lines. The resulting hybrids contain truncated versions of the initial target chromosome or chromosomes.

Pulse-field gradient electrophoresis (PFGE) allows a restriction map to be established over several megabases of DNA in the region of interest (van Ommen and Verkerk, 1986). This technique has the additional advantage that CpG-rich islands (CPIs) can be identified and located, the significance of which is discussed below.

FISH is a useful and quick method for establishing the order of loci along a chromosome. Several probes can be examined at any time, making use of the wide variety of fluorochromes that are spectrally separable (Lengauer et al, 1993). The sensitivity of FISH is also increased by the application of cooled charge-coupled detectors, although these expensive items are by no means necessary for the majority of FISH-based techniques. Metaphase analyses are used for markers separated by more than 2 Mb. Interphase nuclei have proved particularly useful in the diagnosis of chromosomal aneuploidy both in congenital defects and neoplasia, but also provide a means of ordering and distancing linked markers. It is possible to use markers separated by a known distance (determined perhaps by PFGE, or YAC size) to calibrate distance in microns versus distance in kilobases, and then use this calibration to measure distances between test markers (van den Engh et al, 1992; Lindsay et al, 1993). Interphase analysis offers resolution up to 50 kb. Greater resolution is provided by the application of extended DNA analysis. Free DNA can be released from nuclei by treatment with detergent (halo preparations; Wiegant et al, 1992). The released DNA can be stretched across a slide in the **direct visualization hybridization** (DIRVISH) technique to provide linear DNA for hybridization (Parra and Windle, 1993). These procedures can be used to map small fragments, cosmids or YACS and multicolour hybridization used to detect overlaps. The resolution is of the order of a few kilobases. Mechanically stretched chromosome preparations can be used for intermediate resolutions (Laan et al, 1995).

The aim of both physical and genetic mapping is often to identify markers that flank the locus of interest. Then an overlapping array of genomic clones is established that links the two flanking markers. Several vector systems and libraries are available for this purpose. Most commonly the genomic walk takes place in YACs. **YAC libraries** may be screened by PCR-based or hybridization-based methods. In PCR-based approaches pools of YACs are screened with various subsequent steps employed to identify a single positive recombinant. Several YAC libraries have been robotically arrayed and are available as filters for hybridization (Zehetner and Lehrach, 1994). Chromosome-specific YAC libraries are being generated and are conveniently analysed by hybridization to gridded arrays. Contiguous arrays of clones, **contigs**, may be generated by using YAC end-fragments as probes for the next step of the walk, or by hybridization of YAC Alu-PCR products to gridded arrays of Alu-PCR products from the library. Chimerism, where two or more non-contiguous genomic sequences are joined in a clone, can be assessed using FISH, which can also be used to monitor the map position of the clones: for example the position of the YAC with respect to a balanced translocation breakpoint. At any stage, the YACs can be tested for the presence of microsatellites that may be polymorphic. New markers can then be used in association studies, or in the analysis of recombination events close to the disease locus which pinpoint its position.

Cosmid libraries may be used for shorter walks and again, for many chromosomes, the workload is mitigated by the availability of gridded arrays (Zehetner and Lehrach, 1994). Occasionally, researchers find that their region of interest is absent or poorly represented in YAC and cosmid libraries. Several more recently developed vector systems have been used in these situations: for instance fosmids, bacterial artificial chromosomes (BACs) P1 phage and P1 artificial chromosomes (PACs) (Kim et al, 1992, 1994; Ioannou et al, 1994). Shuttling between different libraries is not uncommon.

If the region to be covered is relatively large and poorly covered by existing markers, it might be advantageous to isolate new markers from the region. Marker chromosomes may be flow-sorted to provide PCR template, or the DNA may be cloned directly. Specific pulse-field fragments may be excised from gels and cloned (Michiels et al, 1987). Alu-PCR may be used to generate clones and sequence-tagged sites (STSs) from subchromosomal regions using somatic cell hybrid DNA as template. Region-specific probes can also be generated by microdissection and microcloning. The microdissected material can be enzymatically amplified, labelled and used directly as probe (Meltzer et al, 1992) for the study of chromosome rearrangement (microFISH).

IDENTIFICATION OF CODING SEQUENCES

Genetic mapping, physical mapping and chromosome walking techniques may combine to implicate an area of tens of kilobases as the region containing the disease gene locus. The next task is to isolate novel candidate genes from these genomic sequences, and there is no shortage of methods to choose from. The simplest procedure is the direct screening of cDNA libraries with genomic clone inserts, and success has even been achieved with whole YACs (Elvin et al, 1990). However, the technique suffers from a relatively low sensitivity and problems related to incomplete suppression of repeat-sequence hybridization. More commonly, the genomic sequences are subcloned and these new markers hybridized to **zoo blots** which aim to detect the presence of sequence similarity between the human sequences and those of other species. Detection of such hybridization may indicate a sequence conserved during evolution and therefore a potential coding sequence. Northern analysis and cDNA library screening follow.

The 5', and occasionally the 3', end of genes often contains regions rich in CpG dinucleotides in which the C is unmethylated. Therefore several cloning strategies aimed at identification of potential CPIs have been devised including detection of clusters of rare-cutting restriction endonuclease sites and direct cloning (Estivill et al, 1987). In the future it may be possible to use genomic clones to screen whole genome or single chromosome CPI gridded arrays as it has been shown that CPIs may be isolated using a methylated-DNA affinity column (Cross et al, 1994). The CPIs are then used to screen cDNA libraries.

Another strategy, **exon trapping** or **exon amplification**, makes use of the splicing reaction to identify exons within coding DNA. Genomic sequences are cloned into plasmid vectors, transfected into mammalian cells and mature mRNAs cloned or PCR amplified. There are two types of vector. In one the system selects for sequences with single splice sites (Duyk et al, 1990), and therefore is susceptible to artefacts generated by cryptic splice sites. In the second system the vector pSPL3 requires the presence of both donor and acceptor splice sites, and cryptic products are removed by restriction endonuclease digestion prior to amplification (Church et al, 1994) (see Figure 3.3).

Exon trapping or exon amplification has the advantage that one need not know where or when a particular gene is expressed before embarking on the experiments. However, cDNAs still have to be isolated using the trapped products. An alternative is the cDNA selection procedure (Lovett et al, 1991; Parimoo et al, 1991). Short cDNA fragments (often amplified products) are

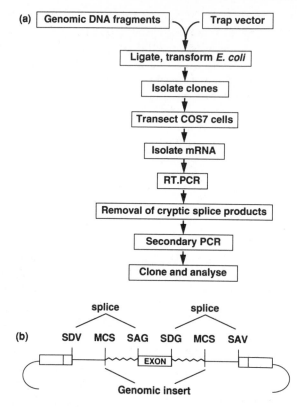

Figure 3.3   (a) Experimental steps involved in exon amplification using the pSPL3 vector (PCR polymerase chain reaction). (b) The vector. SDV, splice donor site vector; SAG, splice acceptor site genomic insert; SDG, splice donor site genomic insert; SAV, splice acceptor site vector; MCS, multiple cloning site. Splicing in vivo removes the intervening sequences delineated by the 'splice' brackets. The exon can then be PCR amplified using flanking primers

hybridized to genomic DNA immobilized on nylon membranes or beads. Repeated sequence hybridization is suppressed by competitive hybridization. Bound cDNA is eluted, reamplified and rehybridized to the genomic DNA through two or three cycles. The final cDNA products are then checked to confirm that they are encoded by sequences within the target genomic DNA, and full-length cDNAs obtained.

Finally, the increasing automation of DNA sequencing protocols has led to several large-scale genomic sequencing projects. Computer programs, such as Grail, are then employed to scan the sequence for potential exons (Uberbacher and Mural, 1991). The sequence from such potential exons is then used to design primers for **exon connection** (PCR between candidate exons) or **RACE PCR** (rapid amplification of cDNA ends) experiments, the latter having the potential to isolate full-length cDNA sequences.

GENE CHARACTERIZATION

Once a cDNA has been isolated certain basic characterization is undertaken. Northern analysis gives some indication as to transcript size (is the cDNA full length?), the number of transcripts detected (is the gene a member of a family? is there alternate splicing?), the relative abundance in various tissues or at various times in development, and the presence of aberrant transcripts or absence of transcription in samples from affected individuals. The sequence of the gene is also vital for mutation detection, database searching and secondary structure prediction.

MUTATION DETECTION

Identification of mutations within a candidate gene is generally regarded as proof that a disease locus has been identified. A reasonable first step is Southern analysis of patient versus control DNAs to rapidly scan for rearrangements or, in the most serendipitous cases, point mutations. In some instances it is possible to sequence the corresponding cDNA from affected individuals, although access to an expressing tissue is often problematic, and in some cases only one allele may be represented. If the intron–exon structure of the gene has been established, PCR may be used to amplify exons for direct sequencing (Gyllensten and Erlich, 1988). It is also possible to use the PCR reaction, usually with nested primers, to amplify overlapping cDNA fragments for sequencing from tissues that do not apparently express the gene. This procedure utilizes 'illegitimate' transcripts which, depending on the gene, are present at low levels in cells such as Epstein–Barr virus-transformed lymphoblastoid lines (Chelly et al, 1989).

Mutations can be detected by various methods not involving DNA sequencing. Each of these methods has distinct advantages and disadvantages, and each makes use of PCR. In the simplest method, single-strand conformational polymorphism (SSCP), control and patient DNAs (genomic or cDNA) are amplified, and the products denatured and electrophoresed by non-denaturing **polyacrylamide gel electrophoresis** (PAGE) (Orita et al, 1989). The single-stranded products adopt a three-dimensional conformation dependent on the primary sequence of the strand; thus a heterozygote would produce four bands, with two seen in wild-type samples. Several studies have examined the efficiency of various parameters that affect the ability to detect mutations, and the sensitivity is quoted to be 70–90% (Glavac-Ravnik et al, 1994).

In **denaturing gradient gel electrophoresis** (DGGE) dsDNA products from normals and affecteds are mixed, reannealed and electrophoresed in a denaturing gradient (chemical or temperature gradients may be used) (Sheffield et al, 1989; Tee et al, 1992). In a mutant/wild-type mix there is differential melting of the hetero- and homoduplexes and a consequent alteration in the distance each product migrates. Computer algorithms have been devised to predict the efficacy of various primers within the target sequence, as the method works best in domains of comparatively low melting temperature (Lerman and

Silverstein, 1985). If no such domains are present, a GC clamp can be applied to the ends of the primers (Sheffield et al, 1989).

Differential mobility of heteroduplexes forms the basis for another technique named, naturally enough, heteroduplex analysis (White et al, 1992). Patient and control templates are amplified together which allows the heteroduplexes to form. The differential mobility is best detected using specialized matrices such as Hydrolink[R] and MDE™, available commercially. Sensitivity is close to that provided by SSCP.

In the procedures outlined above, should a potential mutation be detected, no information as to its position within the amplified fragment is available. However, it is possible to cleave heteroduplexes at the mismatch position. The relative sizes of the resolved cleavage products then indicate the site of the mismatch. One technique uses the enzyme RNase A to cleave RNA–DNA heteroduplexes, the RNA being a radioactively labelled riboprobe, but sensitivity is only about 50% (Myers et al, 1985). Chemical methods of cleaving heteroduplexes are much more sensitive (approaching 100%). Various chemicals are available that modify the base(s) at the mismatch site and thus identify the site at which the cleavage agent acts. One drawback of this approach is the toxicity of many of the compounds used in the reactions (Cotton et al, 1988).

Finally, changes detected by any of the above mechanisms have to be checked by sequencing. Sequence alterations may cause frame shifts or premature termination, but amino-acid substitutions may be polymorphisms. Usually, a large appropriate population of control DNAs is scanned for absence of the change, or an incidence compatible with carrier frequency (recessives) or non-penetrance (dominants). Demonstration that the alteration is de novo may provide additional evidence that the change is actually a mutation, and functional studies are useful in some cases. In cystic fibrosis, for example, transfection of the wild-type gene into cell lines with a homozygote affected genotype results in complementation of a physiological defect (Rich et al, 1990).

The subsequent steps in the molecular genetic analysis of the gene and its mutant counterpart(s) depend to a great extent on the type of protein the gene encodes. In general, work often involves attempting to correlate genotype with phenotype, resolving questions of genetic heterogeneity and creating mouse models for the disorder using gene knockouts. The last may also shed light on gene function (see Chapter 4).

It has to be remembered that positional cloning experiments do not always lead to an immediate increase in the understanding of pathophysiological or developmental mechanisms. Where sequence database searches shed little light on the nature of a protein product, elucidating the likely function of a protein can be one of the most challenging subsequent problems. With a working hypothesis concerning protein function it is then possible to explore the role of the gene product in a wider context, using the newly identified protein as an entry point into a developmental pathway for example. One approach which is increasingly followed is the identification of proteins that interact with the protein initially isolated. For example, different subunits of transcriptional factors or holoenzymes may be isolated in this way. Screening for interacting proteins may be conducted in vitro or in vivo. In-vitro methods centre on screening expression libraries with labelled or tagged protein (Blackwood and Eisenman, 1991; Blanar and Rutter, 1992; Ayer et al, 1993). In order to obviate the problems associated with altered conformational states in this type of experiment, in-vivo approaches based on that described by Fields and Song (1989) are increasingly used (see Figure 3.4). In one such system a yeast strain is established in which the expression of a GAL1-LacZ reporter gene is under the control of a GAL4-activated promoter. This activation is dependent upon a reconstitution of GAL4 activity via protein–protein interaction. The GAL4 protein contains discrete modules with a DNA-binding domain and a transcriptional activation domain. In the dihybrid system these two modules are brought into apposition by the interaction of two polypeptides fused to each domain. The production of β-galactosidase allows colonies containing interacting peptides to be detected by colour reaction. In the experiment, a vector containing the GAL4 binding domain is fused to the probe domains, and a cDNA library is constructed using mRNA from a source of likely target proteins such that the candidate interacting proteins are fused to the GAL4 DNA activation domain or vice versa. The test protein construct is transfected into yeast that contains the reporter gene. The resulting strain is then transfected with the cDNA library containing the potential interactors. Transfectants are tested for β-galactosidase activity by

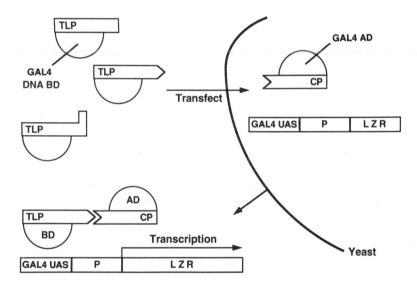

Figure 3.4 Interaction cloning in vivo. The candidate protein (CP) represents the protein for which interacting proteins will be isolated. It is expressed in a yeast strain fused to the GAL4 activation domain (GAL4 AD). A cDNA library is created which, when transfected into yeast, will direct synthesis of GAL4 DNA binding domain (GAL4 DNA BD)/target library protein (TLP) fusion products. If any TLP interacts with CP, then the GAL4 AD and BD are brought into apposition. The complex then binds to the GAL4 upstream activating sequence (GAL4 UAS) of the GAL4 promoter (P), activating transcription of the reporter gene (LZR, bottom left), which is then detected by colony filter assay. Clones encoding the TLP can then be isolated and sequenced

colony filter assay in order to identify interacting proteins. One example of the successful application of this technique was the isolation of proteins reacting with the *Jun* leucine zipper (Chevray and Nathans, 1992).

CONCLUSION

It should be evident from this chapter that there is a bewildering array of technologies available for positional cloning. Many methods have not been discussed: for instance chromosome jumping, differential display and the use of comparative maps of other species. The choice of technique is somewhat dependent on the resources available for the region of interest and on local expertise. While this review has concentrated on techniques that have been applied successfully to human disorders, from the developmental point of view it may be that the identification of mutations in other animals will be more important. While the mouse genome mapping programme is advancing apace, it could be that newer technologies such as RDA, GMS and microFISH will also allow faster mapping in organisms such as the rat, dog, pig and zebrafish.

REFERENCES

Ayer, D.E., Kretzner, L. and Eisenman, R.N. (1993) Mad: a heterodimeric partner for Max that antagonizes Myc transcriptional activity. *Cell* 72, 211–222.

Ballabio, A. (1993) The rise and fall of positional cloning? *Nature Genetics* 3, 277–279.

Blackwood, E.M. and Eisenman, R.N. (1991) Max: a helix-loop-helix zipper protein that forms a sequence-specific DNA-binding complex with Myc. *Science* 251, 1211–1217.

Blanar, M.A. and Rutter, W.J. (1992) Interaction cloning: identification of a helix-loop-helix zipper protein that interacts with c-Fos. *Science* 256, 1014–1018.

Brown, P.O. (1994) Genome scanning methods. *Curr. Biol.* 4, 366–373.

Carey, A.H., Kelly, D., Halford, S. et al (1992) Molecular genetic study of the frequency of monosomy 22q11 in DiGeorge syndrome. *Am. J. Hum. Genet.* 51, 964–970.

Chelly, J., Concordet, J.P., Kaplan, J.C. and Kahn, A. (1989) Illegitimate transcription: transcription of any gene in any cell type. *Proc. Natl. Acad. Sci. USA* 86, 2617–2622.

Chevray, P.M. and Nathans, D. (1992) Protein interaction cloning in yeast: identification of mammalian proteins that react with the leucine zipper of Jun. *Proc. Natl. Acad. Sci. USA* 89, 5789–5793.

Church, D.M., Stotler, C.J., Rutter, J.L. et al (1994) Isolation of genes from complex sources of mammalian genomic DNA using exon amplification. *Nature Genetics* 6, 98–105.

Collins, F.S. (1992) Positional cloning: let's not call it reverse anymore. *Nature Genetics* 1, 3–6.

Cotton, R.G., Rodrigues, N.R. and Campbell, R.D. (1988) Reactivity of cytosine and thymine in single-base-pair mismatches with hydroxylamine and osmium tetroxide and its application to the study of mutations. *Proc. Natl. Acad. Sci. USA* 85, 4397–4401.

Cross, S.H., Charlton, J.A., Nan, X. and Bird, A.P. (1994) Purification of CpG islands using a methylated DNA binding column. *Nature Genetics* 6, 236–244.

Davies, J.L., Kawaguchi, Y., Bennett, S.T. et al (1994) A genome-wide search for human type 1 diabetes susceptibility genes. *Nature* 371, 130–135.

Dib, C., Faure, S., Fizames, C. et al (1996) A comprehensive genetic map of the human genome based on 5264 microsatellites. *Nature* 380, 152–154.

du Manoir, S., Speicher, M.R., Joos, S. et al (1993) Detection of complete and partial chromosome gains and losses by comparative genomic in situ hybridisation. *Hum. Genet.* **90**, 590–610.

Duyk, G.M., Kim, S., Myers, R.M. and Cox, D.R. (1990) Exon trapping: a genetic screen to identify candidate transcribed sequences in cloned mammalian genomic DNA. *Proc. Natl. Acad. Sci. USA* **87**, 8995–8999.

Elvin, P., Slynn, G., Black, D. et al (1990) Isolation of cDNA clones using yeast artificial chromosome probes. *Nucleic Acids Res.* **18**, 3913–3917.

Estivill, X., Farrall, M., Scambler, P.J. et al (1987) A candidate for the cystic fibrosis locus isolated by selection for methylation-free islands. *Nature* **326**, 840–845.

Farr, C.J., Stevanovic, M., Thomson, E.J., Goodfellow, P.N. and Cooke, H.J. (1992) Telomere-associated chromosome fragmentation: applications in genome manipulation and analysis. *Nature Genetics* **2**, 275–282.

Farrall, M. (1993) Homozygosity mapping: familiarity breeds debility. *Nature Genetics* **5**, 107–108.

Fields, S. and Song, O.-K. (1989) A novel genetic system to detect protein–protein interactions. *Proc. Natl. Acad. Sci. USA* **340**, 245–246.

Glavac-Ravnik, M., Glavac, D. and Dean, M. (1994) Sensitivity of single-strand conformation polymorphism and heteroduplex method for mutation detection in the cystic fibrosis gene. *Hum. Molec. Genet.* **3**, 801–807.

Gyllensten, U.B. and Erlich, H.A. (1988) Generation of single-stranded DNA by the polymerase chain reaction and its application to direct sequencing of the HLA-SQA locus. *Proc. Natl. Acad. Sci. USA* **85**, 7652–7656.

Hudson, T.J., Stein, L.D., Genety, S.S. et al (1996) An STS-based map of the human genome. *Science* **270**, 1945–1954.

Ioannou, P.A., Amemiya, C.T., Garnes, J. et al (1994) A new bacteriophage P1-derived vector for the propagation of large human DNA fragments. *Nature Genetics* **6**, 84–88.

Itzhaki, J.E., Barnett, M.A., MacCarthy, A.B. et al (1992) Targeted breakage of a human chromosome mediated by cloned human telomeric DNA. *Nature Genetics* **2**, 283–287.

Jorde, L.B., Watkins, W.S., Carlson, M. et al (1994) Linkage disequilibrium predicts physical distance in the adenomatous polyposis coli region. *Am. J. Hum. Genet.* **54**, 884–898.

Kim, U.-J., Shizuya, H., de Jong, P., Birren, B. and Simon, M.I. (1992) Stable propagation of cosmid sized human DNA inserts in an F factor based vector. *Nucleic Acids Res.* **20**, 1083–1085.

Kim, U.-J., Shizuya, H., Birren, B. et al (1994) Selection of chromosome 22-specific clones from human genomic BAC library using a chromosome-specific cosmid library pool. *Genomics* **22**, 336–339.

Knight, S.J.L., Flannery, A.V., Hirst, M.C. et al (1993) Trinucleotide repeat amplification and hypermethylation of a CpG island in FRAXE mental retardation. *Cell* **74**, 127–134.

Korenberg, J.R., Bradley, C. and Disteche, C.M. (1992) Down syndrome: molecular mapping of congenital heart disease and duodenal stenosis. *Am. J. Hum. Genet.* **50**, 294–302.

Laan, M. Kallioniemi, O.-P., Hellsten, E. et al (1995) Mechanically stretched chromosomes as targets for high-resolution FISH mapping. *Genome Res.* **5**, 13–20.

Lander, E.S. (1993) Finding similarities and differences among genomes. *Nature Genetics* **4**, 5–6.

Lengauer, C., Speicher, M.R., Popp, S. et al (1993) Chromosomal bar codes produced by multicolour fluorescence in situ hybridisation with multiple YAC clones and whole chromosome painting probes. *Hum. Molec. Genet.* **2**, 505–512.

Lerman, L.S. and Silverstein, K. (1985) Computational simulation of DNA melting and its application to denaturing gel electrophoresis. *Meth. Enzymol.* **155**, 482–501.

Lindsay, E.A., Halford, S., Wadey, R., Scambler, P.J. and Baldini, A. (1993) Molecular cytogenetic characterisation of the DiGeorge syndrome region using fluorescence in situ hybridisation. *Genomics* **17**, 403–407.

Lisitsyn, N.A., Lisitsyn, N.M. and Wigler, M. (1993) Cloning the differences between two complex genomes. *Science* **259**, 946–951.

Lisitsyn, N.A., Segre, J.A., Kusumi, K. et al (1994) Direct isolation of polymorphic markers linked to a trait by genetically directed representational difference analysis. *Nature Genetics* **6**, 57–63.

Lovett, M., Kere, J. and Hinton, L.M. (1991) Direct selection: a method for the isolation of cDNAs encoded by large genomic regions. *Proc. Natl. Acad. Sci. USA* **88**, 9628–9632.

Mears, A.J., Duncan, A.M.V., Budarf, M.L. et al (1994) Molecular characterisation of the marker chromosome associated with cat eye syndrome. *Am. J. Hum. Genet.* **55**, 134–142.

Meltzer, P.S., Guan, X.-Y., Burgess, A. and Trent, J.M. (1992) Rapid generation of region specific probes by chromosome microdissection and their application. *Nature Genetics* **1**, 24–28.

Michiels, F., Burmeister, M. and Lehrach, H. (1987) Derivation of clones close to MET by preparative pulsed field gel electrophoresis. *Science* **236**, 1305–1308.

Myers, R.M., Larin, Z. and Maniatis, T. (1985) Detection of single base substitutions by ribonuclease cleavage at mismatches in RNA : DNA duplexes. *Science* 230, 1242–1246.

Nelson, S.F., McKusker, J.H., Sander, M.A. et al (1994) Genomic mismatch scanning: a new approach to genetic linkage mapping. *Nature Genetics* **6**, 11–17.

Orita, M., Suzuki, Y., Sekiya, T. and Hayashi, K. (1989) Rapid and sensitive detection of point mutations and DNA polymorphism using the polymerase chain reaction. *Genomics* **5**, 874–879.

Parimoo, S., Patanjali, S.R., Shukla, H., Chaplin, D.D. and Weissman, S.M. (1991) cDNA selection: efficient PCR approach for the selection of cDNAs encoded by large genomic regions. *Proc. Natl. Acad. Sci. USA* **88**, 9623–9627.

Parra, I. and Windle, B. (1993) High resolution visual mapping of stretched DNA by fluorescent hybridization. *Nature Genetics* **5**, 17–21.

Rack, K., Harris, P.C., MacCarthy, A.M. et al (1993) Characterization of three de novo derivative chromosomes 16 by reverse chromosome painting and molecular analysis. *Am. J. Hum. Genet.* **52**, 987–997.

Ramsay, M., Williamson, R., Estivill, X. et al (1993) Haplotype analysis to determine the position of a mutation among closely linked genetic markers. *Hum. Molec. Genet.* **2**, 1007–1014.

Reiner, O., Carrozzo, R., Shen, Y. et al (1993) Isolation of a Miller–Dieker lissencephaly gene containing G protein beta-subunit-like repeats. *Nature* **364**, 717–721.

Rich, D.P., Anderson, M.P., Gregory, R.J. et al (1990) Expression of cystic fibrosis transmembrane conductance regulator corrects defective chloride channel regulation in cystic fibrosis airway epithelial cells. *Nature* **347**, 358–363.

Robinson, W.P., Binkert, F., Gine, R. et al (1993) Clinical and molecular analysis of five inv dup(15) patients. *Eur. J. Hum. Genet.* **1**, 37–50.

Schalling, M., Hudson, T.J., Buetow, K.H. and Housman, D.E. (1993) Direct detection of novel expanded trinucleotide repeats in the human genome. *Nature Genetics* **4**, 135–139.

Sheffield, V.C., Cox, D.R., Lerman, L.S. and Myers, R.M. (1989) Attachment of a 40-ase-pair G + C-rich sequence (GC-clamp) to genomic DNA fragments by the polymerase chain reaction results in improved detection of single base changes. *Proc. Natl. Acad. Sci. USA* **86**, 232–236.

Tee, M.K., Moran, C. and Nicholas, F.W. (1992) Temperature gradient gel electrophoresis: detection of single base substitution in the cattle beta-lactoglobulin gene. *Anim. Genet.* **23**, 158–160.

Telenius, H., Pelmear, A.H., Tunnacliffe, A. et al (1992) Cytogenetic analysis by chromosome painting using degenerate oligonucleotide-primed-polymerase chain reaction amplified flow-sorted chromosomes. *Genes Chromosomes Cancer* **4**, 257–263.

Uberbacher, E.C. and Mural, R.J. (1991) Locating protein-coding regions in human DNA sequences by a multiple sensorineural network approach. *Proc. Natl. Acad. Sci. USA* **88**, 11261–11265.

van den Engh, G., Sach, R. and Trask, B.J. (1992) Estimating genomic distance from DNA sequence in cell nuclei by a random model. *Science* **257**, 1410–1412.

van Ommen, G.J.B. and Verkerk, J.M.H. (1986) Restriction analysis of chromosomal DNA in a size range up to two million base pairs by pulse field gradient electrophoresis. In *Human Genetic Diseases: A Practical Approach* (Ed.: K.E. Davies), pp. 113–133. IRL Press: Oxford.

Verkerk, A.J.M.H., Pieretti, M., Sutcliffe, J.S. et al (1991) Identification of a gene (*FMR-1*) containing a CGG repeat coincident with a breakpoint cluster region exhibiting length variation in fragile X syndrome. *Cell* **65**, 905–914.

White, M.B., Carvalho, M., Derse, D., O'Brien, S.J. and Dean, M. (1992) Detecting single base substitutions as heteroduplex polymorphisms. *Genomics* **12**, 301–306.

Wiegant, J., Kalle, W., Mullenders, L. et al (1992) High-resolution in situ hybridisation using DNA halo preparations. *Hum. Molec. Genet.* **1**, 587–591.

Wilson, D.I., Cross, I., Goodship, J.A. et al (1992) Prospective cytogenetic study of 36 cases of DiGeorge syndrome. *Am. J. Hum. Genet.* **51**, 957–963.

Woodage, T., Prasad, M., Dixon, J.W. et al (1994) Bloom syndrome and maternal uniparental disomy for chromosome 15. *Am. J. Hum. Genet.* **55**, 74–80.

Zehetner, G. and Lehrach, H. (1994) The reference library system: sharing biological material and experimental data. *Nature* **367**, 489–491.

4 Transgenic Technology as a Tool

RUDI BALLING

Institut für Säugetiergenetik, GSF Forschungszentrum Neuherberg, Neuherberg, Germany

The discovery that genetic information is based on the sequence of nucleotides in a DNA molecule resulted in an explosion of knowledge in almost all fields of biological and medical sciences. The ability to read and translate the genetic code has become routine in today's biological research, and the number of diagnostic procedures that involve the use of DNA analysis is increasing at an exponential rate. Very soon we will have the complete sequence of the human genome available in our databases. However, even if we know the complete sequence of our genome, this does not automatically provide the answer to questions such as how the form of an embryo is established, why a genetic disease results in a specific phenotype or how our brain functions. The most powerful strategy available to understand such biological mechanisms is the use of genetics.

A central theme in genetics is the analysis of mutants. Indeed, the deciphering of the genetic code was made possible by the production and analysis of mutant phage. Important insights into the mechanisms of gene regulation were obtained because of the availability of bacterial mutants with defects in metabolic pathways such as glucose metabolism. A growing number of human genetic diseases are now understood because the genes responsible have been isolated and sequenced from affected patients (see Chapter 2). In these instances, the patient can be considered the 'mutant'. Generally, the mutants analysed have arisen spontaneously in nature and have been recognizable because of the externally visible characteristics of the phenotype. The discovery by H. Muller in 1923 that X-rays could be used to increase the mutation rate had a major impact on genetics, particularly for the study of the fruitfly *Drosophila melanogaster*.

During the last decade a genetic approach has also been applied to the analysis of mammalian development. The model of choice has been the mouse. The reason for this has been the availability of a large number of mouse mutants which have emerged from breeding colonies all over the world in the last hundred years (Lyon and Searle, 1989). Like *Drosophila*, most of these mutants arose spontaneously or were induced by chemical or physical means. This chapter will describe recent technological advances that will allow the production of mutants in the mouse at will. Genes can now be introduced systematically into the genome of mice or they can be effectively deleted. The DNA sequence of individual genes can even be changed and the developmental consequences analysed. Transgenic technology

Embryos, Genes and Birth Defects. Edited by P. Thorogood.
© 1997 John Wiley & Sons Ltd.

will not only be a major research tool in the future but also establish a basis for the development of new therapeutic procedures, such as gene therapy.

BASICS OF MOUSE PRE-IMPLANTATION EMBRYOLOGY AND REPRODUCTIVE BIOLOGY

Mice live on average about 2 to 3 years. Their gestation period is about 20 days and embryonic development takes place entirely within the body of the mother. Embryonic development of mice can be divided into two phases:

- **pre-implantation development,** from fertilization up to the blastocyst stage, and
- **post-implantation development,** from implantation into the uterus up to birth (Hogan et al, 1986).

Understanding transgenic mouse technology inevitably requires a familiarity with the early stages of mouse development. Mouse embryogenesis begins with fertilization of the ovulated egg by a spermatozoon. Fertilization takes place in the upper part of the oviduct, from where the zygote is transported through the action of the ciliated epithelial lining into the uterus. During this time a number of **cleavage divisions** take place which increase the number of blastomeres, but not the overall size of the pre-implantation embryo (Figure 4.1). At that time the

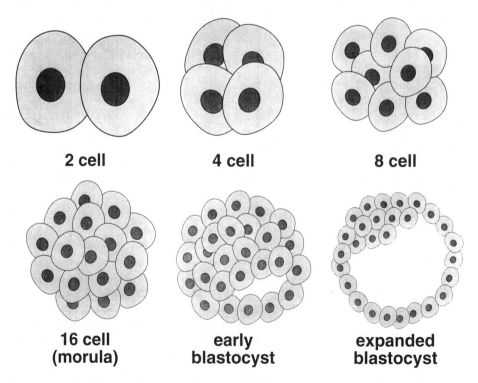

| 2 cell | 4 cell | 8 cell |

| 16 cell (morula) | early blastocyst | expanded blastocyst |

Figure 4.1   Early stages of mouse embryogenesis

embryo is surrounded by an acellular transparent layer, the **zona pellucida**. However, there is no direct contact with the maternal blood vascular system. Approximately 2 days after fertilization a **morula** is formed consisting of about 16 blastomeres. These blastomeres look identical and are **totipotent**, which means that they are still able to form all kinds of cell types. The first differentiation event takes place around 3.5 days after fertilization, with the formation of the **blastocyst**. At that time a fluid-filled cavity, the blastocyst cavity, can be seen between the compacted blastomeres. This is followed by the first appearance of two different cell types of the developing embryo: an **inner cell mass** (ICM) and an outer layer, the **trophectoderm**. Whereas the trophectoderm becomes specialized for the nutritional supply of the embryo and for implanting into the epithelium of the uterine wall, the ICM cells retain their developmental totipotency. In addition to the trophectoderm, an additional cell layer is now formed, the **primitive endoderm**, which covers the ICM. This cell layer will also form parts of the **extraembryonic tissues** (i.e. the yolk sac) but does not contribute to the final **embryo proper**. At 4.5 days of development the embryo implants into the uterus, establishing contact with the maternal blood system. Following implantation, the embryo rapidly increases in cell number and size.

Post-implantation development starts with the process of **gastrulation**, which is characterized by the formation of the three definite germ layers: **ectoderm**, **mesoderm** and **endoderm**. Gastrulation not only establishes the different germ layers that are required for the later stages of organogenesis, but also marks the time when the first polarity of the embryo along the anteroposterior axis becomes visible. The **primitive streak** is the midline structure through which epiblast cells internalize, in a progressive anteroposterior sequence, as the point of most active internalization – the 'node' – regresses in a posterior direction. Through a number of complicated tissue interactions and cell migrations the **final body plan** is established and **organogenesis** proceeds, leading to the formation of the heart, nervous system and all the other organs (see Chapters 7 to 15). During the last third of pregnancy the developing organs grow in size and the special cell types of each organ continue to differentiate.

IN-VITRO CULTURE, CHIMERAS AND EMBRYONIC STEM CELLS

One of the major breakthroughs leading to today's transgenic technology was the development of techniques enabling the culture of pre-implantation embryos **in vitro**. Through the refinement of culture media and conditions it is now possible for a fertilized egg to develop completely in vitro from fertilization up to the blastocyst stage (Hogan et al, 1986). Even earlier stages of oocyte maturation and fertilization can be accomplished in vitro, as is routinely practised in the clinical application of in-vitro fertilization. In-vitro culture allows access to these early embryos, which would not otherwise be possible in their normal environment of the oviduct and uterus. After in-vitro culture, embryos can be transferred back into the oviduct or the uterus of a **pseudopregnant foster mother**. (A pseudopregnant state can be created in female mice by mating them to a vasectomized male; this leads to endocrinological changes that mimic a pregnant state and allows implantation and a successful pregnancy provided embryos are transferred into the uterus from outside; Hogan et al, 1986.)

As stated earlier the blastomeres of early cleavage-stage embryos, and the ICM cells of the blastocyst, are still totipotent. If one removes blastomeres from an early embryo, the resulting loss of cells can be compensated, so that **size regulation** is achieved. Similarly, ICM cells from one embryo can be added to the ICM of another embryo. Cells from both are thereby integrated into a single embryo, which now is composed of cells from two genetically different individuals. Such a 'mixed' embryo is called a **chimera**. Chimeras can be produced either by aggregating two morula-stage embryos or by injecting cells from the ICM of one embryo into the blastocoelic cavity of a second embryo. In the latter case, the injected ICM cells attach to the ICM cells of the host embryo, intermingle and become part of a chimera.

Before and during gastrulation extensive cell mixing occurs which leads to a contribution of cells from both embryos to most, if not all, tissues. There is an important distinction between chimerism in somatic tissues alone and those instances where there is a contribution of donor-derived cells to the germ line of the host. The latter will result in a chimeric individual producing individual gametes of both donor and host embryo genetic constitution. The successful production of such a **germ-line chimera** can be monitored if the two embryos used for chimera production differ in some **genetic markers** that can be scored. The easiest marker is a difference in coat colour. Combining cells from early embryos of white and black mice would result in a chimera that has a mixture of patches of white and black hairs. However, such a marker alone is only useful to detect chimerism in those tissues in which pigmentation is expressed (chiefly skin and retina) and cannot be used to detect germ-line chimerism. In order to assess the existence and extent of chimerism in other, non-pigmented tissues (including gametes), other markers are needed. A frequently used marker is the enzyme glucophosphoisomerase which occurs in two isoforms that can be separated electrophoretically. In this case only homogenized tissue can be analysed. However, a difference in DNA sequence, be it a deletion, an insertion or only a point mutation, can also be followed as a polymorphic marker to determine the genetic origin of a specific cell.

Although the in-vitro culture of pre-implantation embryos has become a routine procedure in reproductive biology and embryology, the number of embryos that can be manipulated at any given time is limited. This is of significant, practical importance in any kind of genetic manipulation in which screening of a large number of cells is required in order to find a rare event, such as a particular mutation. This problem of limited numbers of embryonic cells for analysis has been solved by the discovery that ICM cells can be put in culture and, if handled appropriately, maintain their totipotent state (Evans and Kaufman, 1981; Martin, 1981; Robertson, 1987; Bradley, 1990). These cells are called **embryonic stem cells** (ES cells). One of the most important features of ES cells is the fact that, after in-vitro culture, they can still contribute to the formation of chimeras if they are aggregated with a morula or injected into a host blastocyst. This means that all those manipulations suitable for cell culture, including the use of selection markers and genetic manipulations, can be applied to ES cells and that, out of such manipulated cells, mice can be produced via the generation of chimeras. (Further details on the culture of ES cells, and their use in making chimeras, is given later.)

PRODUCTION OF TRANSGENIC MICE

The core of any genetic analysis is the question of gene function. As discussed earlier, this is best approached by the analysis of mutants in which a specific gene or gene function is missing, so that the consequences of its lack can be analysed. In addition to the loss of gene function it can be very useful to study the consequences of adding additional copies of a gene or an altered gene to the genome, in order to have genes expressed inappropriately at specific stages of development or at ectopic sites. Transgenic mice are mice that have exogenous DNA integrated into their genome by experimental procedures. If this integration has occurred into functional germ cells, the foreign DNA will be transmitted from generation to generation, becoming part of the normal genetic make-up of this mouse line. The two main techniques for making transgenic mice are DNA microinjection and the use of ES cells (see later).

DNA MICROINJECTION

Currently the quickest way to produce a transgenic mouse is to inject the exogenous DNA of interest directly into the **pronucleus** of a fertilized egg (Figure 4.2; and see Hogan et al, 1986). For this purpose fertilized eggs are removed from the oviduct about 24 h after fertilization. At this time the embryos are still surrounded by a cloud of **cumulus cells**. In order to remove the cumulus cells a short application of hyaluronidase is given and the freed embryos are put into in-vitro culture medium. In order to obtain a large number of fertilized embryos, female donor mice are often pretreated with hormones (follicle-stimulating hormone, luteinizing hormone), which results in artificial maturation of eggs and induction of ovulation (**superovulation**). Once in culture the embryos can be observed using a stereomicroscope, but all subsequent manipulations necessitate the use of specialized equipment such as micromanipulators, attached to a compound microscope equipped with differential interference contrast optics. For a few hours the individual pronuclei are clearly visible before they fuse and form the zygote. During this time a solution of DNA can be directly injected into one of the **pronuclei** through a finely drawn glass micropipette; usually the male pronucleus is used as a target of injection because of its larger size (Figure 4.3). In terms of quantity, about 100–10 000 copies of the foreign DNA are injected; the actual volume of injected DNA is monitored by the degree of swelling of the pronucleus. After microinjection the embryos are kept in culture for a short time so that any damaged embryos can be identified and discarded.

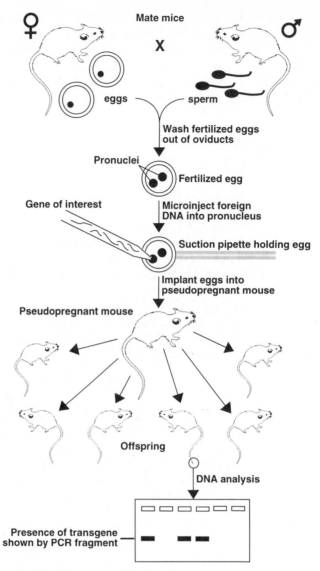

Figure 4.2 Production of a transgenic mouse using DNA microinjection (redrawn after Sedivy and Joyner, 1992)

After DNA microinjection the embryos are transferred to the reproductive tract of the **pseudopregnant foster mothers**. Following anaesthesia a small incision is made in the back skin of the foster mother to make the oviduct accessible for transfer of the injected embryos. Using a small glass pipette the eggs are transferred into the opening of the oviduct, the infundibulum. Typically, between 10 and 20 embryos are transferred back into a single foster mother. Approximately 50% of the embryos survive the injection procedure and about 20% survive to term; out of these, 10–30% are usually transgenic.

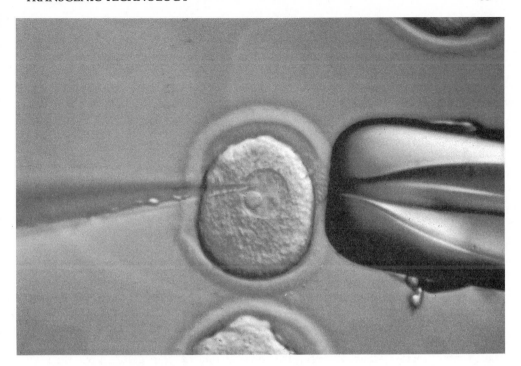

Figure 4.3 Microinjection of DNA into pronucleus

Integration into the genome of the injected embryos occurs at random. In most cases a variable number of transgene copies inserts into one integration site in a head-to-tail concatemer fashion. It is important to note that the strategy of DNA microinjection can only allow DNA to be added to the genome; endogenous DNA cannot be modified or deleted in a directed way by this procedure. However, in about 10% of transgenic mice transgene insertion has occurred into an endogenous gene, resulting in an **insertional mutation** event (Kuehn and Stoye, 1992). Often this can be detected by the occurrence of a phenotype with visible mutant characteristics amongst the offspring. Depending upon the nature of the phenotype, transgene-induced insertional mutation events can be very informative, since the affected gene can be cloned using the transgene as a probe for recovery.

Transgenic mice made by DNA microinjection are often used in order to study various aspects of **gene regulation**. For this purpose, fusion constructs between potential regulatory sequences (i.e. promoter regions) and a **reporter gene** (i.e. *β*-**galactosidase**) are injected and the expression of the reporter gene is analysed. Using specific deletions or mutations in the regulatory sequences, important information can be gained on the kind of regulatory elements that are necessary for correct expression of the gene in question. Often this kind of information cannot be obtained by tissue culture experiments simply because it may be almost impossible to reconstruct in vitro the precise cellular interactions that control gene expression in vivo. In addition to gene regulation studies, investigations aimed at elucidating the function of genes can be made by DNA microinjection transgenics. Thus, genes can be expressed ectopically under the control of various promoters, or mutated genes can be expressed under their own or foreign regulatory sequences. Recently techniques have been developed to introduce large DNA fragments of up to a few hundred kilobases as **yeast artificial chromosomes** (YACs; see Chapter 3) by DNA microinjection into the germ line of mice (Schedl et al, 1992, 1993; Jacobovits et al, 1993).

RETROVIRAL INFECTION

Producing transgenic mice by retroviral infection makes use of the natural life cycle of retroviruses. Retroviruses are able to integrate their viral genome into the genome of the infected host cell. However, not all retroviral sequences are necessary for this integration event and some of these sequences can be deleted and substituted with exogenous DNA. The lack of certain retroviral sequences, however, then prevents the production of infectious retroviral particles. These can be supplied by the use of certain helper cell lines. The recombinant retrovirus is then able to serve as a vector to introduce foreign DNA into cells (Stewart et al, 1987). The technique of inserting foreign DNA by retroviral infection has the advantage that only one copy of foreign DNA is inserted as compared to as many as 50 copies after DNA microinjection. However, a serious drawback is the limited size of foreign DNA (less than 10 kb) that can be packaged into a retroviral vector. Consequently, the production of transgenic mice through retroviral infection has not developed into a widely used procedure to date. However, many research laboratories are developing the use of retroviral or modified DNA virus vectors (i.e. adenovirus) as tools for somatic gene therapy.

GENE TARGETING BY HOMOLOGOUS RECOMBINATION

DNA microinjection and retroviral infection share one serious drawback. With both techniques, DNA can only be added to the mouse genome but endogenous sequences cannot be removed or altered in a specific, directed way. In many cases this restricts the kind of mutations that can be introduced into a mouse to **gain-of-function** mutations. Furthermore, the integration site of the transgene cannot be controlled and consequently position effects of genomic flanking sequences can exert influence on the expression of the transgene. In order to take full advantage of the power of genetics, **loss-of-function** mutations are required where genes are inactivated and the consequences of a lack of the gene product can be analysed.

Due to the progress in the isolation of genes and to the information that is coming out of the Human Genome Project, we will soon have a tremendous number of gene sequences at hand, but with little idea about their function. Therefore, it would be highly desirable to have techniques available which allow a directed, specific and efficient inactivation of any gene that has been cloned. Such a technique has recently been developed, originally in yeast but now also for mice – **homologous recombination** (Capecchi, 1989, 1994; Joyner, 1991, 1993; Sedivy and Joyner, 1992; Wagner and Keller, 1992).

The term homologous recombination, was originally used to describe a reciprocal exchange of genetic information between the maternal and paternal chromosomes during meiosis. However, it was soon realized that in principle such an exchange can also take place in somatic mammalian cells (Bollag et al, 1989). Of particular importance was the observation, first made in yeast, that foreign, episomal DNA can undergo homologous recombination with endogenous, chromosomal DNA. Studies in yeast also showed that foreign DNA is able to integrate at high frequency into endogenous DNA, if homologous sequences between incoming and endogenous DNA exist. Interestingly, efficient recombination with the chromosomal target requires a double-stranded break in the homologous sequences of the vector. The possibility of directly integrating foreign DNA into endogenous genes could therefore be used to specifically disrupt endogenous genes by insertional mutations and opened up the era of **gene targeting** (Capecchi, 1989, 1994; Sedivy and Joyner 1992). The successful development of gene targeting via homologous recombination as a routine technique in yeast genetics stimulated similar work on mammalian cells. In the late 1980s, research teams led by Mario Capecchi and Oliver Smithies were successful in working out the strategies whereby this goal could be accomplished.

One of the main differences in homologous recombination between yeast and mammalian cells is the frequency of homologous compared to non-homologous recombination. Whereas in yeast, non-homologous recombination occurs rarely, in mammalian cells the vast majority of recombination events are non-homologous. Therefore, it was necessary to develop techniques that could find the rare cells that had undergone homologous recombination among those in which the incoming DNA had integrated randomly somewhere in the genome. The solution to this problem came with the development of **polymerase chain reaction** (PCR) technology (see Chapter 3). Using pools of DNA from transfected cells and a protocol of **sib selection**, a single cell in which homologous recombination had occurred can be discovered among 1000–10 000 cells with non-homologous recombination events. To facilitate gene targeting by homologous recombination, a number of different vectors and strategies have been developed, the most important ones of which will now be described.

TARGETING VECTORS

The two most frequently used vectors are **gene insertion vectors** and **gene replacement vectors** (Sedivy and Joyner, 1992).

Gene insertion vectors

Based on the observation in yeast that homologous recombination is stimulated by a **double-strand break**, insertion vectors are linearized once within the homologous DNA sequence. After transfection or electroporation of this DNA into the host cell, the cellular recombination machinery leads to an integration of the vector sequences into the endogenous gene. The end result is a **duplication**

of the homologous sequences and the interruption of the endogenous gene. Usually these vectors contain a **selectable marker** (i.e. the neomycin resistance gene), which is also integrated into the endogenous gene. This strategy produces rather crude mutations, in most cases gene inactivations through insertion.

Gene replacement vectors

In order to create more subtle mutations, other vectors were developed that allow the introduction of very subtle, specific mutations, i.e. point mutations. For this purpose gene replacement vectors are used. In this case two double-stranded breaks are introduced into the targeting vector, one on either side of the homologous sequences. Through two reciprocal crossovers the fragment produced by the two double-stranded breaks is substituted into the chromosome for the corresponding endogenous gene. In contrast to gene insertion vectors, gene replacement vectors do not result in duplication of homologous sequences.

Because of the low frequency of homologous versus non-homologous recombination, specific techniques had to be developed to make gene targeting feasible in mammalian cells. PCR technology, which allows the detection of a rare recombination event on the high background of non-homologous recombination, has already been mentioned. The use of isogenic DNA in which the DNA used for construction of the targeting vectors and the genome of the ES cells are of the same genetic background results in a significant improvement in the targeting frequency (te Riele et al, 1992). Additional increases in the frequency of homologous recombination were achieved by employing **promoterless selection**. In this case, the selectable marker neomycin does not have its own promoter. Expression of *neo* can only be activated either when targeting occurs correctly into the endogenous gene so that its promoter drives expression of *neo* (and at the same time inactivates the endogenous gene by insertional mutation), or when a non-homologous integration event places the sequence next to an arbitrary cellular promoter. Treatment with G418/neomycin eliminates all other clones during the selection procedure so that this procedure enriches for homologous recombination events.

Another improvement to achieve enrichment of successful homologous recombination events was the introduction of **negative selection** against integrations at non-homologous positions (Sedivy and Joyner, 1992; Capecchi, 1994). The rationale of this strategy is the hypothesis that whereas replacement vector-based homologous recombination requires two reciprocal crossover events somewhere in the homologous regions, non-homologous recombination occurs primarily through the ends of the transfected molecules. If a negatively selectable marker is attached to the ends of a targeting construct, it will be lost if integration occurs through homologous recombination but retained if integration occurs non-homologously. A combination of positive selection to screen for cells that have integrated DNA at all and negative selection to screen for cells that have undergone homologous recombination (**positive–negative selection**), leads to an enrichment of successfully targeted cells.

PRODUCING KNOCKOUT MICE

ES cell culture

ES cells that have retained their totipotency have been established by a number of laboratories during recent years, and therefore they do not need to be re-established each time a gene targeting experiment is planned. ES cells can be grown in culture similar to other cell lines (Robertson, 1987). The most important difference, however, is their tendency to differentiate in vitro into all sorts of derivatives (Figure 4.4). This differentiation can be prevented by growing ES cells on feeder layer cells, i.e. primary embryonic fibroblasts or rat STO fibroblast cells. Apparently these feeder layer cells produce a factor or factors that prevent differentiation and, instead, maintain proliferation and a state of totipotency. A few years ago an important factor that is able to substitute for feeder layer activity was isolated. This factor is called LIF (leukaemia inhibitory factor), as it was originally described to have a role in the differentiation of haematopoietic cells. Using LIF supplementation, ES cells can now be maintained or even established in the absence of feeder layers, which makes the logistics of gene targeting experiments more simple. Nevertheless many researchers still use feeder layers in their experiments because there are indications that the success rate of maintaining totipotent ES cells remains higher when feeder cells are used. ES cells maintained in culture also have a tendency to accumulate deleterious mutations, i.e. aneuploidies or other chromosomal abnormalities. Therefore, it is essential to regularly check the karyotype of ES cells and to try to minimize the number of times they are passaged and maintained in culture before they are used for gene targeting experiments.

Homologous recombination in ES cells

The first step in a gene targeting experiment is designing and constructing the appropriate targeting vector (see above). After electroporation or transfection of the appropriate vector into ES cells a selection procedure is carried out in order to screen for ES clones that have successfully undergone gene targeting through homologous recombination (Figure 4.5a). This is usually done by a combination of culturing the cells in the appropriate selection media and screening by PCR for positive clones. A typical screen can take weeks due to the slow growth rate of ES cells and the labour-intensive screening procedure. However, once a positive clone has been identified the production of chimeras with these ES cells can proceed. If possible, a number of different ES clones in which the gene of interest has been targeted are isolated in parallel because often there are some ES clones that will fail to contribute to the germ line although they are derived from the same parental clone.

Chimera production

In order to make chimeras, ES cells are treated with trypsin to make a single cell suspension. At the same time blastocysts are isolated from pregnant female mice.

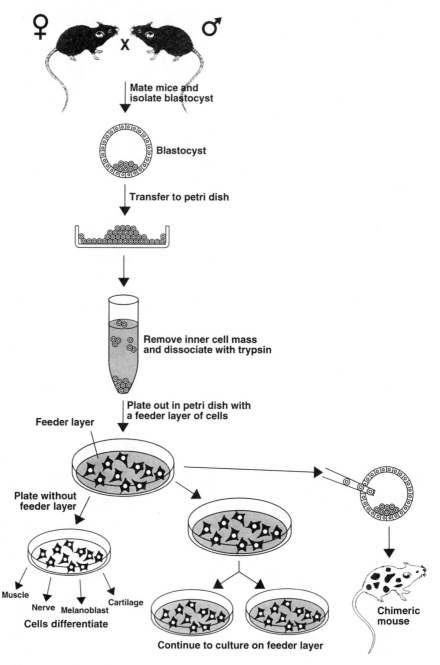

Figure 4.4 Culture of embryonic stem (ES) cells on feeder layer cells prevents differentiation and maintains totipotency (redrawn after Sedivy and Joyner, 1992)

Between 5 and 10 ES cells are injected into the blastocyst cavity of each blastocyst, using standard microinjection techniques (Figure 4.5b) and, again, the resultant blastocysts are transferred into the uterus of pseudopregnant foster mothers.

An alternative procedure to make chimeras with ES cells involves the aggregation of morulae with ES cells (Wood et al, 1993). Clumps containing between 5 and 10 ES cells are added to each zona pellucida-free morula. During a 1-day culture period the ES cells and the blastomeres of the morulae form single aggregates and develop into large blastocysts. These are then transferred back into pseudopregnant mothers in a fashion similar to that used for blastocysts derived from ES cell injection. The main advantage of using the aggregation method is the large number of chimeras that can be produced in a short time and the lack of expensive equipment needed for the microinjection procedure. The skills necessary for successful aggregation are also easier to learn compared to mastering ES cell injection.

Germ-line transmission

After birth, chimeras can be recognized by the mosaic of coat colours that results from the different coat colour genotypes of the ES cells and the host blastocysts (Figure 4.5b). The chimeras are mated to non-transgenic mice to achieve germ-line transmission of the ES cell allele. The offspring of the chimeras are then tested by PCR or Southern blotting analysis in order to determine if they have inherited the mutated allele. Positive mice will be heterozygous for the mutation introduced by homologous recombination into the ES cells. As can be seen from this brief account, the production of a knockout mouse line can easily take up to one year, taking into consideration the time needed for vector construction, ES cell electroporation, clone selection up to the stage of chimera formation and, finally, breeding to heterozygous offspring.

FUTURE APPLICATIONS OF GENE TARGETING IN MICE

The *Cre/loxP* system

The most frequently used application of gene targeting in ES cells is the complete inactivation of specific genes in ES cells and through this in mice. The creation of such **null alleles** is a very important first step in the analysis of gene function. However, future research will need further improvements in the kind of mutations that can be introduced into the genes under study (Valancius and Smithies, 1991). Consider for example a gene that is required during two phases in embryonic development, the first during gastrulation and the second in the late stages of kidney formation. Mice that would be homozygous for a null allele of such a gene might die during or after gastrulation, which would make it impossible to analyse the consequences of a loss of gene function on kidney development. A solution to this dilemma would be the possibility of inactivating the function of this gene only in cells that give rise to the kidney (somatic mutation). Currently a number of approaches are being developed that are directed to achieve such **tissue-specific knockouts**. One of them that is very promising is the *Cre/loxP* system (Ramirez-Solis and Bradley, 1994; Sauer, 1994). *Cre* (cyclization recombination) recombinase

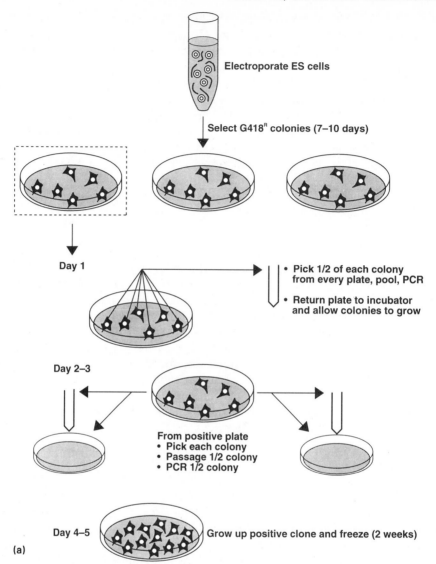

Figure 4.5 (a) Screening for embryonic stem (ES) clones that have successfully undergone gene targeting. (b) Production of chimeras, and germ-line transmission of ES cell allele (redrawn after Sedivy and Joyner, 1992)

has been found in the bacteriophage P1. *Cre* is able to recombine DNA recognizing 34-bp sites called *loxP* (locus of crossover of P1). Each *loxP* site consists of two 13-bp inverted repeats flanking an 8-bp core region. DNA between two *loxP* sites can be deleted by the activity of *Cre* recombinase through intramolecular recombination if the sites are directly repeated. If the two *loxP* sites are in an opposite orientation DNA, an inversion results. Recently it was found that *Cre* recombinase

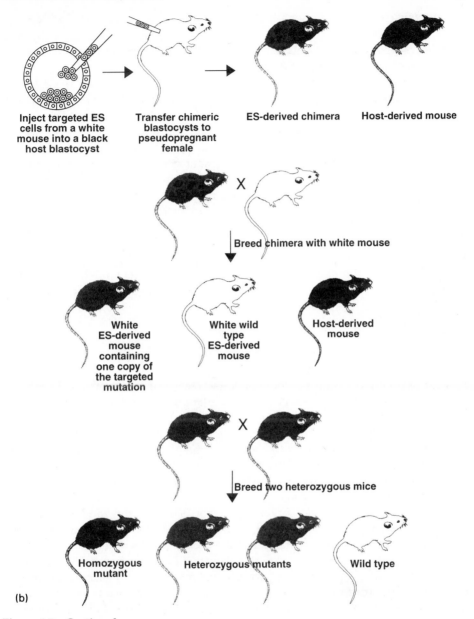

Figure 4.5 *Continued*

can recognize and recombine *loxP* sites not only in phage but also in yeast and even in mammalian cells (where they normally do not occur). This led to the design of a strategy in which cell lineage specific gene inactivation could be achieved by the production of two independent transgenic mouse lines. The first line would be one in which *Cre* recombinase is expressed from a tissue-specific promoter, i.e. only in kidney cells. The second one would be a line that has been engineered by homologous recombination such that the gene of interest is flanked by two *loxP* sites. Neither line itself shows an aberrant phenotype. Crossing the two lines, however, would result in kidney-specific excision of the gene under study, leading to inactivation of that gene only in the kidney cell lineage.

A similar strategy to the *Cre/loxP* system makes use of the *FLP* recombinase originally isolated from 2 μm circle of *Saccharomyces cerevisiae* (Ramirez-Solis and Bradley, 1994; Sauer, 1994). The recognition sites for the *FLP* recombinase (*FRT* sites) are similar to the *loxP* sites but contain an additional 13-bp repeat. Instead of inactivating genes at specific stages during development; the *Cre/LoxP* strategy could also be used to activate dormant genes at specific times. In this case the gene of interest would contain a STOP sequence flanked by *loxP* sites. Expression of *Cre* recombinase would then allow excision of the STOP sequence and expression of the gene. This strategy could also provide a useful way to mark cells for cell lineage analysis: thus, if a reporter gene such as β-galactosidase could be released from a dormant state by the expression of *Cre* recombinase at a specific time during development, marking would occur of all daughter cells of the cell in which expression of *Cre* had mediated β-galactosidase transcription and such cells could be followed in a cell lineage analysis.

Enhancer/gene trap

The total number of genes in the mammalian genome is estimated to be between 50 000 and 100 000. Only a fraction of these genes have been cloned and, of these, the expression patterns and function are known for only a minority . In *Drosophila*, saturation mutagenesis approaches have been applied to produce a large number of mutants in a specific pathway (e.g. segmentation), such that almost every gene that is involved in a certain pathway can be identified. Saturation mutagenesis in the mouse is not feasible, due to the large costs and logistics involved in maintaining the necessary mouse lines. An alternative strategy called **gene trapping** has recently been developed which is designed to identify and isolate new genes with interesting expression patterns (Gossler et al, 1989; Skarnes et al, 1992; Forrester et al, 1996). A β-galactosidase-containing vector is introduced randomly into the genome of ES cells by electroporation. The β-galactosidase gene does not contain its own promoter, so that expression only occurs if integration occurs into an endogenous gene (Figure 4.6). Through the production of chimeras, ES clones with the most interesting expression patterns can be preselected and germ-line chimeras produced. This approach yields simultaneously the expression pattern of the 'trapped' gene, the possibility of cloning this gene via isolation of the flanking sites of the gene trap vector, as well as a mutant for the gene, because integration into the gene often results in an insertional mutation.

OUTLOOK

The importance of mutants for the study of biological processes such as embryonic development cannot be overemphasized. Being able to mutate any gene that has been cloned has already revolutionized experimental biological

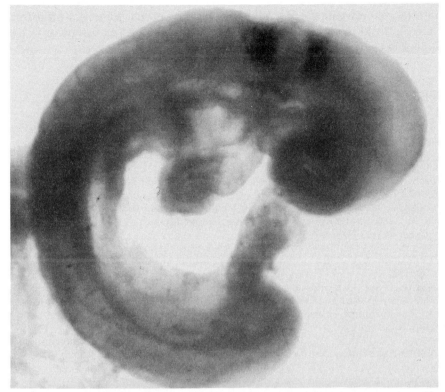

Figure 4.6 LacZ-gene trap embryo showing expression of a gene restricted to thrombomeres 3 and 5 in the hindbrain

research. With respect to the study of birth defects, it will now be possible to establish animal models for genes found to be responsible for human congenital diseases. Phenotypes that are the result of gene knockout experiments in mice will help to identify candidate genes for human congenital diseases for which the molecular basis is not yet known. Undoubtedly, gene targeting is the most powerful approach to decipher the function of genes during development. Insight into developmental pathways, gene regulatory hierarchies and networks, as well as into the structure–function relationships of individual proteins, will rise exponentially during the next few years. It is already clear that one of the major challenges will be the development of the necessary information-handling technology (computer hardware and software, databases) to keep track of the vast amount of information that is already being generated. Making null mutations will be only the first step in the analysis of a specific gene. We will be able to make very subtle 'designer mutations' (Valancius and Smithies, 1991). Even complicated genomic rearrangements, such as chromosomal translocations, which are known to be involved in a number of human genetic diseases, will be 'recreated' in transgenic mice. Past experience has shown that not all mutations in mice result in the same phenotype as in humans. This is not a reason for disappointment or frustration. 'Treasure the odds' is an old saying in genetics. Understanding the molecular mechanisms that lead to differences in phenotypic manifestation between species might tell us a lot about biological mechanisms. Transgenic technology has given us a tool that will be at the heart of much biological research for the foreseeable future.

REFERENCES

Bollag, R.J., Waldman, A.S. and Liskay, R.M. (1989) Homologous recombination in mammalian cells. *Annu. Rev. Genet.* **23**, 199–225.

Bradley, A. (1990) Embryonic stem cells: proliferation and differentiation. *Curr. Opin. Cell Biol.* **2**, 1013–1017.

Capecchi, M. (1989) Altering the genome by homologous recombination. *Science* **244**, 1288–1292.

Capecchi, M. (1994) Targeted gene replacement. *Scientific American* **270**, 34–41.

Evans, M.J. and Kaufman, M.H. (1981) Establishment in culture of pluripotent cells from mouse embryos. *Nature* **292**, 154–156.

Forrester, L., Nagy, A., Stevenson, L. et al (1996) An induction gene trap screen in ES cells: identification of genes that respond to retinoic acid in vitro. *Proc. Natl. Acad. Sci. (USA)* **93**, 1677–1982.

Gossler, A., Joyner, A.L., Rossant, J. and Skarnes, W.C. (1989) Mouse embryonic stem cells and reporter constructs to detect developmentally regulated genes. *Science* **244**, 463–465.

Hogan, B., Costantini, F. and Lacy, E. (1986) *Manipulating the Mouse Embryo: A Laboratory Manual.* Cold Spring Harbor Laboratory: Cold Spring Harbor, NY.

Jacobovits, A., Moore, A.L., Green, L.L. et al (1993) Germ-line transmission and expression of a human-derived yeast artificial chromosome. *Nature* **362**, 255–258.

Joyner, A.L. (1991) Gene targeting and gene trap screens using embryonic stem cells: new approaches to mammalian development. *BioEssays* **13**, 649–656.

Joyner, A.L. (1993) *GeneTargeting: A Practical Approach.* IRL Press: Oxford.

Kuehn, M.R. and Stoye, J.P. (1992) Insertional mutagenesis and mouse development. In *Development: The Molecular Genetic Approach* (eds: V.E.A. Russo, S. Brody, D. Cove and S. Ottolenghi, Ch. 29. Springer Verlag: Berlin.

Lyon, M. and Searle, A. (1989) *Genetic Variants and Strains of the Laboratory Mouse.* Oxford University Press: Oxford.

Martin, G.R. (1981) Establishment of pluripotential cell lines from embryos cultured in medium conditioned by teratocarcinoma stem cells. *Proc. Natl Acad. Sci. USA* **78**, 7634–7638.

Ramirez-Solis, R. and Bradley, A. (1994) Advances in the use of embryonic stem cell technology. *Curr. Opin. Biotechn.* **5**, 528–533.

Robertson, E.J. (1987) *Teratocarcinomas and Embryonic Stem Cells: A Practical Approach.* IRL Press: Oxford.

Sauer, B. (1994) Site-specific recombination: developments and applications. *Curr. Opin. Biotechn.* **5**, 521–527.

Schedl, A., Beerman, F., Thies, E. et al (1992) Transgenic mice generated by pronuclear injection of a yeast artificial chromosome. *Nucleic Acids Res.* **20**, 3073–3077.

Schedl, A., Montoliu, L., Kelsey, G. and Schütz, G. (1993) A yeast artificial chromosome covering the tyrosinase gene confers copy number-dependent expression in transgenic mice. *Nature* **362**, 258–261.

Sedivy, J.M. and Joyner, A.L. (1992) *Gene Targeting.* W.H. Freeman: New York.

Skarnes, W.C., Auerbach, B.A. and Joyner, A.L. (1992) A gene trap approach in mouse embryonic stem cells: the lacZ reporter is activated by splicing, reflects endogenous gene expression, and is mutagenic in mice. *Genes Dev.* **6**, 903–918.

Stewart, C.L., Schuetze, S., Vanek, M. and Wagner, E.F. (1987) Expression of retroviral vectors in transgenic mice obtained by embryo infection. *EMBO J.* **6**, 383–388.

te Riele, H., Maanadag, E.R. and Berns, A. (1992) Highly efficient gene targeting in embryonic stem cells through homologous recombination with isogenic DNA constructs. *Proc. Natl Acad. Sci. USA* **89**, 5128–5132.

Valancius, V. and Smithies, O. (1991) Testing an 'in–out' targeting procedure for making subtle genomic modifications in mouse embryonic stem cells. *Molec. Cell. Bio.* **11**, 1402–1408.

Wagner, E.F. and Keller, G. (1992) The introduction of genes into mouse embryos and stem cells. In *Development: The Molecular Genetic Approach* (eds: V.E.A. Russo, S. Brody, D. Cove and S. Ottolenghi, Ch. 30. Springer Verlag: Berlin.

Wood, S.A., Pascoe, W.S., Schmidt, C. et al (1993) Simple and efficient production of embryonic stem cells-derived chimeras by coculture. *Proc. Natl Acad. Sci. USA* **90**, 4582–4584.

5 Chemical Teratogens: Hazards, Tools and Clues

NIGEL A. BROWN

Department of Anatomy and Developmental Biology, St George's Hospital Medical School, London, UK

Individual chemicals, a single drug or food contaminant for example, cause only a small proportion of birth defects, perhaps less than 5%. Nevertheless, since this represents a significant health burden, there is no excuse for not making every effort to avoid such exposures, and this chapter will review some of these human teratogens. However, the contribution of chemicals to human birth defects may be much wider, and studies of chemical teratogens can certainly contribute more to understanding both normal and abnormal development. This chapter will consider how chemical teratogens can phenocopy birth defects for which there are no convenient genetic models; can be used as tools to manipulate development; can reveal unknown components of normal development; and have generated general principles applicable to human malformation.

When Étienne Geoffroy Saint-Hilaire concocted the term 'teratology' in the early 19th century he meant the study of birth defects, in a broad and all-encompassing sense. However, in the 1960s, the thalidomide tragedy generated a new field of investigation dedicated to ensuring that we are not exposed to environmental influences that cause birth defects. This study of chemical and physical agents, largely an aspect of toxicology, assumed the name **teratology**. That this field is now termed **developmental toxicology** (and teratology has reverted to its original meaning) provides the first general principle. It is clear from experimental studies that chemically induced effects on prenatal development are manifest in many more ways than the 'monstrous' defects of Hilaire. Pre- and perinatal death, growth retardation, behavioural and functional impairment, germ cell mutation, and adult-onset disease are all parts of the spectrum. There was no scientific reason to consider structural defects separately when studying the consequences of embryonic chemical insults, and there is equally no reason to be blinkered about wider effects when considering human birth defects.

Prevention of environmental (non-genetic) causes of birth defects requires methods to detect teratogens (**hazard identification**) and to predict their human effect (**risk characterization**). Testing is a thorny issue, particularly as society

Embryos, Genes and Birth Defects. Edited by P. Thorogood.
© 1997 John Wiley & Sons Ltd.

increasingly questions the use of animals. Eventually, we will understand mechanisms of teratogenesis and the conservation of developmental processes between species. Until then, there is no choice but to do the best we can to devise tests that balance the conflicting needs for sensitive detection and for humanity to animals. To characterize risk, we need to know about the exposure, absorption, disposition, metabolism and elimination of a chemical, both in the test system and in humans. All these aspects are essential for the active **prevention** of birth defects, but are outside the scope of this book.

TERATOGENS AND HUMAN MALFORMATIONS

Lists of human teratogens are dangerous, and have undoubtedly resulted in the deaths of many normal fetuses, through needless therapeutic abortion. They are also notoriously contentious, and for good reasons. Should a list give what we know has happened, or what might happen? Many chemicals probably would cause human malformation, given sufficient exposure. Should a list include only agents that cause structural defects? What about miscarriage, functional effects, and so on? Should a list include pharmacological effects, like the congenitally heroin-addicted baby, or neonatal meconium ileus after anticholinergics? What evidence is required to place chemicals on the list? Most importantly, what about dose? Ionizing radiation and ethanol are undoubtedly human teratogens but all embryos are exposed to both from natural sources. Lest there be any doubt: just because a pregnant woman has been exposed to a chemical listed as a human teratogen does not necessarily justify a termination of pregnancy, and just because a chemical is not on the list does not guarantee safety.

So, Table 5.1 is offered with caution. These are chemicals that certainly have disrupted human prenatal development, meeting objective criteria for identification (Shepard, 1992). The list is not comprehensive, but selected to illustrate the range of effects and chemical classes. Perhaps the most important aspect of this list is that we have no plausible molecular mechanism for over half of these teratogens. However, successful investigation of those with known mechanisms has revealed previously unknown processes in development, as discussed below.

It is sometimes said that all human teratogens have been identified by astute clinical observation. This is both a truism and misleading. A truism in that, of course, the only conclusive proof of human teratogenicity is an affected baby. Misleading in that several human teratogens were known animal teratogens before any human exposure (valproate, retinoids, lithium and angiotensin-converting enzyme inhibitors in Table 5.1). Indeed, there have been no human teratogens identified over the past 20 years that were not already under suspicion from experimental studies. Who knows how many more human teratogens there might be were it not for current testing? The pharmaceutical industry has shelves full of prospective drugs abandoned because of teratogenicity in animals.

Table 5.1 Teratogens that have caused human birth defects

Chemical	Use	Effects	Molecular site of action
ACE inhibitors: captopril, enalapril, etc.	Antihypertensive	Patent ductus arteriosus, oligohydramnios, renal abnormalities and dysfunction, skull hypoplasia	ACE (kininase II)
Androgens, including synthetic progestins	Anti-miscarriage	Masculinization of female external genitals and urogenital sinus	Androgen receptor
Cytotoxic agents: cyclophosphamide, busulphan, etc.	Cancer chemotherapy	Multiple malformations: most organ systems	DNA integrity?
Diethylstilboestrol	Anti-miscarriage	Multiple defects of female (and male less often) reproductive tract, vaginal adenocarcinoma	Oestrogen receptor
Diphenylhydantoin	Anticonvulsant	Nail and digit hypoplasia, fetal hydantoin syndrome	?
Ethanol	Recreational drug	Growth and mental retardation, craniofacial and CNS defects, fetal alcohol syndrome	?
Folic acid antagonists: aminopterin, methotrexate, etc.	Abortifacient, cancer chemotherapy	Multiple malformations: most organ systems	DNA synthesis?
Lithium	Antidepressant	Cardiac defects: Ebstein's anomaly	?
Mercury, organic	Food contaminant	Cerebral palsy, microcephaly	?
Polychlorinated biphenyls	Food contaminant	Intrauterine growth retardation, skin discoloration	?
Retinoids: isotretinoin, etretinate, etc.	Anti-acne	Multiple malformations: craniofacial, CNS, cardiac, thymic aplasia	Retinoid receptors
Streptomycin	Antituberculous	Deafness	?
Tetracyclines	Antibiotic	Tooth and bone discoloration	?
Thalidomide	Sedative	Phocomelia, external ear defects, oesophageal and duodenal atresia, tetralogy of Fallot, renal agenesis	?
Trimethadione	Anticonvulsant	Cleft palate and other craniofacial defects, cardiac defects	?
Valproic acid	Anticonvulsant	Spina bifida, cardiac defects, fetal valproate syndrome	?
Warfarin	Anticoagulant	Nasal hypoplasia, bone stippling	Vitamin K-dependent bone matrix protein?

ACE, angiotensin-converting enzyme.
See Shepard (1992) and Schardein (1993) for comprehensive listings, and Buyse (1990) for full descriptions of syndromes.

GENERAL STRATEGY IN CHEMICAL TERATOGENESIS

The approach to discovering a mechanism of teratogenesis obviously depends upon the properties of the chemical and the nature of the birth defects, but a general strategy is shown in Figure 5.1. This has been a well-worn path for some 30 years, but there are still few complete journeys, perhaps only for TCDD (2,3,7,8-tetrachlorodibenzo-*p*-dioxin) and the glucocorticoids (see below) in

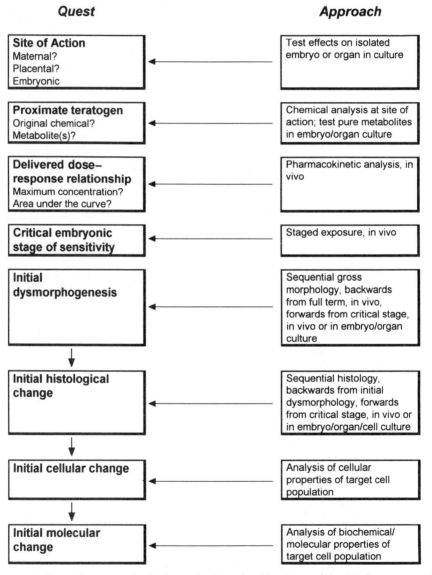

Figure 5.1   General strategy for the investigation of mechanisms of chemical teratogenesis

addition to those in Table 5.1. The major impact of the advances in developmental biology that fill this book has been to introduce a much more solid background in which to take the final two steps towards cellular and molecular mechanisms. The teratogenicity of the antiepileptic valproic acid (VPA; Depakene®, Epilim®) illustrates the general strategy.

VALPROIC ACID

VPA is a short-chain carboxylic acid, 2-propyl pentanoic acid (Figure 5.2). It was first identified as a teratogen by orthodox animal testing. The site of action is embryonic and the unchanged drug is the proximate teratogen, as shown by direct effects on mammalian embryos in culture, which also showed effective

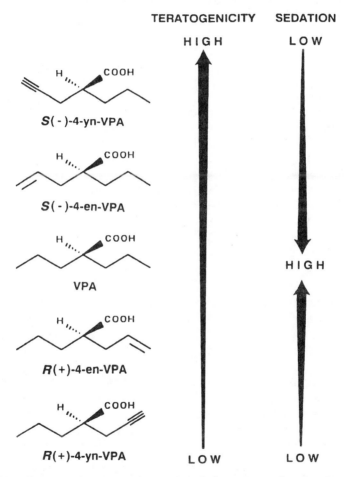

Figure 5.2 Structure of valproic acid (VPA) and derivatives, showing stereoselectivity and the separation of teratogenic and anticonvulsant activities. Sedation measured in adult mice, as an index of anticonvulsant activity. Teratogenicity measured as the induction of exencephaly in mice. (Figure provided by Nau; see review by Nau, 1994)

concentrations close to clinical plasma levels (Kao et al, 1981). This, and teratogenic doses well below those toxic to the maternal animal, characterized VPA as a likely human teratogen (Brown et al, 1980). Clinically, the drug was first shown to cause spina bifida but it can also induce malformations of the heart, craniofacies, axial skeleton and limb (Shepard, 1992). A fetal valproate syndrome has been described, with facial features in common with the fetal hydantoin syndrome (Buyse, 1990).

Several antiepileptic drugs appear to cause birth defects: carbamazepine and trimethadione, and perhaps some barbiturates, as well as valproate and the hydantoins (Shepard, 1992). This suggests a relationship between the mechanisms of pharmacological and teratological effects, but may simply reflect the fact that anticonvulsants are one of few classes of drug that women of child-bearing age take chronically. The pharmacological mechanisms vary widely across the chemical classes, but modulation of neurotransmitter levels is a feature in common. Some neurotransmitters function in other capacities during development, and indeed this may have been their primary role in early evolution (Lauder, 1993). The action of valproate may be a clue to such a process. However, it is clear that the pharmacological and teratological activities of VPA are separable (Figure 5.2).

Studies of the relationship between delivered dose (the amount that reaches the site of action – the embryo in this case) and response for VPA were instrumental in establishing the importance of pharmacokinetics in teratogenesis (Nau and Scott, 1987). In the case of VPA, it is peak plasma concentration (C_{max}), not duration of exposure (AUC), that correlates with teratogenic effect (see Nau and Scott, 1987). For other chemicals, cyclophosphamide for example, the opposite is true. The fact that not only dose, but also kinetics, determine teratogenic response has important implications for clinical management in pregnancy. For example, divided doses are preferable for VPA in women of child-bearing age. These studies also generated the general principle that much of the often observed variation in species sensitivity to teratogens is pharmacokinetic in origin, with wide variation in delivered dose after the same administered dose (reviewed by O'Flaherty and Clarke, 1994).

Small structural changes to VPA have a profound effect on teratogenicity (see Nau, 1994). Two aspects are particularly interesting: separation of pharmacological and teratological properties, and chirality (Figure 5.2). A metabolite of VPA, 2-ene-VPA, retains anticonvulsant activity but is not teratogenic and is a candidate replacement drug (Nau, 1994). Introducing a terminal triple bond in one of the carboxyl side-chains is one of the few modifications that enhances the teratogenicity of VPA. This produces a molecule with an asymmetric centre, and the two enantiomers (R-4-yn-VPA and S-4-yn-VPA) differ markedly in their teratogenic (and pharmacological) potency. This is due to intrinsic activity, since both enantiomers distribute equally into the embryonic compartment (Nau, 1994), and is suggestive of a receptor-mediated action, but this remains enigmatic. Short-chain carboxylic acids, in general, may share a common mechanism of teratogenicity (Coakley et al, 1986). The teratogenicity of the glycol ethers, widely used industrial solvents, is mediated by their stable alkoxyacid metabolites. For example, methoxyacetic acid is responsible for the effects of ethyleneglycol monomethyl ether, and the structure–activity relationship of these alkoxyacids is reminiscent of VPA.

The critical stage for VPA induction of spina bifida in the mouse is gestational day 9 (Nau, 1994) and the initial dysmorphogenesis may involve the neural suture and presomitic mesoderm (Brown et al, 1991). Initial histological changes have been described, including cell death in the neuroepithelium (Turner et al, 1990), but the molecular mechanism of VPA teratogenicity remains unknown. Early effects on lipid synthesis, intracellular pH, or on zinc or neurotransmitter metabolism have been suggested (reviewed by Nau, 1994), but perhaps most plausible is an effect on folate metabolism. Supplementation with some folates can reduce the incidence of VPA-induced defects, and VPA alters folate metabolism, perhaps by inhibition of glutamate formyltransferase. However, folates also reduce the incidence of malformation from other genetic and chemical causes. This is clinically important and several programmes are under way to supplement food with folate to reduce the risk of neural tube defects, following the clear demonstration of its effectiveness in controlled trials (see Chapter 8). However, the mechanism of this folate protection remains obscure (reviewed by Bock and Marsh, 1994).

GENE–TERATOGEN INTERACTION

The susceptibility to VPA teratogenesis varies markedly across different inbred mouse strains (Nau, 1994). The molecular basis of this genetic modification of VPA teratogenicity is unknown, but the phenomenon is very common and introduces the general principle of **gene–teratogen interaction**. We do not know the causes of most human birth defects, but it is clear that only a small proportion, perhaps 20%, are Mendelian genetic syndromes. It is a salutary thought that even when all the mutations responsible for McKusick's (1994) compendium are identified, it will not explain the vast majority of human malformation. It is often said that most birth defects are multifactorial, that is the result of environmental action on a susceptible genotype. Some would say this is not profoundly helpful, since if we exclude genotype and the environment there is nothing left but chance, and it is too depressing to conclude that random developmental 'error' is responsible for most human malformation. On the other hand, the principle of gene–teratogen interaction has been formalized in the **multifactorial/threshold hypothesis** of Fraser (1977) and this provides a useful conceptual model (Figure 5.3).

Using the development of the palate as an example (Ferguson, 1988; see Chapter 10), Fraser (1977) suggested that the palatal shelves must become horizontal before a critical stage, otherwise they will be unable to fuse and a cleft will result. Any population of embryos will be distributed around a mean stage of shelf development, due to usual biological variation. Many aspects of head development (tongue motility, shelf growth, and so on) will contribute to this process, and each will be influenced by both genetic and environmental factors. The proportion of embryos that fall beyond the threshold depends upon this complex interaction. The search for genetic variations in the human population

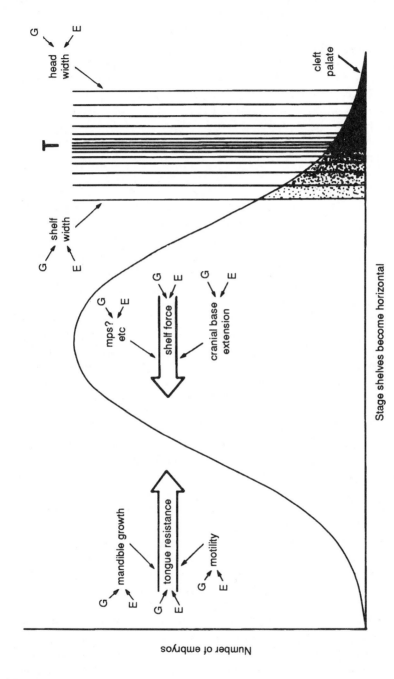

Figure 5.3 Multifactorial/threshold model of teratogenesis. Cleft palate is proposed to result if palatal shelves do not become horizontal before a certain threshold (T) embryonic stage. A population of embryos is distributed normally about a mean stage of shelf elevation, with a small proportion falling beyond the threshold. Many developmental processes (cranial base extension, extracellular matrix accumulation, etc.) either shift the distribution of stages, or the position of the threshold. Each of these processes can be influenced by both genetic (G) and environmental (E) factors. (After Fraser, 1977)

that determine sensitivity to particular environmental agents represents a major challenge for the future.

TERATOGENS AND PHENOCOPIES

An understanding of the pathogenesis, that is the sequence of cellular and tissue changes leading to a particular malformation, can help to design the best approach to corrective surgery, may suggest potential cellular and molecular changes, and can identify critical aspects of normal development. As discussed throughout this book, there are very many genetic animal models of human malformation, and new transgenic knockout models are being generated rapidly (see Chapter 4). Nevertheless, there are some important abnormal phenotypes for which there are no genetic models, but which chemical teratogens **can** phenocopy. It is also useful to be able to compare the pathogenesis of two different insults that lead to the same malformation.

Chemical phenocopies have a long history (Landauer, 1948) but a couple of examples are sufficient to illustrate the approach. The ideal phenocopy is one in which the chemical induces a single malformation in all treated embryos. As a model for the most common human cardiac malformation, ventricular septal defect (VSD), the anticonvulsant trimethadione (TMD) comes very close to these criteria (Veuthey et al, 1990). VSD can be induced in 98% of rat fetuses treated with TMD, and the critical changes appear to be in the proximal parts of the conotruncal ridges, particularly the septal ridge. Bisdiamine can also induce close to 100% incidence of cardiac malformation (Veuthey et al, 1990) and, although more varied in morphology, this may be a phenocopy of the heart defects in the catch-22 syndrome and prove to be a useful tool in the examination of candidate genes.

The herbicide nitrofen (2,4-dichlorophenyl 4'-nitrophenyl ether) is an interesting experimental teratogen that has been used to phenocopy several malformations, including diaphragmatic hernia (Wickman et al, 1993). Nitrofen can also induce a 100% incidence of absence of the Harderian gland, a lacrimal gland prominant in some species but rudimentary in man (reviewed by Manson, 1986). Its mechanism is not established, but may involve thyromimetic activity and it should be a useful tool to study the role of the hypothalamic/pituitary/thyroid axis in development. One area for which chemical phenocopies would be valuable is the gut atresias, both oesophageal and anorectal. These are amongst the most common life-threatening birth defects, and there are no convenient genetic animal models. Several chemical teratogens can induce gut atresias, currently only at low incidences, but systematic research should yield a working model.

One problem with the gene knockout approach to studies of developmental mechanisms is that the normal function of the affected gene is prevented in all tissues and at all stages of development, which can considerably complicate the analysis of effects, since the resultant phenotype will include secondary and tertiary effects of gene elimination. Antisense oligonucleotides can be considered as the ultimate in designer teratogens, and are an alternative to knockouts that may allow both spatial and temporal control over interference in gene function (Sadler and Hunter, 1994).

TERATOGENS AS MANIPULATIVE TOOLS

There is a distinguished history of advances in understanding mechanisms of development by following the consequences of induced abnormalities. Early studies, around the turn of the century, usually used surgical tools, like the cautery needle of Roux and hair loop of Spemann (see Oppenheimer, 1967, and Barow, 1971, for historical perspectives), but chemical treatments were also common in those heydays of experimental embryology. Experiments using lithium to induce transformation of the germ layers of echinoderms, performed by Herbst in the 1890s, and expanded by both Horstadius and von Ubisch in the 1920s were seminal studies, as were 'animalization' treatments with cyanide and other respiratory inhibitors by Lindhal in the 1930s.

Clearly, early teratology contributed much to our understanding of development, but are chemicals useful tools today? I believe they can be, but with the usual caveat that one does not know all the consequences of treatment. When Roux killed a blastomere to examine its influence on the neighbouring cell, he did not know that the dead cell would have a mechanical constraint on further development. So even killing a cell, the easiest thing for an experimentalist to do, may induce an effect more complex than is immediately apparent.

Early mammalian development is a progressive hierarchy of regional specification by inductive interactions, rather than by autonomous cellular mechanisms. This enables mammalian embryos to be highly regulative and, at least in theory, able to repair damage. Very little is known of the mechanisms and capabilities of mammalian embryos to regulate, and it is here that chemical teratogens could be very useful tools, but ironically are not being extensively utilized. In contrast, there are currently some elegant studies of embryonic response to physical damage (Martin et al, 1994).

The only extensive studies of regulation following chemical insult concern the recovery of mouse embryos from mitomycin C (MMC) treatment (reviewed by Snow, 1987). This yielded important information on mechanisms of development and suggested a novel mechanism of teratogenesis. MMC is an alkylating agent that kills cells and arrests cell division. A single injection of MMC at primitive streak stages in mice results in massive cell death so that 12 h later the neural plate stage embryos contain only 10–15% of the normal number of cells. Despite this, most (>85%) embryos survive and by the end of organogenesis are overtly normal and of usual size. This is remarkable, given that many populations of cells are specified by primitive streak stages, and suggests extensive respecification during recovery from damage. At the end of organogenesis, less than 10% of embryos show gross malformation, the most common defect being microphthalmia.

However, these apparently normal embryos harbour covert defects. Newborn animals have severe neurological defects and few (<30%) survive to weaning. Even the healthy survivors have reduced fertility. Snow (1987) showed that the synchrony in development of individual organ systems was not normal during organogenesis, and suggested that this asynchrony is responsible for the subsequent abnormalities. Organs could be grouped into those that showed little or no retardation in their appearance, those with a moderate delay (5–6 h), and those delayed by more than 10 h. Derivatives of all three germ layers were found in all groups, but cells already committed to a particular tissue at the time of treatment (neural ectoderm, heart, germ cells, hindgut, allantois) appeared least delayed. No more is known, but further study is surely called for.

The precise relationship between the start of sensitivity of a tissue or organ to chemical disruption and its stage of development is another area where teratogens are under-utilized as tools. In broad terms, the variation in sensitivity with gestational age has long been documented. For example, the peak sensitivity for thalidomide-induced defects was 21–27 days post-conception for external ears, 27–30 days for arms, and 30–33 days for legs (Shepard, 1992). The start of sensitivity must often relate to the allocation of cells to a particular fate, but this is poorly studied. An excellent example of what can be learned is the startling limb duplications following retinoic acid treatment at pre-implantation stages in the mouse, suggesting allocation even before gastrulation (Rutledge et al, 1994).

Programmed cell death is an important mechanism of morphogenesis. In many phases of development, too many progenitor cells are produced; subsequently, numbers are regulated by programmed death. The numbers of neurones in the optic stalk are an example of this (Raff, 1992). It is possible to manipulate regions of cell death by chemical treatment. It has long been observed that cell death is a common feature in the pathogenesis of chemically induced malformation (Scott, 1977). Furthermore, several teratogens, such as ethanol and retinoic acid, increase the areas of normal programmed cell death (Sulik et al, 1988). This provides an opportunity to vary, systematically, the proportion of cells in a particular region that die, then study subsequent development.

The mechanisms of teratogen expansion of regions of cell death are unknown, but the view (Raff, 1992) that death is the fate of all cells, unless they receive sufficient survival factors, provides a potential explanation. Competition for limited quantities of survival factors from target cells may control the degree of 'programmed' death. Such conditions would involve a fine balance between the production of sufficient versus insufficient factor by a group of signalling cells, with the population of responding cells on a knife-edge of survival. Any action that reduced the amount of factor would expand the proportion of responding cells that died. One can imagine many mechanisms by which a chemical teratogen could, rather unspecifically, reduce the amount of survival factor: metabolic or growth inhibition, or killing of signalling cells for example. This would also provide a means whereby chemical teratogens of diverse mechanism might act additively at one site.

TERATOGENS AS CLUES

When an exogenous chemical has an unexpected potent teratological effect, particularly when a reproducible syndrome of defects is induced with a high frequency, then suspicions should be raised that a fundamental developmental process is being disrupted. In several such cases, the search for the teratogenic mechanisms has provided valuable clues to normal mechanisms, whilst many others remain to be solved.

RETINOIDS

No chemical has received more attention, nor contributed more to understanding development over the past 20 years, than vitamin A (retinol) and its derivatives (see Chapters 7, 10 and 13). The first demonstration that mammalian development could be profoundly affected by an environmental manipulation was Hale's (1933) observation of pigs born without eyeballs to sows on a vitamin A-deficient diet. The very wide range of defects that could be caused by deficiency were beautifully described by the fathers of modern teratology, Wilson and Warkany (see Wilson et al, 1953), and they unknowingly provided phenocopies of recent multiple retinoic acid receptor (RAR) and retinoid X receptor (RXR) targeted mutations. Subsequently, vitamin A excess was shown also to be a teratogen with a remarkable spectrum of dysmorphic effects. More recent experience shows that the synthetic retinoids, isotretinoin and etretinate, are perhaps the most effective human teratogens known (Shepard, 1992).

It is now appreciated that retinoids play a widespread and critical role in developmental control, but it is still not clear exactly how exogenous retinoids induce some of their teratogenic effects. For example, the archetypal morphological effect of retinoid treatment at late gastrulation/early neurulation is abnormal branchial arch development (Webster et al, 1986). Treatment at this time can cause anterior shifts in the expression domains of Hox genes (see Chapters 10 and 13) and the most profound result of this seems to be the homeotic transformation of hindbrain rhombomeres (Marshall et al, 1992). However, this does not seem to be involved in the development of abnormal arches since the critical stage for their induction is slightly later, when no shifts in Hox expression are seen. The roles of extended cell death and inhibited cell migration, which do occur in specific cell populations (Sulik et al, 1988), are not clear and are of unknown molecular mechanism.

DIOXINS

2,3,7,8-Tetrachlorodibenzo-p-dioxin (TCDD; dioxin) is the most potent of the halogenated aromatic hydrocarbons. It is a contaminant of many industrial mixtures, most famously the Agent Orange herbicide sprayed on Vietnam. Concern over the developmental effects of TCDD began with the demonstration that birth defects induced by 2,4,5-T (a component of Agent Orange) in rats and mice were actually caused by contaminating TCDD (reviewed by Peterson et al, 1993). The usual model of TCDD teratogenicity is cleft palate induction in mice, but kidney, brain and other organs are also affected. It is thought that the ectodermal dysplasia syndrome in offspring of women from Yusho and Yu-Cheng who consumed contaminated rice oil was caused by TCDD but many other contaminants were present (Peterson et al, 1993).

The extraordinary potency of TCDD led to studies of molecular mechanisms that have provided one of the most complete descriptions of chemical teratogenesis. Postnatal behavioural and neuroendocrine functions are among the most TCDD-sensitive developmental processes. Significant effects on reproductive function have been found in male rat offspring after a single dose of 64 ng/kg on day 15 of gestation (Mably et al, 1992). The offspring of rhesus monkeys exposed to less than 1 ng/kg/day before pregnancy were reported to have measurable behavioural changes (Schantz and Bowman, 1989).

TCDD has an unusual cellular mechanism of cleft palate formation (Abbott and Birnbaum, 1989, 1990a, 1991). The palatal shelves of treated mice grow and make contact normally, but the subsequent loss of periderm, shelf adhesion, and medial epithelium to mesenchyme transformation does not occur. Rather than transforming, TCDD-treated medial epithelium cells proliferate and differentiate into a stratified epithelium. This occurs in palate cultures from mouse, rat and human embryos, although the mouse is most sensitive. It is possible that this effect is mediated by an interference with epidermal growth factor (EGF) or transforming growth factor (TGF) functions (Abbott and Birnbaum, 1990b), and an effect on the regulation of EGF receptors may also be involved in TCDD actions on kidney development (Abbott and Birnbaum, 1990c). It is clear that palate epithelium cells have a high-affinity receptor for TCDD, the aryl hydrocarbon receptor (AhR; Abbott et al, 1994a).

The mouse *AhR* gene encodes an 89-kDa transcription factor of the basic helix-loop-helix (bHLH) family (Figure 5.4; reviewed by Whitlock, 1993). It has a DNA-binding domain, a glutamate-rich activation domain, and a 'PAS' domain, named after homology with *Per* (encoding the *Drosophila* circadian rhythm protein), *Arnt* (encoding a protein that dimerizes with Ah, see below) and *Sim* (encoding a CNS development regulator in *Drosophila*), which may be involved in ligand binding. When unbound by ligand, AhR resides in the cytoplasm and is translocated to the nucleus on TCDD binding. Arnt is an 86-kDa nuclear protein, which also has bHLH and PAS domains (Whitelaw et al, 1993). It has no affinity for TCDD nor the unbound AhR, but forms a heterodimer with activated AhR. Neither activated AhR nor Arnt have substantial DNA binding activity as monomers. By analogy with other bHLH proteins, and other classes of transcription factor, it is possible that the diversity in biological effects of TCDD is the result of differential gene regulation mediated by heterodimers of AhR with as yet uncharacterized proteins. AhR associates with the 90-kDa heat-shock protein (Hsp90) in cytoplasm, which is thought to maintain the receptor in a conformation optimal for ligand binding, and to prevent the inappropriate binding to the unliganded receptor to DNA (Pongratz et al, 1992).

The genes that the AhR regulates are largely unknown, but TCDD is a strong inducer of the expression of the cytochrome P450 1A1 isozyme (*CYP1A1* gene). Studies of this gene have identified the dioxin-responsive element (DRE), a hexanucleotide core recognition sequence that is present in multiple copies (probably six) within the enhancer region (Saatcioglu et al, 1990; Wu and Whitlock, 1993). DREs have been identified upstream of other TCDD-inducible genes (Pimental et al, 1993).

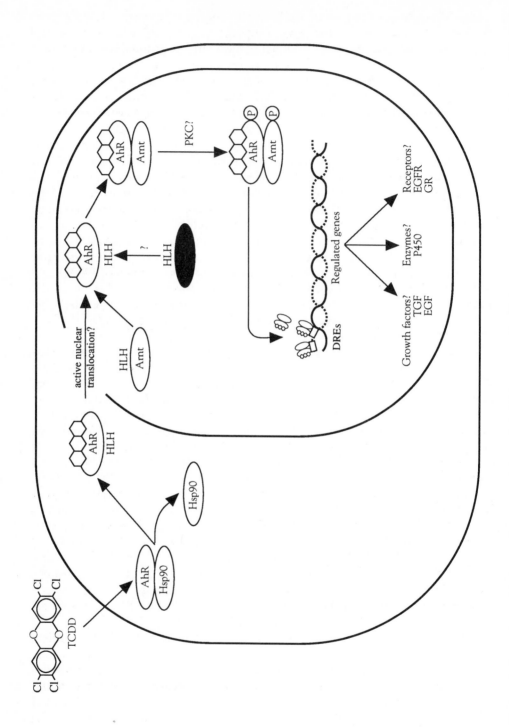

The link between TCDD–AhR mediated changes in gene expression and abnormal development has yet to be established. *AhR* mRNA and protein are expressed in mouse palate, particularly in the epithelium (Abbott et al, 1994a). There is tissue and spatial variation in intracellular distribution of the protein: perinuclear in the mesenchyme, and cytoplasmic and nuclear in the medial fusing epithelium. Changes in the levels of TGF-α and -β, and of EGF and its receptor, have been observed following TCDD exposure, presumably mediated by AhR regulation (Abbott and Birnbaum, 1989, 1990b). These growth factor changes are compatible with the abnormal proliferation of medial epithelia cells, but the link is not established. TCDD synergizes with excess glucocorticoids in the induction of cleft palate in the mouse, and it has been proposed that there is a cycle of mutual induction involving the AhR and glucocorticoid receptor (Abbott et al, 1994b). Because TCDD affects neuroendocrine development, there may also be interactions between the AhR and oestrogen and/or androgen receptor-mediated regulation (Whitlock, 1993).

The natural ligand for the AhR is not known. There are naturally occurring chemicals with a high affinity for the receptor, particularly in plants, so it is possible that the receptor evolved to induce the enzymes responsible for the metabolism of some ingested lipophilic chemicals. If this were the case, however, it is not clear why the receptor would be expressed during embryogenesis. A more attractive hypothesis is that there is an unidentified natural ligand which has an important role in normal development. The identification of this ligand and of AhR-regulated genes are exciting prospects for the immediate future.

XENOESTROGENS

Diethylstilboestrol (DES) was synthesized as a synthetic oestrogen and used for almost 30 years, until the 1970s, for the prevention of threatened miscarriage and other complications of pregnancy. DES acts by binding to the oestrogen receptor, a cytoplasmic protein that translocates to the nucleus on ligand-induced activation and acts as a transcription factor. The discovery of a rare form of cancer in the reproductive tracts of women who were exposed to DES in utero is now well known. However, vaginal adenocarcinoma was a rare (perhaps 1 in 1000) outcome of prenatal DES exposure, whilst structural and functional defects of both the male and female reproductive organs were much more common (reviewed by Edelman, 1986).

Figure 5.4 TCDD (2,3,7,8-tetrachlorodibenzo-*p*-dioxin) regulation of gene expression. TCDD binds to the aryl hydrocarbon receptor (AhR) which is held in an accessible conformation in the cytoplasm by a 90-kDa heat-shock protein (Hsp90). Binding activates the AhR, releasing Hsp90 and translocating into the nucleus. Here, it dimerizes with other basic helix-loop-helix (HLH) proteins including the Arnt protein and other unidentified factors. The dimer is phosphorylated, possibly by protein kinase C (PKC), before binding to dioxin-responsive elements (DREs) in the enhancer regions of regulated genes. TGF, transforming growth factor; EGF, epidermal growth factor; EGFR, EGF receptor; GR, glucocorticoid receptor (After Whitlock, 1993)

Human exposure to DES is no longer a problem, but there are a very large number of man-made and natural chemicals that have oestrogenic activity. Many of these bear no overt structural resemblance to oestradiol-17β (Figure 5.5), the natural ligand for the oestrogen receptor, but nevertheless have sufficient affinity to activate the receptor. There is currently concern that the complex mix of **xenoestrogens** in the environment may be affecting the reproductive health of wild animals and humans alike. For example, polychlorinated biphenyls (PCBs)

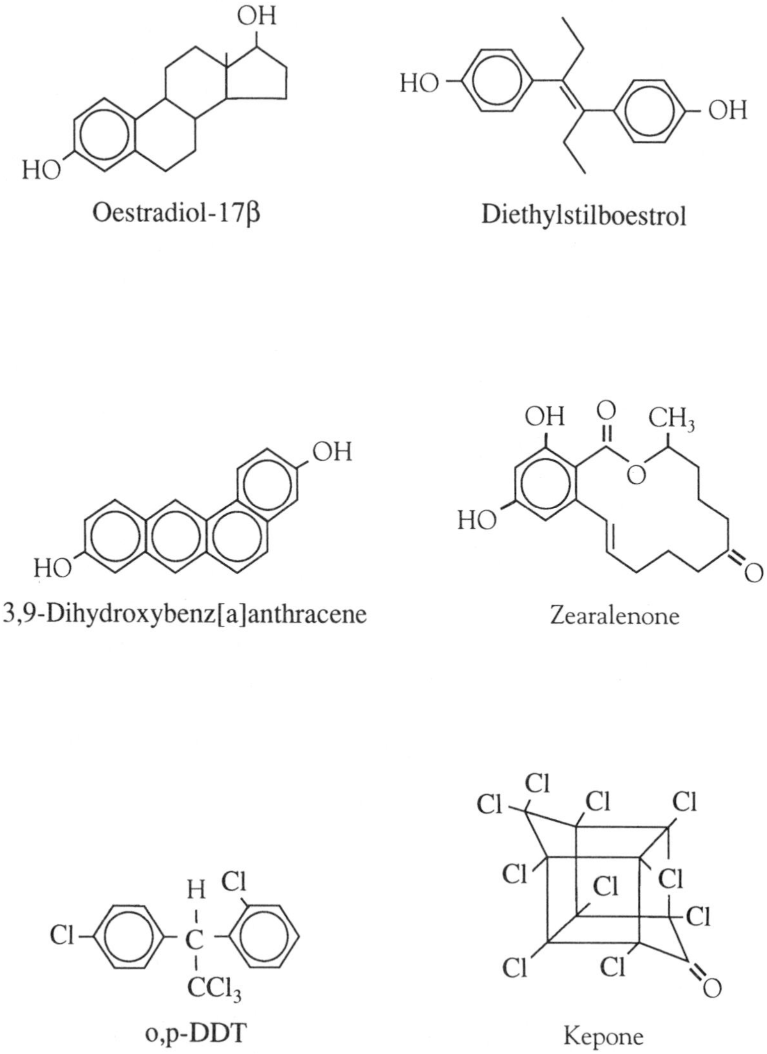

Oestradiol-17β   Diethylstilboestrol

3,9-Dihydroxybenz[a]anthracene   Zearalenone

o,p-DDT   Kepone

Figure 5.5 Diverse chemical structures that bind to the oestrogen receptor. Oestradiol, natural ligand; diethylstilboestrol, synthetic oestrogen; dihydroxybenzanthracene, metabolite of environmental combustion product; zeralenone, mycotoxin product; DDT, pesticide; kepone, flame retardant. (After McLachlan, 1993)

can cause gonadal sex-reversal in animals that exhibit temperature-dependent sex determination (Bergeron et al, 1994). It has been suggested that the apparent decline in sperm counts, and increases in gonadal abnormalities, of men in Europe and the USA over the past 50 years is caused by environmental oestrogens (Sharpe and Skakkebaek, 1993). The studies of DES teratogenicity in mouse provide a model for xenoestrogens, and have revealed interesting features of normal reproductive tract development.

Because the development of the reproductive tract is hormone-dependent it is not surprising that DES is disruptive. Structural abnormalities of the uterus and oviducts in females, testicular and epididymal defects in males, and reproductive dysfunction in both sexes are consequences of prenatal DES exposure in mice (reviewed by Mori and Nagasawa, 1988). The molecular correlates of these actions are now being characterized. Lactoferrin is the major oestrogen-inducible uterine protein in mice, and is not normally expressed in the male. Prenatal DES exposure results in constitutive and inducible expression of lactoferrin in the seminal vesicle epithelium of adult offspring, without affecting the normal response to androgens (Beckman et al, 1994). This is not an effect on circulating hormones, but appears to be due to an alteration in the differentiation of epithelial cells by oestrogen imprinting. Similarly, in the uterus of DES-exposed female mice, there is a permanent up-regulation of lactoferrin and EGF expression, independent of normal ovarian oestrogen induction (Nelson et al, 1994). These permanent changes are the molecular analogues of structural birth defects – 'molecular teratogenesis'.

At certain critical stages of gestation, prenatal DES 'masculinizes' the behaviour of female animals (reviewed by Newbold, 1993). This paradoxical effect illustrates the potential impact of chemical teratogens on functional brain development. The explanation for the paradox is that oestradiol is the normal mediator of testosterone imprinting of the developing male brain. Testosterone synthesized by the fetal testis is metabolized to oestradiol within cells of the brain. The brain is normally protected from circulating oestrogens, of maternal or fetal ovarian origin, by alpha-fetoprotein (AFP), which has a high affinity for oestradiol but not testosterone. DES and other xenoestrogens do not bind to AFP so gain access to the brain, subsequently activating oestrogen receptors in an androgenizing manner. Whether there is an equivalent effect of DES in humans is contentious. Although several reports suggest changes in behaviour patterns associated with prenatal exposure to DES, current evidence is not convincing (Newbold, 1993).

FINAL COMMENTS

What does the future hold for chemical teratogenesis? Inventive chemists will continue to synthesize new molecules with surprising effects on development, providing clues for the astute investigator. In the right hands, chemical tools will help to unlock developmental mechanisms. The burgeoning molecular basis of development will make it much easier to identify the initial molecular insults inflicted by chemical teratogens. As these are characterized, we will be better able to detect hazards. We can now reasonably conclude that a chemical with affinity for the retinoid, oestrogen, glucocorticoid, androgen or Ah receptor is a potential teratogen. In time, this array of potential targets will expand and simple reporter–construct tests will be devised to screen new chemicals (McLachlan, 1993). And we will begin to unravel the real contribution of the environment to birth defects.

REFERENCES

Abbott, B.D. and Birnbaum, L.S. (1989) TCDD alters medial epithelial cell differentiation during palatogenesis. *Toxicol. Appl. Pharmacol.* **99**, 276–286.

Abbott, B.D. and Birnbaum, L.S. (1990a) Rat embryonic palatal shelves respond to TCDD in organ culture. *Toxicol. Appl. Pharmacol.* **103**, 441–451.

Abbott, B.D. and Birnbaum, L.S. (1990b) TCDD-induced altered expression of growth factors may have a role in producing cleft palate and enhancing the incidence of clefts after coadministration of retinoic acid and TCDD. *Toxicol. Appl. Pharmacol.* **106**, 418–432.

Abbott, B.D. and Birnbaum, L.S. (1990c) Effects of TCDD on embryonic ureteric epithelial EGF receptor expression and cell proliferation. *Teratology* **41**, 71–84.

Abbott, B.D. and Birnbaum, L.S. (1991) TCDD exposure of human embryonic palatal shelves in organ culture alters the differentiation of medial epithelial cells. *Teratology* **43**, 119–132.

Abbott, B.D., Perdew, G.H. and Birnbaum, L.S. (1994a) Ah receptor in embryonic mouse palate and effects of TCDD on receptor expression. *Toxicol. Appl. Pharmacol.* **126**, 16–25.

Abbott, B.D., Perdew, G.H., Buckalew, A.R. and Birnbaum, L.S. (1994b) Interactive regulation of Ah and glucocorticoid receptors in the synergistic induction of cleft palate by 2,3,7,8-tetrachlorodibenzo-*p*-dioxin and hydrocortisone. *Toxicol. Appl. Pharmacol.* **128**, 138–150.

Barrow, M.V. (1971) A brief history of teratology to the early 20th century. *Teratology* **4**, 119–130.

Beckman, W.C., Newbold, R.R., Teng, C.T. and McLachlan, J.A. (1994) Molecular feminization of mouse seminal vesicle by prenatal exposure to diethylstilbestrol: altered expression of messenger RNA. *J. Urol.* **151**, 1370–1378.

Bergeron, J.M., Crews, D. and McLachlan, J.A. (1994) PCBs as environmental estrogens: turtle sex determination as a biomarker of environmental contamination. *Environ. Hlth Perspect.* **102**, 780–781.

Bock, G. and Marsh, J. (Eds) (1994) *Neural Tube Defects*. Ciba Foundation Symposium, vol. 181. Wiley: Chichester.

Brown, N.A., Kao, J. and Fabro, S. (1980) Teratogenic potential of valproic acid. *Lancet* **1**, 660–661.

Brown, N.A., Clarke, D.O. and McCarthy, A. (1991) Adaptation of post-implantation embryos to culture: membrane lipid synthesis and response to valproate. *Reprod. Toxicol.* **5**, 245–253.

Buyse, M.L. (1990) *Birth Defects Encyclopaedia*. Blackwell Scientific: London.

Coakley, M.E., Rawlings, S.J. and Brown, N.A. (1986) Short chain carboxylic acids, a new class of teratogens: studies of potential biochemical mechanisms. *Environ. Hlth Perspect.* **70**, 105–111.

Edelman, D.A. (1986) *DES/Diethylstilbestrol: New Perspective*. MTP Press: Boston.

Ferguson, M.J.W. (1988) Palate development. *Development* **103** Suppl., 41–60.

Fraser, F.C. (1977) Relation of animal studies to the problem in man. In *Handbook of Teratology* (Eds: J.G. Wilson and F. Clarke-Fraser), vol. 1, pp. 75–96. Plenum: New York.

Hale, F. (1933) Pigs born without eyeballs. *J. Hered.* **24**, 105–106.

Kao, J., Brown, N.A., Schmidt, B., Goulding, E.H. and Fabro, S. (1981) Teratogenicity of valproic acid: in vivo and in vitro investigations. *Teratogen. Carcinogen. Mutagen.* **1**, 376–382.

Landauer, W. (1948) Hereditary abnormalities and their chemically induced phenocopies. *Growth* **12**, 171–200.

Lauder, J.M. (1993) Neurotransmitters as growth regulatory signals: role of receptors and second messengers. *Trends Neurosci.* **16**, 233–240.

Mably, T.A., Bjerke, D.L., Moore, R.W., Gendron-Fitzpatrick, A. and Peterson, R.E. (1992) In utero and lactational exposure of male rats to 2,3,7,8-tetrachlorodibenzo-*p*-dioxin: (3) effects on spermatogenesis and reproductive capability. *Toxicol. Appl. Pharmacol.* **114**, 118–126.

Manson, J.M. (1986) Mechanism of nitrofen teratogenicity. *Environ. Hlth Perspect.* **70**, 137–147.

Marshall, H., Nonchev, S., Sham, M.H. et al (1992) Retinoic acid alters hindbrain Hox code and induces transformation of rhombomeres 2/3 into a 4/5 identity. *Nature* **260**, 756–759.

Martin, P., Nobes, C., McCluskey, J. and Lewis, J. (1994) Repair of excisional wounds in the embryo. *Eye* **8**, 155–160.

McKusick, V.A. (1994) *Mendelian Inheritance in Man*, 11th edn. Johns Hopkins University Press: Baltimore, MD.

McLachlan, J.A. (1993) Functional toxicology: a new approach to detect biologically active xenobiotics. *Environ. Hlth Perspect.* **101**, 386–387.

Mori, T. and Nagasawa, H. (Eds) (1988) *Toxicity of Hormones in Perinatal Life*. CRC Press: Boca Raton.

Nau, H. (1994) Valproic acid-induced neural tube defects. In *Neural Tube Defects* (Eds: G. Bock and J. Marsh), vol. 181, pp. 144–160. Wiley: Chichester.

Nau, H. and Scott, W.J. (Eds) (1987) *Pharmacokinetics in Teratogenesis*, vols 1 and 2. CRC Press: Boca Raton.

Nelson, K.G., Sakai, Y., Eitzman, B., Steed, T. and McLachlan, J. (1994) Exposure to diethylstilbestrol during a critical developmental period of the mouse reproductive tract leads to persistent induction of two estrogen-regulated genes. *Cell Growth Differ.* **5**, 595–606.

Newbold, R.R. (1993) Gender-related behaviour in women exposed prenatally to diethylstilbestrol. *Environ. Hlth Perspect.* **101**, 208–213.

O'Flaherty, E.J. and Clarke, D.O. (1994) Pharmacokinetic/pharmacodynamic approaches for developmental toxicology. In *Developmental Toxicology* (Eds: C.A. Kimmel and J. Buelke-Sam), 2nd edn, pp. 215–244. Raven Press: New York.

Oppenheimer, J.M. (1967) *Essays in the History of Embryology and Biology*. MIT Press: Cambridge, MA.

Peterson, R.E., Theobald, H.M. and Kimmel, G.L. (1993) Developmental and reproductive toxicity of dioxins and related compounds. *Crit. Rev. Toxicol.* **23**, 283–335.

Pimental, R.A., Liang, B., Yee, G.K. et al (1993) Dioxin receptor and C/EBP regulate the function of the glutathione S-transferase Ya gene xenobiotic response element. *Molec. Cell. Biol.* **13**, 4365–4373.

Pongratz, I., Mason, G.G.F. and Poellinger, L. (1992) Dual roles of the 90 kDa heat shock protein hsp90 in modulating functional activities of the dioxin receptor. *J. Biol. Chem.* **267**, 13728–13734.

Raff, M.C. (1992) Social controls on cell survival and cell death. *Nature* **356**, 397–400.

Rutledge, J.C., Shourbaji, A.G., Hughes, L.A. et al (1994) Limb and lower-body duplications induced by retinoic acid in mice. *Proc. Natl Acad. Sci. USA* **91**, 5436–5440.

Saatcioglu, F., Perry, D.J., Pasco, D.S. and Fagan, J.B. (1990) Multiple DNA-binding factors interact with overlapping specificities at the aryl hydrocarbon response elements of the cytochrome P4501A1 gene. *Molec. Cell. Biol.* **10**, 6408–6416.

Sadler, T.W. and Hunter, E.S. (1994) Principles of abnormal development: past, present and future. In *Developmental Toxicology* (Eds: C.A. Kimmel and J. Buelke-Sam), 2nd edn, pp. 53–56. Raven Press: New York.

Schantz, S.L and Bowman, R.E. (1989) Learning in monkeys exposed perinatally to 2,3,7,8-tetrachlorodibenzo-p-dioxin (TCDD). *Neurotox. Teratol.* **11**, 13–19.

Schardein, J.L. (1993) *Chemically Induced Birth Defects*, 2nd edn. Marcel Dekker: New York.

Scott, W.J. (1977) Cell death and reduced proliferated rate. In *Handbook of Teratology* (Eds: J.G. Wilson and F. Clarke-Fraser), vol. 2, pp. 81–98. Plenum Press: New York.

Sharpe, R. and Skakkebaek, N.E. (1993) Are oestrogens involved in falling sperm counts and disorders of the male reproductive tract? *Lancet* **341**, 1392–1395.

Shepard, T.H. (1992) *Catalog of Teratogenic Agents*, 7th edn. Johns Hopkins University Press: Baltimore, MD.

Snow, M.H.L. (1987) Uncoordinated development of embryonic tissue following cytotoxic damage. In *Approaches to Elucidate Mechanisms in Teratogenesis* (Ed: F. Welsch), pp. 83–107. Hemisphere: London.

Sulik, K.K., Cook, C.S. and Webster, W.S. (1988) Teratogens and craniofacial malformations: relationships to cell death. *Development* **103** Suppl., 213–232.

Turner, S., Sucheston, M.E., de Philip, R. and Paulson, R.B. (1990) Teratogenic effects on the neuroepithelium of the CD-1 mouse embryo exposed in utero to sodium valproate. *Teratology* **41**, 421–442.

Veuthey, S., Pexieder, T. and Scott, W.J. (1990) Pathogenesis of cardiac anomalies induced by trimethadione in the rat. In *Developmental Cardiology: Morphogenesis and Function* (Eds: E.B. Clark and A. Takao), pp. 453–465. Futura: New York.

Webster, W.S., Johnston, M.C., Lammer, E.J. and Sulik, K.K. (1986) Isotretinoin embryopathy and the cranial neural crest: an in vivo and in vitro study. *J. Craniofac. Genet. Dev. Biol.* **6**, 211–222.

Whitelaw, M., Pongratz, I., Wilhelmsson, A., Gustafsson, J.A. and Poellinger, L. (1993) Ligand-dependent recruitment of the Arnt co-regulator determines DNA recognition by the dioxin receptor. *Molec. Cell. Biol.* **13**, 2504–2514.

Whitlock, J.P. (1993) Mechanistic aspects of dioxin action. *Chem. Res. Toxicol.* **6**, 754–763.

Wickman, D.S., Siebert, J.R. and Benjamin, D.R. (1993) Nitrofen-induced congenital diaphragmatic defects in CD1 mice. *Teratology* **47**, 119–125.

Wilson, J.G., Roth, C.B. and Warkany, J. (1953) An analysis of the syndrome of malformations induced by vitamin A deficiency: effects of restoration of vitamin A at various times during gestation. *Am. J. Anat.* **92**, 189–217.

Wu, L. and Whitlock, J.P. (1993) Mechanism of dioxin action: receptor–enhancer interaction in intact cells. *Nucleic Acids Res.* **21**, 119–125.

6 Uses of Databases in Dysmorphology

MICHAEL BARAITSER

Mothercare Unit of Molecular Genetics and Fetal Medicine, Institute of Child Health, London, UK

Clinical geneticists and especially dysmorphologists have, as one of their main tasks, the recognition of the large number of malformation syndromes. There are a number of reasons why making a precise diagnosis is essential. First, it is necessary to establish whether the combination of malformations is genetic and, if so, determine the mechanism of inheritance and assess the subsequent recurrence risks. Secondly, a precise diagnosis is needed in order to establish a prognosis and to direct the clinician to investigate other organs that might be involved. Thirdly, a syndrome diagnosis may lead to prenatal diagnosis with the possibility of increasing parental choice regarding the continuation of a subsequent pregnancy. Finally, many people simply want to know the diagnosis. In some instances this opens up the possibility of meeting others with the same condition, together with their families. Indeed, there are lay societies dedicated to specific syndromes and parents join in order to discuss mutual problems. Many parents express the difficulty they have when friends ask them what is wrong with their child and many feel they would be able to cope better if they had a name they could use.

A clinical geneticist faces a number of problems in making a diagnosis. There are at least two thousand known dysmorphic syndromes. 'Known' in this sense means a syndrome that has been described before, although perhaps only once in a single case report, and the literature each month contains reports of new syndromes not thought to have been described previously.

The reports of syndromes are widely spread among many different specialist journals. As familial occurrence of malformations has always intrigued clinicians, the literature stretches back for many years and there is considerable difficulty in remembering or finding older reports, which indeed might be the only relevant descriptions. The vast majority of these conditions can only be recognized by using clinical and radiological criteria so that there is a constant need to look at the detail of previous cases of children thought to have the same problem.

All children with multiple disabilities will need a chromosomal analysis and diagnosis may be confirmed in this way, without needing to use a database in order to find a match. Thus far, other specialized blood tests, be they biochemical or molecular, have not made a significant contribution to syndrome diagnosis, although there are developments in these areas.

Embryos, Genes and Birth Defects. Edited by P. Thorogood.

Syndrome identification can be extremely difficult. A **syndrome** is defined as a group of malformations that tend to occur together. Syndromes are variable and are easier to define if they occur in siblings or in previous generations, especially if the combination is unusual, making the likelihood of separate conditions in the same family small. Familial cases also allow the clinician to define the variability of a condition, as the spectrum of a single disorder can be wide. More difficult is the recognition of a new syndrome that always occurs as a sporadic condition, as this necessitates the recollection of previous single case reports, some of which might have occurred in the distant past. It is not unusual for the clinician to vaguely remember a previous patient with the same condition, either reported somewhere in the literature or seen previously at the clinic, but finding documentation can be a daunting task. Additionally, it is clear that each clinical genetics unit is seeing patients not reported previously and possibly, for that unit, unique, but only by consulting a database will the clinician ascertain if there is a literature to consult.

DYSMORPHOLOGY DATABASES

Dysmorphology databases have a major clinical function in aiding doctors seeking a differential diagnosis for a patient presenting with a given array of signs. They can provide a list of all conditions with a combination, for example, of mental handicap, deafness and retinal dystrophy. The emphasis tends to be on a differential diagnosis – a manageable list of possible diagnoses – and although this might not seem as desirable as an exact diagnosis, searching a database for an exact diagnosis may lead to the correct condition being missed. This is because many unique features, or **handles**, will need to be entered in order to retrieve only one possibility, and for this to happen other possibilities will be excluded. In clinical dysmorphology too many syndromes overlap and it is better to view a short list of the possible diagnoses (not too many) and then reject those which seem on inspection not to fit than to be so exclusive at the outset that possible diagnoses are missed because the questions asked were too specific.

There are a small number of dysmorphology and related databases that have been developed over the past 10 years to help solve some of these clinical problems. Databases currently available commercially in this field include: the Online Mendelian Inheritance in Man (OMIM) database (McKusick, 1966), the London Dysmorphology Database (Winter and Baraitser, 1996) with its partner, the London Neurogenetic Database (Baraitser and Winter, 1995a), POSSUM (an Australian dysmorphology database; Bankier, 1994), and the Human Cytogenetics Database (Schinzel, 1994). A mouse database is currently being developed to help researchers to look for conditions that might match mapped syndromes in mice.

OMIM is based on the McKusick catalogue and includes all conditions showing Mendelian inheritance; it therefore excludes many of the sporadic syndromes. It can only be searched by means of key words, and there is no search strategy for diagnosing a syndrome by using features that are not included in the abstract or reference title. It is an excellent source of reference if the diagnosis is already known.

The **London Dysmorphology Database** and **POSSUM** are widely used and largely cover the same ground. Both contain a comprehensive, alphabetically indexed syndrome list, with each syndrome entry attached to an abstract, a list of features found in the condition, the related references from the literature, a mode of inheritance, a gene localization (if known) and a McKusick number. The abstract describes the main clinical features so that every case suggested in the differential diagnosis need not be consulted in detail. It also includes a discussion of other similar conditions and whether the inheritance pattern is uniform or the condition is heterogeneous. Databases can now provide, on CD-ROM or video disc, an accompanying set of photographs of patients with any condition, in instances where these have been published, and this is especially useful since visual clues are important in dysmorphology (see later).

Most databases have inclusion and exclusion criteria. For the London Dysmorphology Database it was decided to include all clinical reports of patients with multiple malformations, be they clearly genetic or simply sporadic. It was thought unnecessary to include the dysmorphology of all the chromosomal deletions and duplications as these conditions are usually diagnosed on cytogenetic analysis: a computer was not thought to be necessary to diagnose *cri-du-chat* syndrome (5p deletion), for instance. However, this is changing and clinicians have become aware that the cytogenetic laboratory can only detect certain deletions if the clinician gives guidance on where to look. The classic example of this is the Wolf–Hirschhorn syndrome (4p deletion), in which the deletion at the tip of the short arm is so small that it could be missed by routine cytogenetics and only detected after that region is intensively studied. An even finer degree of resolution is needed for some other deletions; for example, the deletion now known to be involved in Williams syndrome can only be detected by fluorescent in-situ hydridization (FISH; see Chapter 3). There is, therefore, a need either to include cytogenetic microdeletions on a dysmorphology database or to establish a separate database for them. The problem has largely been solved by the creation in Zurich of the Human Cytogenetics Database (Schinzel, 1994), using similar programs to those used on the London Dysmorphology Database.

By far the most powerful tool that these databases contain is the **search function**. This search strategy is sufficiently versatile to allow searching on a number of different bases:

(1) a **combination of features**.
(2) **features combined with an inheritance pattern**; e.g. any X-linked disorder with a cleft palate and deafness
(3) **key words**
(4) an **author and a key word**; it is possible that the user has a diagnosis in mind but can only remember the first author's name, or only the journal in which it was published and possibly a rough idea of the year. The programs allow a search on any of these variables.

WHAT IS A SYNDROME?

The first component of a database that a user accesses is a comprehensive list of dysmorphic syndromes. This is constructed from an extensive review of the past and present literature. Syndrome names in the literature are often meaningless (the first author's name on the paper might be used) and it is not uncommon for syndromes to be reported in different journals under separate titles or for clinicians on different sides of the Atlantic to use different names for the same condition. A classic example is the Beckwith–Wiedemann or Wiedemann–Beckwith syndrome. It is also known as the 'EMG syndrome' denoting its main features as exomphalos, macroglossia and gigantism (not very useful as these features might not always be present). On a database each syndrome can carry a number of related synonyms that will access information about the same condition. The syndrome list is indexed alphabetically but it is possible to search using only part of the name – remembering only 'Sheldon' of the Freeman–Sheldon syndrome will still access information about the condition.

One of the biggest problems concerns the definition of any given syndrome. Almost without exception, all syndromes are variable. The extent of the variability can usually be determined by looking at the same condition within a single family. Siblings who have, for instance, Laurence–Moon–Biedl syndrome, which is characterized by post-axial polydactyly, mental retardation, obesity, renal abnormalities and a pigmentary retinopathy, might differ in that one sibling has the complete picture whereas the other might be of normal intelligence, present in renal failure and have only mild obesity, or present with visual problems due to retinopathy and be found to have an extra small toe, or nubbin of tissue on the lateral border of the foot. Because it is likely that both siblings have the same genetic defect (there is too much overlap for them to have different conditions), the boundaries of the syndrome can begin to be delineated.

There is another form of variability that needs to be taken into account. In a given syndrome, even within a single family, a feature might differ in severity. For instance, a child presents with a radial aplasia. Many syndromes in which there are problems down the radial side of the limb are variable to the extent that in the same syndrome there might be a classic radial club hand, or a normal radius but an absent thumb, just a small thumb or, surprisingly, a duplicated thumb. All of these should be in the list of features of a condition such as VATER where the R stands for radial problems. The VATER syndrome is relatively common and there is a reasonably large literature which helps to determine the extent of the malformations. If the syndrome is less well delineated, the variability of the radial lesions might not be known (those updating the database can only put in what has been described) and diagnoses will be missed because the patient might have a malformation not previously described. A further problem arises when a patient has, for instance, two extra malformations not previously recorded and then it becomes difficult to know whether one is dealing with a new syndrome or not.

It is this definition of what is, and what is not, essential to a syndrome that is a major problem in the diagnosis of many of the two thousand syndromes described to date. If it were possible to rank features (i.e. decide what are the **essential** features), then this would be quite easy to incorporate into the database and indeed some have tried to do this. If it were always, or even often, possible to determine the relative or absolute importance of an individual feature to the diagnosis of a syndrome, then syndrome identification would be a lot easier. If 100% of cases of TAR syndrome (another syndrome involving the radius, the AR standing for aplasia of the radius and the T for thrombocytopenia), despite having radial aplasia, always had the thumb present, then clearly a diagnosis could not be made if it were absent and the computer could be programmed to insist on this.

The classic way of approaching the problem of variability in recessive disorders was well demonstrated in a study of Meckel–Gruber syndrome by Fraser and Lytwyn (1981). The main features are polydactyly, polycystic renal disease and a posterior encephalocele. The proband was ignored, as the variability of the condition could have led to considerable ascertainment bias (a series of cases seen and reported by a neurosurgeon would always be found to have a posterior encephalocele as that would be the very reason why they were seen by the neurosurgeon) and only the malformations present in the second affected were considered. In this way it was shown that 100% had polycystic renal disease, which is therefore essential for the diagnosis. The other features could likewise be ranked. The problem is that many of the recessive syndromes are so rare that a sib–sib study has not been performed and data are not available. The other major problem concerning ranking is that many syndromes seem to be on the whole sporadic events, as seen with both De Lange syndrome and the CHARGE association. In the latter syndrome, patients might present to a cardiologist (H is for heart defects); an ear, nose and throat specialist (A is for atresia choanae and E is for ear); or to a paediatrician, for growth failure (R stands for retardation of growth or development). Thus, depending on who collects and reports the data, bias will enter and the ranking of individual features becomes a problem.

A further problem about syndrome diagnosis is that new features are constantly being added. This might be because the syndrome is rare and the extent of the manifestations is not yet known, or because the underlying mechanism of causation is a chromosomal deletion, in which case a bigger or smaller piece missing might slightly alter the phenotype whilst retaining the facial features and hence the recognizable gestalt. The underlying aetiology might also depend on the timing of an insult and result in similar but not necessarily identical phenotypes. All of the above make syndrome recognition difficult and yet further complications might arise from the occurrence of a feature not described before.

One of the other major problems is that syndromes can evolve. Some features are present at birth but are not recognized because they are not looked for, whereas others evolve with time. Consider the following scenario:

- **At birth** a baby is found to have a post-axial polydactyly (an extra digit on the small toe side of the foot). At this stage no conclusions can be drawn and indeed there might be nothing more to the situation than that. If the baby is black, then the experienced clinician might decide at this stage that this is a common, unimportant, autosomal dominant finding in those of African origin, and be cautiously optimistic. If the database were to be used at this stage, a total of 114 conditions would be displayed and each one would be found to have additional features.

- **Nine months later** it might be noticed that the infant's development is slightly behind and causing concern. If a search were done at this stage, there would be 39 possibilities. Certainly Laurence–Moon–Biedl syndrome should be considered but the evidence from the patient would be inconclusive.
- **At 14 months** the child appears obese. The main problem at this stage is clinical judgement. The clinician might decide with some justification that the child is a little 'chubby' and not regard this new feature as significant. However, if the computer has prompted the clinician to consider Laurence–Moon–Biedl syndrome, then the weight gain might be considered in another light. If suspicion has now been raised, then it would be appropriate to ask for a renal scan to look for cystic dysplasia and to ask the ophthalmologists to investigate retinal function. If both series of tests are normal, the clinician would wait.
- **At 2 years** the retinal test would be repeated. If the retina is found to be abnormal, then the diagnosis is secure. If not, a further period of cautious waiting is appropriate.
- During this process the computer has made other suggestions that need to be followed. In the list of possibilities, given an entry of mental retardation, obesity and a retinal dystrophy, is found another condition – Cohen syndrome. To date, no one has described polydactyly in that condition, but all dysmorphic syndromes are rare and therefore the possibility has at least to be considered.

It is sometimes not possible to know whether one of the dysmorphic features is part of the clinical picture or not. It could just be that in a patient with learning difficulties and a bulbous nasal tip, the latter feature is not part of the condition, but is inherited from a parent who is perfectly normal but just happens to have a broad, bulbous nasal tip.

Variability also encompasses changes that occur with age, as the passage of time may alter the phenotype, and dysmorphologists are accustomed to recognizing faces at a particular age. For instance, the faces of patients with Williams syndrome change with age (the face becomes coarser) but provided that the feature list includes all the features, whatever the age, this should not be a problem. In addition, with the advent of pictures on the database, a sequential series of images showing these changes with age is very valuable.

In summary, the problems faced by the clinician, and which have to be addressed by database design, are as follows:

(1) Not only are syndromes rare, they are variable.
(2) Because there is mostly no test to confirm the diagnosis, no precise criteria can be formulated.

(3) Syndromes change with age.
(4) Some dysmorphic signs are familial and not relevant.

CLINICAL SIGNS, FEATURES OR 'HANDLES'

For a dysmorphology database to be useful, a comprehensive list of dysmorphic features needs to be constructed covering every possible malformation. The list of malformations can then be ordered in such a way that they can be accessed system by system or by entering a key word. A thesaurus can be incorporated to list similar features if the one being looked for is not found. (If, for example, the user enters the feature 'ante-mongoloid eye-slant', which is synonymous with 'downslanting palpebral fissures', the thesaurus will link the two terms together.)

In the London Dysmorphology Database, the feature list is biased towards signs rather than symptoms, as the former are more important to the dysmorphologist. As a result, certain features will not be found. For instance, diarrhoea might occasionally be an important feature of a condition but it is not included in the feature list – though it is still possible to search on the word 'diarrhoea' if it appears in the syndrome title or abstract. Similarly, 'vomiting', 'headache', and 'abdominal pain' are excluded, as these are of more importance to the paediatrician than to the dysmorphologist. However, the handles used in making a diagnosis are changing all the time. For instance the behavioural phenotype is an important part of Williams syndrome, in that the children are friendly and tend to want to engage with strangers. Angelman syndrome was previously called the 'happy puppet' syndrome in order to emphasize the happy disposition that is an integral part of the diagnosis, and it might be that some mentally handicapped, non-dysmorphic children will in future only be characterized by patterns of behaviour.

Features are accessed in two main ways. If the patient has cataracts, then it is quickest to simply write in the word in order to perform the search. However, it is often safer and easier to browse through the feature list. The London Dysmorphology Database has a three-tier system. The initial subdivisions are 'build', 'stature', 'head', 'neck', 'ears', 'eyes', 'thorax' and so on. Each of the above is then broken down into the next level of complexity. For example, the first level might be 'eye'. A search on this will search for anything abnormal with the eye.

The next level divides the eye into:

> – Anterior chamber
> – Conjunctiva
> – Cornea
> – Iris
> – Retina etc.

A search on this level will search on anything wrong with the anterior chamber, the cornea, or whichever subdivision is chosen. If the user is sure that the ophthalmic problem is a coloboma of the iris, then it is better to search at the third level which will look like this:

> – Iris
>   – Aniridia
>   – Brushfield spots
>   – Coloboma of the iris
>   – Heterochromia of the iris
>   – Pigmentary abnormalities of the iris
>   – Iris atrophy/dysplasia

The user simply chooses 'coloboma of the iris' and performs a search using this single criteria.

Not only, as seen earlier, are there problems with syndrome definition, there can also be difficulties with the definition of features (or **handles** as they are sometimes termed). As an example, take the case of a child with Coffin–Lowry syndrome. The main clinical features are mental retardation (a reasonable handle, but there are approximately a thousand syndromes with this feature), downslanting palpebral fissures and a prominent lower lip. But there are categories for 'full lips', 'everted lips', and 'prominent lips' and this can be confusing. If you search on 'full lips', those conditions with thick lips or everted lower lips will be missed and one can never be certain whether the lip in the original case reports was correctly described or not.

This problem can be overcome by using a search function that allows you to search on 'either/or' and, in the example given above, the computer will locate all syndromes with prominent, full *or* everted lips, in combination with downslanting palpebral fissures and mental retardation. This problem would not, of course, have arisen if these features had not been presented as separate categories, but some would argue that there is a difference between full lips and prominent lips. The 'either/or' technique is used in a similar way to the three-tier system: that is, by exploiting the ability to search on a general category such as 'lip–general', the second-level tier incorporating anything to do with the lip. Similarly, a patient is short but the clinician might be uncertain which limb segment is affected. The user could then search using 'either rhizomelic or mesomelic or acromelic' to cover all possibilities or, alternatively, merely search on 'short stature – general', which will pick up everything to do with short stature. Both strategies will give the same end result.

Database searches are not useful if the user loads the search with non-essential trivia. It is necessary to pick out the essential dysmorphic features – that is, the 'gross and unusual' features. Absent fingers are strikingly unusual features. Extra fingers and toes are gross and unusual (for gross and unusual, the words **good handles** are used), provided family background is taken into account. Syndactyly between toes 2 and 3 is an important feature in a condition called Smith–Lemli–Opitz syndrome, but in this condition there are also severe mental retardation and genital problems. In fact, syndactyly between toes 2 and 3 is a common familial trait of no particular significance and is therefore not a

particularly good handle in the vast majority of situations in which it is encountered. It is therefore of little use to detail all the abnormal features, starting as some
do at the top of the body and working in an obsessively thorough way to the
bottom, and then present this list to the computer. Far better to look carefully at
everything and then select out the best handles before using the database.

The most unusual feature should be entered first. If this happens to be, for
instance, arrhinia – an absent nose – then there is little point in following this
with three or four more features, as there are only two or three syndromes
known in which the nose is absent, and it would be worthwhile looking at all
three. When one browses through the feature list, the computer displays the
number of syndromes to which each feature is attached, so a user entering
'arrhinia' will realize that only a short differential diagnosis list is going to be
generated. Furthermore, whatever the variability of the condition, if another
condition matches on four other features but does not have an absent nose as a
feature, then it probably is not worth looking at, as one would guess that
arrhinia is such a cardinal feature that it should be present. However, if 'absent
nose' is only providing a very small list of syndromes, and none of these gives a
good match for the patient under consideration, the next step is to try
'hypoplastic nose'. The user can then go to the relevant references and look at the
pictures in the published papers, since a very small nose might just have the
same significance as an absent nose if all other features match. Thus, in order to
overcome the variability problem, it is best not to be too precise.

There is an alternative strategy to overcome the problem of variability. Consider
a further example. A patient has the following features: mental retardation, post-
axial polydactyly, obesity, retinal dystrophy, scoliosis and renal cysts. The patient
appears to have Laurence–Moon–Biedl syndrome but, in addition, has a severe
scoliosis. If the user includes this feature in the search as well as all the more usual
features, then the correct diagnosis will not be made by the computer because the
feature list attached to the Laurence–Moon–Biedl syndrome does not contain
scoliosis. There is, however, a mechanism allowing the user to select, from the
features entered, those which should be mandatory, and then to search on a
selection of the rest. Instead of selectively choosing 'good handles' to enter, the
user can enter all of the features a patient has, but mark, in this case, mental
retardation, post-axial polydactyly and retinal dystrophy as mandatory, asking
the computer to search on these three with one or two of the other three non-
mandatory features. If the user searches on any four out of the six features above,
the correct diagnosis will be made. If he or she searches on any three, then the
correct diagnosis will be made, but another problem arises in that the list of
possibilities becomes so long that the correct diagnosis might be hidden.

Having said that a good handle is an unusual feature not common to many
conditions, there are exceptional features which, although common, are essential
in dividing children into broad categories and these should always be entered.
Mental retardation is one of these, and severe short stature is another. Mild short
stature (someone just under the 3rd centile for height) might not be an essential
handle but, if someone with a syndrome is very short indeed, then this is
important and, is obligatory to the diagnosis.

In general, those conditions most likely to be diagnosed by the computer are those that are strikingly dysmorphic. The differential diagnosis list will, in this type of situation, be short. A child with microphthalmia (small eyes) and a smooth brain (lissencephaly) will produce a list of eight possible diagnoses, whereas microphthalmia combined with mental retardation is much less unusual and the list is long. The experienced clinician will manipulate the feature list until satisfied that all hope of making a diagnosis has gone. If, for instance, a child is born with no eyes (rather than small eyes) and a smooth brain, and the search for syndromes with a combination of anophthalmia and lissencephaly reveals none, then the clinician must think of the possibility that 'small eyes' are in the spectrum of 'no eyes' and should change the search to use microphthalmia in place of anophthalmia.

Most databases can be readily modified and additions to the list of features can easily be made. The only problem is that any change might necessitate the reclassification of an enormous amount of data. For instance, if it is shown that children with cleft lip and palate can be usefully separated according to whether the cleft is on the left or the right, the recoding by rechecking all syndromes in the literature might be a necessary but formidable task. It is much easier if a new diagnostic tool such as magnetic resonance imaging becomes frequently used, since extra categories can just be added and only new data need to be entered.

THE ROLE OF PICTURES

There are many disabled individuals, especially those with mental retardation, in whom the handles or dysmorphic features seem very mild or subtle. Simply entering on to the database a combination of a 'big head' and 'mental retardation' is not a useful search strategy as there are over a hundred syndromes with this combination. By viewing the visual records, the eye can detect subtle similarities and differences and this phenomenon of 'gestalt' recognition, together with textual information, can allow a diagnosis to be made. Perhaps even new syndromes can be delineated in this way.

Dysmorphology is an essentially visual subject and most databases will have a method of displaying pictures either by using CD-ROM or by using a separate screen and a video disc (e.g. Baraitser and Winter, 1995b). The pictures are accessed by syndrome and the system is especially useful when the original pictures cannot be viewed because the local library does not carry the relevant journals. Clearly, electronic means of image archiving together with the advent of digital cameras for the creation of clinical records facilitate the ready incorporation of visual records into databases. Furthermore, electronic means of communication allow images to be transmitted between clinical centres and the use of the Internet could permit (regulated) access to databases from a distance. As a result, the nature of dysmorphology databases, and the ease with which we use them, are likely to evolve dramatically as new modes of information technology are developed.

REFERENCES

Bankier, A. (Ed.) (1994) *POSSUM*. The Murdoch Institute, Royal Children's Hospital, Victoria, Australia.

Baraitser, M. and Winter, R.M. (Eds) (1995a) *London Neurogenetic Database*. Oxford University Press: Oxford.

Baraitser, M. and Winter, R.M. (Eds) (1995b) *Dysmorphology Photolibrary on Compact Disc*. Oxford University Press: Oxford.

Fraser, F.C. and Lytwyn, A. (1981) Spectrum of anomalies in the Meckel syndrome, or: 'maybe there is a malformation syndrome with at least one constant anomaly'. *Am. J. Med. Genet.* **9**, 67–73.

McKusick, V.A. (1966) *Online Mendelian Inheritance in Man*. Johns Hopkins University Press: Baltimore, MD.

Schinzel, A. (Ed.) (1994) *Human Cytogenetics Database*. Oxford University Press: Oxford.

Winter, R.M. and Baraitser, M. (Eds) (1996) *London Dysmorphology Database*. 3rd edn. Oxford University Press: Oxford.

7 The Limbs

PATRIZIA FERRETTI[1] and CHERYLL TICKLE[2]

[1]Developmental Biology Unit, Institute of Child Health, London, UK and [2]Department of Anatomy and Developmental Biology, University College London, London, UK

DEVELOPMENTAL ANATOMY OF THE HUMAN LIMB

Both upper and lower limbs originate from the lateral plate mesoderm which aggregates in discrete regions of the flank of the embryo. The primordium of the upper limb is first apparent 26 days after fertilization (stage 12 according to Moore, 1988) at the level of the cervical somites, while the lower limb bud appears 1 to 2 days later, at the beginning of stage 13, opposite the lumbar and upper sacral somites (Figure 7.1). Apart from this delay in the appearance of the lower limb anlage and its subsequent development, early stages of lower and upper limb development are fundamentally the same. For simplicity, the stages discussed here will refer to development of the upper limb.

The emerging limb bud consists of a rapidly proliferating mass of mesenchymal cells covered by an epithelium which will thicken at the tip of the bud along the anteroposterior axis to form the **apical ectodermal ridge**. The interactions between the apical ectodermal ridge and the underlying mesenchyme are of fundamental importance for proper progression of development, and will be discussed in detail in the section concerned with the cellular and molecular interactions underlying normal development of the limb. Limb buds grow rapidly and in a co-ordinated way. A few days after formation of buds (stage 13–14), spinal nerves start to grow into the mesenchyme of the bud and innervation follows a segmental pattern. Initially the limb bud is supplied by a capillary network which, through processes that are still poorly understood, will transform into a main stem artery and its branches which drain into a marginal vein. The limb bud continues to grow and elongate, and 32–34 days after fertilization (stage 14) a paddle-shaped hand plate has formed. Prechondrogenic condensation of mesenchyme becomes apparent in the regions where the cartilaginous skeletal elements will form in a proximal to distal direction and, towards the end of the fifth week after fertilization (stage 15), overt **chondrogenesis** is in progress. Myoblasts aggregate to form two **muscle masses** dorsal and ventral to the developing skeletal elements. The muscle masses will split to give rise to extensor muscles in the dorsal part of the limb and to flexors ventrally. At the end of the sixth week (stage 17), all of the limb skeletal structures are cartilaginous, digital rays are present, notches appear at the tip of

Embryos, Genes and Birth Defects. Edited by P. Thorogood.
© 1997 John Wiley & Sons Ltd.

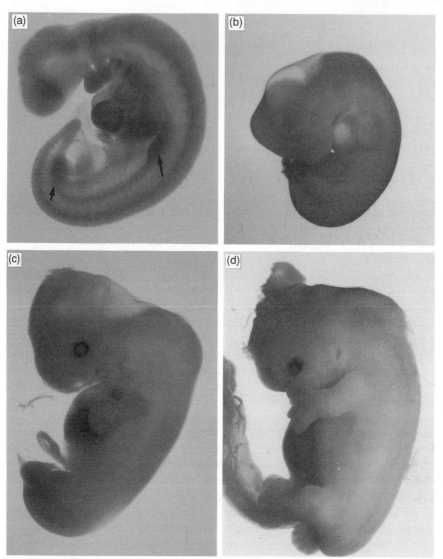

Figure 7.1 Limb development in human embryos at different times after fertilization. (a) Both forelimb (long arrow) and hindlimb (short arrow) buds are apparent in a 28-day-old embryo, but the forelimb bud is more pronounced. (b) In a 35-day-old embryo a hand plate has formed, but the hindlimb bud is still paddle shaped. (c) Finger rays are visible (arrows) and a foot plate has formed in a 38-day-old embryo. (d) Short webbed fingers are present and notches are starting to form between the digital rays of the foot of a 50-day-old embryo

the inter-ray mesenchyme, and the hand plate starts to assume a webbed appearance (44–50 days, stage 18–19). At the same time (48–50 days, stage 19), rotation of upper limbs begins and bending of the elbow occurs. The limb will rotate 90° laterally on the longitudinal axis to assume the adult position with the palm of the hand facing anteriorly. Appropriate positioning of the lower limb, with the knee facing anteriorly, is achieved through a medial rotation of 90° a few days later. Meanwhile, ossification begins and digital separation is accomplished by destruction of the interdigital tissue, probably through a process of programmed cell death as described in other species. By the end of the eighth week both upper and lower limbs appear as miniatures of the adult limb, but not all of the centres of primary ossification have yet formed, and ossification will continue throughout the fetal life.

MAIN CLASSES OF LIMB DEFECTS

Given the numerous events that must be spatiotemporally synchronized in order to develop a normal limb, it is not surprising that limb abnormalities are frequently encountered, and that their severity depends on the stage at which their development is affected. Gradually we are learning how impairment of specific cellular and molecular interactions can result in different limb abnormalities (see later). Limb defects can be caused by environmental factors, either chemical or mechanical, gene mutations and chromosomal abnormalities, or a combination of such factors. As the most important events in limb development occur between the fourth and eighth week post-fertilization, this is also the period of higher susceptibility to teratogens or defective expression of developmentally regulated genes. However, limb defects can also occur as a consequence of trauma once development of all of the limb structures has been accomplished. For example, secondary destruction, so called 'intrauterine amputation', is thought to be caused by constriction of the developing limb by amniotic bands.

Although many of the limb defects observed are quite minor and easily corrected by surgery, major limb abnormalities are observed in 2 out of every 1000 births (Moore, 1988). **Amelia**, which is total absence of the limb, can occur, but it is a fairly rare condition. In contrast, partial absence of one or more of the limbs, **meromelia**, is frequently observed. Meromelia is often associated with other types of limb defects, such as **oligosyndactyly** (fusion of digits), **club foot** (deformity of the ankle) and bowed limbs. A large number of limb deficiencies occurred in the 1960s as a consequence of the antinauseant drug thalidomide, which produced a wide range of bilateral limb deficiencies, including extreme cases of quadruple amelia. More commonly, prenatal exposure to thalidomide resulted in various deficiencies of long bones.

Limb defects are often associated with other malformations, affecting, for example, craniofacial, kidney, cardiac and skin development (Stevenson and Meyer, 1993). Limb defects associated with other abnormalities are often heritable either as autosomal recessive or autosomal dominant traits. X-linked inheritance of limb defects is observed only in a few syndromes. The various causes believed to lead to each syndrome displaying limb abnormalities, including rare ones, can be found in the review by Stevenson and Meyer (1993). An extrapolation of these data for syndromes where either meromelias or synostoses (fusion of various bones) are observed is shown in Table 7.1.

Since the classification of limb abnormalities is rather complex and has been extensively covered elsewhere (Stevenson and Meyer, 1993; Winter et al, 1993), we will give only a few examples of the type of defects that can occur (Table 7.2; Figure 7.2). As already mentioned, limb deficiencies, amelias and meromelias, represent an important group of limb abnormalities. In other cases, instead of deletions of structures, the presence of supernumerary structures such as fingers

Table 7.1 Summary of causation of limb abnormalities in syndromes displaying meromelias and synostosis

	Meromelias (%)	Synostosis (%)
Autosomal recessive	25.8	18.6
Autosomal dominant	25.8	52.1
X-linked dominant	3.2	4.3
Chromosomal abnormalities	4.8	1.4
Sporadic/maternal diabetes	9.6	5.7
Drug (thalidomide, alcohol)	1.6	2.9
Trauma	1.6	1.4
Unknown/uncertain	27.4	12.8

These values have been extrapolated from Stevenson and Meyer (1993). Rare syndromes are also included.

Table 7.2 Classification of limb defects

Limb defects	Prominent features	
Amelia	Complete absence of a limb	
Meromelia	Partial absence of a limb	• terminal • intercalary • transverse • longitudinal
Brachydactyly	Shortening of digits	• single digit (one or more bones involved) • multiple digit (one or more bones involved)
Polydactyly	Supernumerary digits	• incomplete extra finger/toe • complete extra finger/toe • mirror hand/foot
Synostosis	Fusion of bones	• bones normally separated by joint space • bones of different rays • bones of different limbs
Syndactyly	Fusion of digits	• cutaneous • osseous (synostosis)
Skeletal dysplasia	Abnormal growth, organization and density of cartilage and bone	• epiphysis • metaphysis • diaphysis

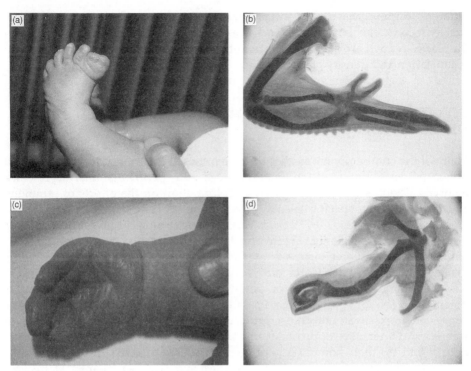

Figure 7.2 Human congenital limb abnormalities (a, c) and experimentally manipulated chick limbs (b, d) can have similar phenotypes. These examples were chosen to illustrate the close resemblance between the results of experimental manipulations in chick embryos and human limb abnormalities, although the mechanisms that produce these phenotypes are not thought to have the same basis in these cases. (a) Greig cephalopolysyndactyly with additional pre-axial toes and fusions between toes. (b) Chick limb with extra digit 2 produced by grafting small number of polarizing region cells to anterior margin of limb bud. (c) Complete fusion of digits (syndactyly) in Apert syndrome. (d) Chick limb that developed after apical ridge removal and application of fibroblast growth factor to posterior margin. The bunched digits are thought to result because the apical ridge has been removed and dorsoventral flattening of the bud is no longer maintained

or toes (polydactylies) is observed (Figure 7.2a). **Polydactyly** occurs fairly frequently and the extra digits formed are usually incomplete. In contrast, mirror hands and feet (i.e. mirror-imaging of digits on either side of a proximodistal-oriented midline of the digital array), which are usually unilateral, are very rare. Most polydactylies (both isolated and associated with other anomalies) are heritable. They are mainly inherited as an autosomal trait, but a few recessive X-linked cases have also been reported. Other limb defects are the consequence of fusion of structures, either bones (synostosis) or cutaneous. Soft-tissue **syndactyly** is a defect in which the web between the rays does not break down during development, and is usually an autosomal dominant abnormality. Another set of defects are the brachydactylies, where shortening of digits occurs;

different digits, phalanges, metacarpals and metatarsals can be affected. **Brachydactyly** can be familial and present in many syndromes and skeletal dysplasias, which are skeletal abnormalities originating from abnormal growth, organization and density of cartilage and bone.

CONTEMPORARY STUDIES ON MECHANISM OF LIMB DEVELOPMENT

Many of the contemporary studies that have shed light on mechanisms involved in normal development of the limb are based on experimental analysis of chick embryos. There is an extensive body of information on the effects of removing and transplanting specific pieces of tissue in developing chick limb buds (reviewed by Saunders, 1977). Such classical embryological investigations have defined cell interactions that are involved in limb patterning. More recently some of the molecules involved in these interactions have been identified (reviewed by Tickle and Eichele, 1994; Cohn and Tickle, 1996). Some of these molecules were first identified from analysis of patterns of gene expression. For example, potential roles of growth factors and homeobox-containing genes were suggested from studies on transcript localization in developing mouse embryos (see later). Other developmentally important genes expressed in the limb have been found by their homology with genes that are affected in developmental mutants of insects, such as, *hedgehog*, *engrailed* and *Wnt* (see Chapter 1). Insights into the roles of these genes have been gained from the effects of gene over-expression, limb bud manipulations and application of defined chemicals in chick embryos, and from creating transgenic mice with specific mutations. In very few cases has the molecular basis of mammalian limb mutants been elucidated (see later, Table 7.3).

CELL INTERACTIONS

Work on chick embryos has revealed three major sets of interactions in the developing limb bud (Figure 7.3): an epithelial–mesenchymal interaction at the tip of the limb bud between the **apical ectodermal ridge** (the thickened rim of epithelium) and the underlying mesenchyme; a second epithelial–mesenchymal interaction in the tip region of the bud which involves the covering ectoderm of the limb bud and underlying mesenchyme; and a mesenchymal–mesenchymal interaction between the **polarizing region** (a region of mesenchyme cells at the posterior margin of the limb bud) and mesenchyme cells at the tip of the limb bud.

The epithelial–mesenchymal interaction between apical ridge and underlying mesenchyme is required for bud outgrowth (Figure 7.3a). Thus, when the apical ridge is cut away from an early chick limb bud, outgrowth is halted and truncated limbs develop. Conversely, when an apical ridge is grafted to the surface of a bud near the tip, outgrowth is induced. Since structures are laid down along the long axis of the limb in a proximodistal sequence, removal of the

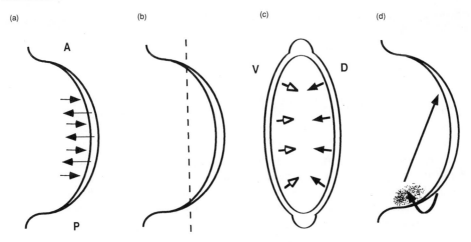

Figure 7.3 Major interactions in the developing limb bud. (a) Arrows indicate reciprocal interactions between the apical ectodermal ridge, the thickened epithelium at the tip of the limb bud and underlying mesenchyme. A, anterior; P, posterior. (b,c) Limb bud sectioned along dotted line and then shown in cross-section. Arrows indicate potential signals from dorsal and ventral ectoderm. V, ventral; D, dorsal. (d) Straight arrow indicates interaction between the polarizing region (stippled) and mesenchyme at the tip of the limb bud. Curved arrow indicates maintenance of the polarizing region by apical ectodermal ridge

ridge at later stages of development gives less severe truncations than removal at early stages. The zone of mesenchyme immediately below the apical ridge consists of undifferentiated cells and is known as the **progress zone** (Summerbell et al, 1973). As cells leave the progress zone, the identity of structures being laid down appears to be controlled by a timing mechanism that operates autonomously in the zone. Cells that leave the progress zone early form proximal structures whereas cells that leave it later form distal ones. The interaction between apical ridge and mesenchyme appears to be reciprocal, in that cells in the progress zone maintain the ridge.

The second epithelial–mesenchymal interaction is between ectoderm covering the tip of the bud and mesenchyme (Figure 7.3b). Signals from the ectoderm appear to control pattern across the dorsoventral axis. When an ectodermal jacket is transplanted from a left limb bud on to a right limb bud, the dorsoventral axis of the part of the limb laid down after the operation (i.e. distal part of the limb) is reversed, as judged by muscle pattern, joint flexure and skin appendages (MacCabe et al, 1974; Akita, 1996). In addition, when an apical ridge is grafted to the surface of a chick limb bud, the outgrowth has a symmetrical pattern, either double-dorsal, when the outgrowth arises from the dorsal surface, or double-ventral, when the outgrowth arises from the ventral surface (Saunders and Errick, 1976).

The ectoderm is thought to play a mechanical role in controlling bud shape. The apical ridge provides a stiffened rim to the tip of the bud and helps to keep the bud dorsoventrally flattened (Figure 7.3b). Furthermore, the length of the apical ridge correlates with the number of digits that subsequently form (Lee and Tickle, 1985).

The mesenchymal–mesenchymal interaction involves signalling by the polarizing region to mesenchyme cells at the tip of the limb bud and this determines the pattern of cell differentiation across the anteroposterior axis of the limb (Figure 7.3c). Signalling by the polarizing region can be demonstrated by grafting the polarizing region from one chick wing bud to the anterior margin of a second bud. In response to the signal from the graft, anterior mesenchyme cells in the host limb bud form an additional set of digits (4,3,2) in mirror-image symmetry with the normal set of digits (2, 3, 4; Saunders and Gasseling, 1968). The strength of the polarizing region signal can be assayed by the character of the additional digits and is dependent on the number of polarizing region cells grafted (Tickle, 1981). With a very small number of polarizing region cells, just an additional digit 2 develops (Figure 7.2b). The polarizing region appears to provide a positional signal and structures that are formed from particular cells depend on the distance of the cells from the polarizing region. When the polarizing region is grafted more posteriorly closer to the host polarizing region, anterior digits do not form and the digit pattern that results is 4, 3, 3, 4. Experiments in which blocks of leg tissue were interposed between graft and responding cells show that the polarizing signal can operate over about 10–30 cell diameters (Honig, 1981).

The polarizing region lies just proximal to the progress zone at the posterior margin of the limb bud and is present throughout the time that the pattern is established. Maintenance of the polarizing region depends on the presence of the apical ectodermal ridge. Assays for polarizing activity after the posterior part of the ridge has been removed show that the ability of posterior mesenchyme to induce digit duplications is reduced (Vogel and Tickle, 1993).

MOLECULES IMPLICATED IN SIGNALLING

Apical ectodermal ridge signals (Figure 7.4)

The signal from the apical ridge that is necessary for bud outgrowth can be substituted by **fibroblast growth factors** (FGFs; Niswander et al, 1993; Fallon et al, 1994). When beads soaked in FGF are placed at or near the margin of a chick limb bud following removal of the apical ridge, outgrowth continues and distal structures are laid down. The most complete patterns have been obtained either by placing two beads, one apically and one posteriorly at the bud margin, or by inserting one bead in distal mesenchyme followed a day later by a second bead. Thus, with appropriate application of FGF beads, a bud with ridge removed, which would normally just give rise to a humerus, can also develop a radius, ulna and set of digits.

Local application of FGF posteriorly maintains the polarizing region, and generation of distal structures when two beads are placed simultaneously at the margin of the limb bud correlates with polarizing activity in the bud. This suggests that the progress zone is only reconstituted when mesenchyme cells are

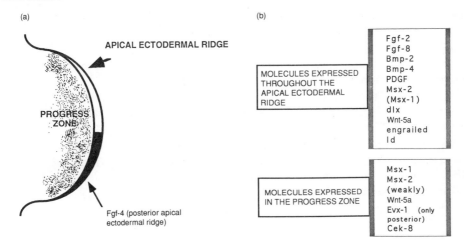

Figure 7.4 Molecules expressed in tissues at the tip of the limb bud and that could be involved in mediating interactions between apical ectodermal ridge and underlying progress zone mesenchyme. (a) Limb bud showing apical ectodermal ridge and progress zone and pattern of expression of *Fgf-4* transcripts. (b) Selected lists of molecules expressed in the two tissues

exposed to both the ridge signal (FGF) and a polarizing signal (Niswander et al, 1993). The effects of application of FGF locally to the anterior part of the bud margin are consistent with this idea. Cell proliferation occurs but only a fat or split humerus develops. Even though FGF can very effectively promote outgrowth, it cannot fulfil the mechanical role of the ridge. When the ridge is removed, buds become bulbous rather than being dorsoventrally flattened. This change in bud shape could account for the bunching of digits that frequently occurs in FGF-treated buds (Figure 7.2d).

It is not clear which member(s) of the FGF family of factors mediate ridge signalling in normal development. FGFs have been shown to be expressed in early chick and mouse limb buds. FGF-2 (basic FGF) has been localized by antibody labelling and is found in mesenchyme and ectoderm, including both ridge and non-ridge ectoderm (Savage et al, 1993; Dono and Zeller, 1994). In contrast, transcripts of another family member, FGF-4, are restricted to the posterior part of the apical ridge in both mouse and chick embryos (Niswander and Martin, 1993; Niswander et al, 1994). FGF-2 and FGF-4 proteins appear to be equally effective in substituting for the ridge and both can operate through the same receptor. Furthermore, the expression of *Fgf-4* transcripts in the apical ridge can be regulated by polarizing region signals (see later). Very recently, it has been shown that yet another member of the FGF family, *Fgf-8* is expressed in the apical ectodermal ridge (Heikinheimo et al, 1994; Ohuchi et al, 1994; Crossley and Martin, 1995).

Apical ridge cells are also known to express other signalling molecules in addition to FGFs, such as **bone morphogenetic proteins** (BMPs) and the product of the *Wnt-5a* gene. *Bmps* and *Wnt-5a* are also expressed in the mesenchyme at the tip of the limb bud (see later). Since FGFs can so completely substitute for apical ridge signal, these other growth factors and other molecules expressed in the ridge appear to be involved in either regulating FGF expression or maintaining mechanical integrity of the ridge. Several different transcription factors are expressed by ridge cells. For example, *Distal-less* (Dollé et al, 1992; Bulfone et al, 1993) and *engrailed* are expressed in ridge (and earlier in ventral limb ectoderm); *Msx* genes (see later) and the *ld* gene are expressed in both ridge and mesenchyme. The *ld* gene is affected in the mouse *limb deformity* mutants. The gene was characterized by identifying the site of an insertional mutation in a transgenic mouse, and encodes a member of a previously unknown family of proteins called 'formins'. Formins are localized in the nucleus and may be involved in gene regulation (Woychik et al, 1990).

Ectoderm signals (Figure 7.5)

Several molecules are now known to be expressed in either dorsal or ventral ectoderm. A striking dorsoventral ectodermal restriction is that of transcripts of the gene *Wnt-7a* which are localized in dorsal ectoderm (Dealy et al, 1993; Parr et al, 1993). *Wnt* genes are a family of genes that comprise vertebrate homologues of the *Drosophila wingless* gene and an *int* gene that is involved in induction of mammary tumours in mice. Since *Wnt* genes encode short-range secreted proteins, the Wnt-7a protein is a good candidate for a signalling molecule secreted by dorsal ectoderm that is involved in controlling dorsoventral patterning. Indeed, it has now been shown that functional inactivation of *Wnt-7a* in mice leads to ventralization of distal limb pattern (Parr and McMahon, 1995). At very early limb bud stages, a number of genes that are later restricted to the apical ridge are expressed in ventral ectoderm, including *engrailed-1* (Figure 7.5). Functional inactivation of *engrailed-1* results in dorsal transformation of ventral

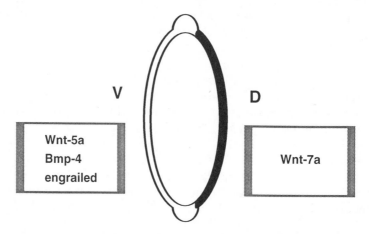

Figure 7.5 Molecules expressed in dorsal and ventral ectoderm. Those expressed in ventral ectoderm are later expressed in apical ectodermal ridge (see Figure 7.4). V, ventral; D, dorsal

paw structures, suggesting a specific role for this gene, in addition to *Wnt-7a*, in dorsoventral patterning of the limb (Loomis et al, 1996).

Polarizing signals (Figure 7.6)

Two molecules have been identified that can mimic signalling of the polarizing region: one is a vitamin A derivative, **retinoic acid** (Tickle et al, 1982) and the other is the product of the *sonic hedgehog* gene (*shh*; Riddle et al, 1993). Beads soaked in retinoic acid, or grafts of fibroblast cells transfected with *shh* gene (or *shh*-soaked beads), placed at the anterior margin of a chick wing bud lead to digit duplications (Tickle et al, 1985; Riddle et al, 1993; Lopez-Martinez et al, 1995). Application of retinoic acid to the anterior margin also induces expression of *shh*, suggesting that the *shh* signal acts downstream of retinoic acid (Riddle et al, 1993; Niswander et al, 1994). Both retinoic acid and *shh* transcripts can be detected in normal limb buds.

Retinoic acid has been extracted from chick and mouse limb buds and is estimated to be present in nanomolar concentrations (reviewed by Hofmann and Eichele, 1994). The posterior part of the bud where the polarizing region is located is enriched in retinoic acid (Thaller and Eichele 1987). Chick limb bud mesenchyme cells can generate retinoic acid from retinol and express a range of molecules that mediate a retinoid response, including nuclear retinoic acid receptors and retinoid binding proteins (reviewed by Mangelsdorf et al, 1994; Kastner et al, 1995).

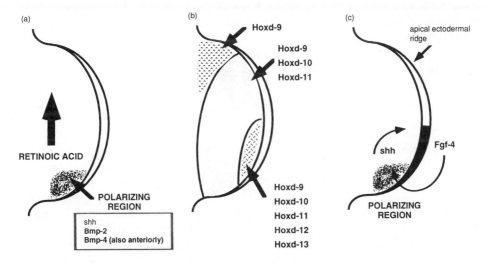

Figure 7.6 Molecules involved in interaction between polarizing region and progress zone mesenchyme at the tip of the bud. (a) Potential signalling molecules; high to low concentration of retinoic acid indicated by large arrow; genes expressed in polarizing region. (b) Pattern of expression of gene members of *Hox-D* cluster across the anteroposterior axis of the limb bud. Changes in expression pattern can be brought about by polarizing signals. (c) Feedback loop between signalling by polarizing region and signalling by posterior ridge. Arrows do not necessarily imply direct action.

Transcripts of the *shh* gene correlate spatially and temporally with the polarizing region in the limb bud. In *Drosophila*, the transmembrane protein encoded by the segment polarity gene **patched** is an immediate downstream regulator of *shh* signalling. Vertebrate *patched* is expressed in the posterior part of vertebrate limb buds and can be induced by *shh* applied ectopically (Goodrich et al, 1996; Hahn et al, 1996a,b; Marigo et al, 1996). Interestingly, *patched* not only plays a crucial role in embryonic axial patterning, but also appears to be a tumour suppressor gene, as mutations of *patched* in humans are frequently associated with basal cell carcinoma (Hahn et al, 1996a,b; Johnson et al, 1996).

Expression of *shh* is maintained by the apical ridge (or FGF) (Niswander et al, 1994). Application of retinoic acid to the anterior margin can activate *Fgf-4* expression. Therefore, in normal limb development, retinoic acid in concert with FGF could activate *shh* expression. However, *shh*-expressing cells can also induce *Fgf-4* expression in overlying ridge epithelium. Once the correct pattern of expression of epithelial and mesenchymal signals has been set up, it appears that a positive feedback loop is then established and links outgrowth with patterning (Figure 7.6; Izpisúa-Belmonte et al, 1992a; Laufer et al, 1994; Niswander et al, 1994). In addition to the feedback loop between *Fgf-4* and *shh*, there is evidence that *Wnt-7a* is necessary for the maintenance of *shh* expression (Parr and McMahon, 1995; Yang and Niswander, 1995). Thus there is interaction between signalling along all three limb axes.

Mesenchyme cells at the posterior margin of the limb bud also contain transcripts of genes encoding BMPs (e.g. *Bmp-2*, *Bmp-4*; Francis et al, 1994), which are signalling molecules of the **transforming growth factor-β** (TGF-β) superfamily (reviewed by Wozney et al, 1993). In *Drosophila* signalling pathways, *hedgehog* activates a gene called *dpp*, which has a patterning function (Basler and Struhl, 1994). This gene, *dpp*, encodes a molecule very closely related to BMP-2 and BMP-4, which suggests, by analogy, that in the vertebrate limb *shh* would activate BMPs and that they could mediate patterning. There is indeed evidence in vertebrates that *shh* can activate *Bmp-2* expression in anterior cells of the limb bud (Francis et al, 1994), but application of neither BMP-2 nor BMP-4 protein, nor of BMP-2 expressing cells, to the anterior margin of the limb bud gives mirror-image digit duplications (Francis et al, 1994; Duprez et al, 1996). However, ectopic expression of human BMP-2 induces *Fgf-4* expression in the apical ectodermal ridge, suggesting that BMP-2 may be involved in the maintenance of the ridge and in the link between patterning and outgrowth of the limb bud. BMP-2 might, therefore, act in a secondary pathway that comes into play after position has been specified. It is also possible that only heterodimers of BMPs can convey a polarizing signal. However, it is likely that BMPs have other roles in limb development. For example, another member of the BMP family, *Bmp-7*, is also expressed in developing limbs, and functional inactivation of this gene results in poly-dactyly (Dudley et al, 1995; Luo et al, 1995). Furthermore, inactivation of a BMP receptor in chick limb buds leads to interdigital webbing (Zou and Niswander, 1996).

Molecules expressed in the progress zone (Figure 7.4)

Genes known to be expressed in mesenchyme at the tip of the limb bud could encode molecules that play roles in controlling cell proliferation, in maintaining cells in an undifferentiated state and in timing mechanisms. Among genes with this expression pattern are those encoding transcription factors and short-range signalling molecules.

Two related homeobox-containing genes, *Msx-1* and *Msx-2* (formerly known as *Hox-7* and *Hox-8*), could be important in maintaining cells in the progress zone in an undifferentiated state (Hill et al, 1989; Robert et al, 1991). Various grafting experiments show that, in chick limb buds, mesenchymal expression of *Msx-1* is regulated by a signal from the ridge, which can be substituted by FGF-4 (Davidson et al, 1991; Robert et al, 1991; Vogel et al, 1995a). The potential role of *Msx-1* in maintaining an undifferentiated cell state is suggested directly by experiments with a potentially myogenic cell line which, when transfected with the *Msx-1* gene, can no longer be induced to differentiate into muscle (Song et al, 1992). Functional inactivation of *Msx-1* in a transgenic mouse has no apparent effect on limb development (Satokata and Maas, 1994), but it is possible that expression of *Msx-2* compensates for it in the limb.

Transcripts of a *Wnt*-gene family member, *Wnt-5a*, are also found at high levels at the tip of the limb bud and could co-ordinate activity of cells at the tip of the limb. In other systems, expression of members of this family of short-range signalling molecules has been shown to be related to cell–cell communication via gap junctions (Olson et al, 1991). This is particularly interesting because distal mesenchyme cells have been shown to be linked by gap junctions (Kelley and Fallon, 1978) and there is evidence from functional blocking studies that gap junctional communication could be important in limb patterning (Allen et al, 1990). In addition, studies of the control of gap junction protein expression in limb bud mesenchyme show that the presence of gap junctions between cells is dependent on ridge signalling (Green et al, 1994).

Recently, expression of a tyrosine kinase receptor, *Cek-8*, has been demonstrated in the tip of the limb mesenchyme (Patel et al, 1996). Signals originating from the apical ridge are required for *Cek-8* early expression, and they can be mimicked by FGF-2 and FGF-4 application.

Molecular response to signalling (Figure 7.6)

Genes involved in this response include gene members of the *Hox-D* cluster. Genes in the part of the *Hox-D* cluster from *Hoxd-9* to *Hoxd-13* are expressed in overlapping domains in vertebrate limb buds, with transcripts of genes located more 5' in the cluster being found more posteriorly (Dollé et al, 1989, 1991; Izpisúa-Belmonte et al, 1991). Thus cells at the very posterior margin of the limb bud express *Hoxd-9* through to *Hoxd-13* whereas cells at the anterior express only *Hoxd-9*. When chick limb buds are manipulated by grafting a polarizing region, or cells constitutively expressing the *shh* gene, or by implanting a bead soaked in retinoic acid, *Hox-D* genes are activated in anterior cells and this results in mirror-image patterns of *Hox-D* gene expression that correlate with the mirror-image patterns of digits that develop (Izpisúa-Belmonte et al, 1991; Nohno et al, 1991; Riddle et al, 1993).

Activation of *Hox-D* genes in anterior cells requires cooperation with a signal from the apical ridge. This fits with the observation that respecification of pattern only takes place in the progress zone (Summerbell, 1974). With defined chemicals now available to provide a polarizing signal (retinoic acid) and a ridge signal (FGF), *Hox-D* genes can be activated in anterior cells in the absence of the ridge quite simply by applying two beads, one soaked in retinoic acid and one soaked in FGF (Niswander et al, 1994; Crossley et al, 1996).

The overlapping expression domains of *Hox-D* genes across the anteroposterior axis of the early bud (Figure 7.6b), and the mirror-image patterns that can be induced with polarizing region signals, suggest that products of these genes may help encode position. Since gene members of another Hox complex, the *Hox-A* cluster, are also expressed in overlapping domains but along the proximodistal axis, this raises the interesting possibility that combination of *Hox-D* and *Hox-A* gene products could specify each of the major elements of the skeleton (Yokouchi et al, 1991). This would map out major regions in the limb and then expression of other downstream genes within each limb region would encode position more finely, as for example *Gnot1* (Ranson et al, 1995).

The idea that Hox genes could encode position in the developing limb is supported by the results of mis-expressing a *Hox-D* gene in chick limb buds. When cells throughout the bud are infected with a retrovirus containing the *Hoxd-11* gene (normally restricted to middle and posterior parts of the bud), changes in anterior pattern are obtained (Morgan et al, 1992). In the leg, the anterior toe develops an additional phalange (giving it the same number of phalanges as a more posterior toe) and, in the wing, an additional digit is produced. However, in mice, in which the most posterior *Hox-D* gene, *Hoxd-13*, has been functionally inactivated, development of the limbs is retarded and phalanges can be missing from several different digits in a pattern unrelated to position, rather than absence of posterior structures as would be predicted (Dollé et al, 1993). These effects are more readily understood in terms of expression pattern of *Hoxd-13* in later limb buds in which, by the time that digits are actually forming, *Hoxd-13* is expressed throughout the tip of the limb bud. Given that it is now known that there is functional redundancy between corresponding Hox genes from different clusters, the lack of severe patterning defects when just one gene is inactivated is not surprising. In double knockouts, such as in the case of *Hoxa-11* and *Hoxd-11*, deletion of entire limb segments occurs (Davis et al, 1995).

Two related vertebrate genes, *Evx-1* and *Evx-2*, homologous to the *Drosophila* pair-rule gene, *even-skipped*, lie just 5' to the end of the *Hox-A* and *Hox-D* gene clusters respectively. Transcripts of *Evx-1* are expressed in mesenchyme at the very posterior tip of the limb bud. This pattern of expression is dependent on a ridge signal that can be supplied by FGF-4 (Niswander and Martin, 1993). It is not clear whether *Evx* gene products operate in concert with products of Hox genes or whether they fulfil an entirely different function, perhaps connected with the progress zone.

It has been recently shown that the transcription factor *Lmx-1* is activated by Wnt-7a signalling in the dorsal chick limb mesenchyme before the bud has emerged and *Hox-A* and *Hox-D* genes are expressed (Riddle et al, 1995: Vogel et al, 1995b). Expression of *Lmx-1* in the ventral mesenchyme leads to formation of ectopic dorsal structures. Thus, the combination of Hox genes and *Lmx-1* expression could specify the approximate three-dimensional pattern of the limb.

INITIATION OF LIMB BUD DEVELOPMENT

The development of two pairs of limbs at different axial levels is a central feature of the vertebrate body plan. There are a number of interesting questions about the plan, including what controls limb number, limb position and limb type (i.e. forelimb versus hindlimb). Recent work suggests that homeobox-containing genes and growth factors may be involved in controlling initiation of limb bud development.

Limb position could be related to the pattern of expression of homeobox-containing genes along the body axis. In vertebrates, genes of the four Hox clusters are expressed in a series of overlapping domains with generally all members of each cluster being expressed posteriorly at the 'tail' end and anterior limits of expression near the 'head' end being staggered, with more 3' genes being expressed more anteriorly. In mouse embryos, forelimb buds arise at the anterior limit of expression of *Hoxb-8*. Recently a transgenic mouse has been created in which the anterior limit of expression of *Hoxb-8* has been shifted by linking the coding region of the gene to the promoter from the *retinoic acid receptor-β* (*RAR-β*) gene, a gene that is expressed in anterior regions of the embryo. Most remarkably, this shift in *Hoxb-8* expression and enhanced expression of *Hoxb-8* at the anterior of the forelimb bud in the transgenic mouse leads to the development of duplicated forelimb patterns (Charité et al, 1994). The duplicated skeletal pattern is preceded in early limb buds by mirror-image expression patterns of *shh* and *Fgf-4*.

An FGF is likely to be the signal that induces formation of the limb bud. In two experimental systems, FGF can initiate limb bud formation. The first clue came from mouse chimeras containing cells that constitutively express FGF-4 (Abud et al, 1996). A striking feature of the chimeric embryos is the development of ectopic 'limb buds' in the flank (the region lying between fore- and hindlimb buds). In chick embryos, a single bead soaked in FGF placed in the presumptive flank can induce development of an ectopic bud that can then give rise to a complete extra limb (Cohn et al, 1995; Ohuchi et al, 1995; Crossley et al, 1996). The type of extra limb induced is related to bead position along the flank: beads placed anteriorly tend to give wings; more posterior beads, legs. An interesting feature of the additional limbs is that they have reversed polarity and this is correlated with a reversed pattern of *shh* expression in ectopic buds. It seems likely that the reversal of polarity is due to an anterior to posterior gradient in polarizing potential in cells of the flank (Hornbruch and Wolpert, 1991). This polarizing potential was assayed by grafting the flank to the anterior margin of chick wing buds and showing that additional digits could be specified. Flank cells will be recruited into an ectopic bud when FGF is applied and cells with highest polarizing potential will be at the anterior of the bud. Ectopic buds also acquire an apical ectodermal ridge and once both signalling regions are established, the bud can then autonomously develop into a limb (Cohn et al, 1995).

LIMB REGENERATION

In the mouse, significant regenerative ability has been observed in the digit tip of the fetus, and it appears to be restricted to levels in which the amputation plane is within the distal region expressing *Msx-1* (Reginelli et al, 1995). The neonate can also regenerate its digit tips, although not always perfectly, and such capability is restricted to the nail bed, where both *Msx-1* and *Msx-2* are expressed. The nail organ has indeed been shown to have inductive ability on bone regrowth (Zhao and Neufeld, 1995). Finally, it has been reported that young children can regenerate their last phalange including the nail (Illingworth and Barker, 1974), but it is only urodele (tailed) amphibians, such as newt and axolotl, that can regenerate functionally and morphologically perfect limbs in adulthood. The regenerating urodele limb represents therefore a valuable model for tackling the complex issue of what mechanisms underlie limb regeneration and why some animals are able to regenerate in adulthood and others not. Numerous cellular and molecular approaches have been developed over the last few years that are proving very useful for tackling molecular mechanisms underlying regeneration, such as availability of specific antibodies (Kintner and Brockes, 1984, 1985; Ferretti et al, 1989), establishment of long-term culture systems (Ferretti and Brockes, 1988), isolation of urodele genes (Casimir et al, 1988; Khrestchatisky et al, 1988; Ferretti et al, 1991, 1993; Onda et al, 1991; reviewed by Géraudie and Ferretti, 1997) and development of transfection techniques (Brockes, 1994).

Limb regeneration proceeds by formation of a **blastema**, a mound of undifferentiated mesenchymal cells (blastemal cells) that accumulate at the stump surface after amputation and start to proliferate after 4–5 days. Innervation and the presence of a specialized **wound epidermis** that lacks a distinct basement membrane are both essential for regeneration in the newt, and they appear to control blastemal growth in the regenerating limb (reviewed by Thornton, 1968; Wallace, 1981; Stocum, 1985). Once a critical mass of blastemal cells has accumulated, differentiation and morphogenesis begin, and in about 10 weeks all the structures distal to the plane of amputation are faithfully replaced. The original pattern, however, can be altered by administration of a class of putative morphogens, vitamin A and its derivatives, among which retinoic acid has been the most widely studied (see earlier). Retinoic acid induces duplication of limb segments in a dose-dependent manner and has been shown to affect all three axes of the regenerating limb under certain experimental conditions (Niazi and Saxena, 1978; Maden, 1982; Brockes, 1990; Stocum, 1991; Bryant and Gardiner, 1992).

DO DEVELOPING AND REGENERATING LIMBS USE THE SAME PATTERNING MECHANISMS?

There is substantial evidence, coming both from classical tissue manipulation and, more recently, from analysis of gene expression, which suggests that developing and regenerating limbs use the same patterning mechanisms. The specialized wound epidermis of the regenerating limb is believed to be homologous to the apical ectodermal ridge in developing limbs (reviewed by Stocum, 1985). Removal of the wound epidermis, like removal of the ectodermal ridge during development, has an inhibitory effect on further development of the regenerate. When formation of wound epidermis is impeded, for example by covering the wound with a skin flap, regeneration does not occur. Regeneration is also impaired in an axolotl mutant, *short-toes*, where, although blastemal cells accumulate following amputation, a thick and convoluted basement membrane forms that is likely to affect interactions between wound epidermis and underlying mesenchyme (Del Rio Tsonis et al, 1992). In the frog, which loses regenerative ability following metamorphosis, a wound epidermis forms after limb amputation in the tadpole, but not in the adult (see review by Thornton, 1968). These observations demonstrate the importance of epithelial–mesenchymal interactions during regeneration, and equivalent interactions in the mammal are probably impaired by the presence of the basement membrane, which rapidly forms after wounding mammalian skin. Interestingly, partial blastema formation has been induced in amputated toes of adult mice in which the presence of a wound epithelium was maintained by repeated surgical skin removal and treatment with sodium chloride (Neufeld, 1980). In addition, some cases of regeneration of fingertips in young children have been observed when the wound was not sutured after injury (Illingworth and Barker, 1974).

During limb development, the polarizing region plays a fundamental role in patterning. However, the regeneration blastema is in direct contact with the mature tissues of the stump, which have 'fixed' positional values. Therefore, re-establishment of a polarizing region in order to trigger the chain of events that will lead to correct patterning of the regenerate may not be necessary. Patterning could instead be determined by mesenchymal–mesenchymal interactions between the blastemal cells and the distal cells of the stump. In order to answer this question it will be important to establish whether signalling molecules normally expressed by the polarizing zone, such as *ssh*, are expressed in the regeneration blastema.

Analyses of gene expression carried out to date further strengthen the claim that many of the mechanisms used to pattern the limb during development and regeneration are the same. The developmentally regulated homeobox genes studied so far are re-expressed following limb amputation, although it has been shown that, at least in the case of the *Hox-A* genes, they are not re-expressed in a co-linear fashion (Brown and Brockes, 1991; Simon and Tabin, 1993; Beauchemin et al, 1994; Gardiner et al, 1995). Interestingly, expression of *Hoxa-6* and *Hoxc-10* is not switched off in the adult newt limb, unlike in vertebrates that cannot regenerate their limbs, suggesting a possible relationship between expression of these genes and maintenance of regenerative ability in adulthood (Savard et al, 1988; Simon and Tabin, 1993; Savard and Tremblay, 1995). In addition, the ability of retinoic acid to affect patterning of regenerating limbs, together with the demonstration that different retinoic acid receptors are expressed in the regenerate and mediate different functions (Pecorino et al, 1994, 1996), supports the view that endogenous retinoids may play a role in limb regeneration, and possibly control the expression of the same set of genes as in the limb bud. It has been recently shown that *Hoxa-13* is down-regulated by retinoic acid treatment (Gardiner et al, 1995). Finally, the presence of FGF and at least three FGF receptor variants in the limb regeneration blastema (Boilly et al, 1991; Poulin et al, 1993; Poulin and Chiu, 1995) further supports the view that the same key molecules are used to build both embryonic and adult limbs. The fact that some regeneration of the embryonic chick limb can be induced by FGF-2 and FGF-4 (Taylor et al, 1994; Kostakopoulou et al, 1996), which can substitute for the apical ectodermal ridge in developing chick limbs (Niswander et al, 1993; Fallon et al, 1994), indicates that the regenerative potential in vertebrates is higher than previously thought, and that, at least in the embryo, it can be stimulated when the right factor (or factors) is provided. Therefore, it will be of fundamental importance to achieve a full understanding of the basic mechanisms underlying limb development and regeneration, if we are to devise strategies aimed at increasing regenerative potential in higher vertebrates, including humans.

DIFFERENCES BETWEEN DEVELOPING AND REGENERATING LIMBS

There are clear differences between development and regeneration concerning the origin of the cells and the control of their division, in particular regarding the role of nerves. While the developing limb bud starts to grow in the absence of innervation, the initial growth of the blastema requires an adequate level of nervous supply (Singer, 1974; Sicard, 1985; Fekete and Brockes, 1987). If the limb is denervated and amputated, blastemal cells can accumulate, but do not proliferate. However, if the limb is denervated after a blastema has formed, regeneration will progress, but the regenerated limb will be smaller in size. Therefore, regeneration depends on the presence of the nerve only during the phase of rapid proliferation of blastemal cells. The factor (or factors) secreted by the nerve (Singer, 1974; Brockes and Kintner, 1986), which either directly or indirectly (Ferretti and Brockes, 1991) controls blastemal cell proliferation, has not yet been identified. Interestingly, some degree of limb regeneration has been induced in young opossums by transplantation of nervous tissue (Mizell and Isaacs, 1970), indicating that the nervous system can also play an important role in limb regeneration in higher vertebrates. It is therefore extremely important to identify the mechanisms underlying the nervous control of limb regeneration.

The other fundamental difference between development and regeneration is the origin of limb progenitor cells in the embryo and in the adult. As discussed earlier, the limb bud originates from the lateral plate mesoderm, whereas the limb blastema originates from the distal tip of the stump. The issue of whether these limb progenitor cells are 'equivalent' and share the same phenotype was neatly addressed when monoclonal antibody technique became available and antibodies against blastemal antigen and markers of the differentiated state were developed. Such antibodies (reviewed by Ferretti and Brockes, 1991; Géraudie and Ferretti, 1996) have allowed the identification of a number of regeneration-associated molecules, analysis of their cellular distribution in developing and regenerating limbs, and isolation of the genes encoding them by screening blastema expression libraries. Two main findings have emerged from these studies. First, a difference in the phenotype of limb progenitor cells in embryos and adult has been revealed, since molecular markers such as 22/18 (Kintner and Brockes, 1985) and the simple epithelial keratins 8 and 18, all of which have been shown to be expressed in the mesenchyme of regenerating limbs, are not detectable during limb development. Secondly, it has become apparent that blastemal cells do not comprise a homogeneous population, as previously believed on the basis of their morphological appearance, but are heterogeneous.

Although many of the events underlying limb regeneration have started to be unravelled, the important issue of how formation of blastemal cells occurs is still unknown. Blastemal cells are believed to originate from the mature tissues of the stump through a process of dedifferentiation. It is generally agreed that, while neither epidermis nor subepidermal glands contribute cells to the blastema, there is a contribution from mesodermal tissues of the stump and from Schwann cells (Maden, 1977). In contrast, the issue of how muscle contributes cells to the blastema has been a matter for debate for many years. Some recent elegant experiments have shown that, when cultured myotubes are injected with a tracing dye and implanted in the blastema in vivo, labelled mononucleate cells can be found in the blastema (Lo et al, 1993), confirming previous work which suggested that muscle fibres contribute to blastema formation through a process of dedifferentiation (Hay, 1959). However, cells equivalent to mammalian satellite cells are present in the newt muscle (post-satellite cells), and these cells proliferate and differentiate into myotubes in vitro (Cameron et al, 1986). It may be that it is these cells which contribute to the blastema, rather than cells produced by dedifferentiation of muscle fibres. Probably both events occur in the regenerating limb: cells produced through muscle dedifferentiation may contribute to the blastema, whereas post-satellite cells may be involved in muscle repair in the stump.

As outlined here, the possibility of inducing at least partial regeneration of limb structures in humans is still in its infancy, and the most formidable challenge ahead of us is to understand how the blastemal cells originate, and in particular how the transition from the differentiated to the undifferentiated state is regulated following amputation.

HOW, WHEN AND WHERE EXPERIMENTAL STUDIES ELUCIDATE ABNORMAL DEVELOPMENT

The cellular and molecular basis of limb development appears to be conserved between vertebrates. For example, the polarizing region from embryonic limb

Table 7.3   Gene defects associated with limb malformations

Gene	Species	Limb phenotype	Reference
Hoxa-11 (over-expression)	Mouse	Skeletal malformations in both forelimbs and hindlimbs, syndactyly, malformed ulna and radius, and tibia and fibula	Small and Potter (1993)
Hoxa-13 (mutation)	Mouse	Hypodactyly (single digit on each limb)	Mortlock et al (1996)
Hoxb-8 (over-expression)	Mouse	Mirror-image duplications in the forelimb	Charité et al (1994)
Hoxc-8 (knockout)	Mouse	Clenched fingers	Le Mouellic et al (1992)
Hoxd-11 (knockout)	Mouse	Short digits, synostosis, malformed ulnar and radial epiphysis	Davis and Capecchi (1994)
Hoxd-13 (knockout)	Mouse	Meromelia, synostosis, synpolydactyly	Dollé et al (1993)
HOXD13 (mutation)	Human	Meromelia, synostosis, synpolydactyly	Muragaki et al (1996)
Hoxa-11/Hoxd-11 (double knockout)	Mouse	Absent radius and ulna, malformed tibia and fibula	Davis et al (1995)
Msx-1 (knockout)	Mouse	No limb defects	Satokata and Maas (1994)
MSX2 (mutation in homeodomain)	Human	Shortened metatarsals triphalangeal thumb	Jabs et al (1993)
En-1 (knockout)	Mouse	Double-dorsal paws	Loomis et al (1996)
Bmp-5 (mutation)	Mouse	No limb defects	Kingsley et al (1992)
Bmp-7 (knockout)	Mouse	Pre-axial polydactyly	Luo et al (1995) Dudley et al (1995)
Gdf-5 (mutation)	Mouse	Brachypodism	Storm et al (1994)
Wnt-7a (knockout)	Mouse	Double-ventral paws	Parr and McMahon (1995)
RAR-$\alpha\gamma$ (double knockout)	Mouse	Various pre-axial malformations in forelimbs; reduction in length and increased diameter of the fibula and other minor defects in ossification in the hindlimb	Lohnes et al (1994)
ld (mutation)	Mouse	Fused forelimb bones, syndactyly in paws and feet	Maas et al (1990, 1991), Woychik et al (1990)

Table 7.3 *Continued*

Gene	Species	Limb phenotype	Reference
Gli-3/GLI3 (mutation)	Mouse Human	Polysyndactyly	Vortkamp et al (1991) Hui and Joyner (1993)
FGFR1 (mutation)	Human	Broad toes and thumbs, syndactyly or brachydactyly in other digits (Pfeifer syndrome)	Wilkie et al (1995)
FGFR2 (mutation)	Human	Broad toes and thumbs, syndactyly or brachydactyly in other digits (Pfeifer syndrome, Apert syndrome)	Rutland et al (1995)
FGFR3 (missense mutation)	Human	Short-limb dwarfism (achondroplasia)	Rousseau et al (1994)
Col2A1 (single-point mutation)	Human	Spondyloepiphyseal dysplasia	Williams et al (1993)

Although only limb defects are described here, other malformations may be associated with these mutations.

buds of a wide range of vertebrates, **including humans,** can lead to additional digit formation in chick wing buds (Fallon and Crosby, 1977). This suggests that the signalling mechanism has been evolutionarily conserved (see Chapter 1) and this conclusion has to some extent been confirmed at the molecular level. For instance, *shh* transcripts have been detected in mouse, chick and fish limb buds (Echelard et al, 1993; Krauss et al, 1993; Riddle et al, 1993) and two human *hedgehog* homologues have been identified (Chang et al, 1994). These and other data suggest that principles of limb patterning that emerge from experimental analysis of chick and mouse embryos can probably be directly applied to consideration of abnormal development and congenital limb abnormalities in humans. In addition, there has been progress in identifying the genetic basis of limb defects in both mice and humans (Table 7.3).

LIMB DEFICIENCIES

Amelia and meromelia

Experimental analysis shows that the apical ectodermal ridge is central to bud outgrowth and this has important implications for interpreting how amelia and terminal meromelic limbs (limbs that lack distal structures) could arise. If the apical ridge does not form at all, limbs will be completely absent and amelia will result. Absence of limbs could result from lack of appropriate initiation signals or failure in response to these signals. Failure of limb bud outgrowth leading to truncated limbs could result from defective signalling: for example, absence of the apical ectodermal ridge and/or FGF production. Changes in apical ridge signalling could either have a genetic basis or be due to damage to the ridge. Another possibility is that there could be a failure in response to ridge signals and, as a consequence, correct patterns of Hox gene expression are not established. In this respect it is interesting that the gene which is affected in the *Hypodactyly* mutant mouse, which has only a single digit on each paw, is *Hoxa-13* (Mortlock et al, 1996).

In some cases of limb meromelia (intercalary or transverse), it is proximal rather than distal structures that are absent. A model for this class of defect is provided by X-irradiation of chick limb buds (Wolpert et al, 1979). As the dose of X-irradiation is increased, proximal limb structures are deleted whereas distal structures develop relatively normally. This result can be understood by reference to the progress zone model. X-irradiation kills cells in the progress zone and the number of cells at the tip of the limb will be reduced. Surviving cells will proliferate to fill the progress zone and, as they do so, they will spend a longer time at the tip and hence give rise to distal rather than proximal structures. Therefore, these ideas suggest that death or killing of mesenchyme cells could be a mechanism that leads to proximal defects. Destruction of mesenchyme cells could be caused directly by cytotoxic drugs or indirectly by interference with the vascular supply. This second mechanism has been suggested for the mechanism of action of thalidomide (Poswillo, 1975). Roberts syndrome, a genetically inherited (autosomal recessive) limb defect is phocomelia-like.

Polydactyly

Experimental analysis shows that the polarizing region is central to anterioposterior patterning. Therefore, defects in anterioposterior patterning could be due either to changes in distribution and/or strength of the polarizing signal or to changes in cellular response to the signal. It may be that both signalling and response could be abnormal. In polydactylous limbs, one might predict that the polarizing signal would be more widespread and produced anteriorly. This could account for extra digits pre-axially or mirror hands/feet but does not explain additional post-axial digits.

In *talpid 3* (polydactylous) chicken mutants, an increased number of morphologically similar digits develop. The limb buds are abnormally broad, and the apical ectodermal ridge is correspondingly extended (Hinchliffe and Ede, 1967). As normal, *shh* expression is restricted to the posterior margin of the broadened buds (Francis-West et al, 1995), but there is a uniform expression pattern of *Hox-D* genes across the tip of early buds instead of the normal progressively posterior restriction of expression (Coelho et al, 1992; Izpisúa-Belmonte et al, 1992b). Both *Bmp* genes and *Fgf-4* are also uniformly expressed, suggesting that there is a change in response to the polarizing signal (Francis-West et al, 1995).

The mouse mutant *Extra toes* (*Xt*), is characterized by pre-axial digit duplications in the hindlimbs, and the gene affected has been identified as *Gli-3*, which encodes a zinc-finger transcription factor (Hui and Joyner, 1993; and see

Chapter 2). In this mouse mutant, ectopic expression of both *shh* and *Fgf-4* has been detected in the anterior region of the limb bud (Masuya et al, 1995). It has now been shown that the homologous human syndrome, Greig cephalopolysyndactyly (Figure 7.2a) is also due to mutations in *GLI-3* (Hui and Joyner, 1993). The basis of another human polydactyly has been recently identified: synpolydactyly is caused by mutations in *HOXD13* (Muragaki et al, 1996).

Synostosis

Synostosis refers to the fusion between successive or adjacent skeletal elements. This could result from defects of patterning or be due to abnormalities in later events such as growth and shaping. Fusion between successive elements and lack of elbow/knee joints have been reported in chick and mice embryos following retinoic acid treatment at a time when chondrogenesis has begun (e.g. Kochhar, 1977). In the mouse mutant *limb deformity* (*ld*, see earlier), there is fusion between adjacent skeletal elements, for example between radius and ulna. The early buds in the mutant are narrower than normal and the apical ridge is patchy (Zeller et al, 1989). It is not clear whether the defect is primarily affecting the epithelial or the mesenchymal component because *ld* is normally expressed in both tissues. In this mouse mutant, *shh* expression is down-regulated posteriorly and *Fgf-4* transcripts cannot be detected in the apical ridge of the limb bud (Chan et al, 1995; Haramis and Brown, 1995)

Syndactyly

Syndactylies are normally thought to be due to failure of programmed cell death. In chick embryos, treatment with Janus Green impairs mitochondrial function and leads to absence of interdigital cell death. Soft-tissue webbing between the digits results. Interdigital cell death can also be inhibited by locally removing the apical ridge between presumptive digits. This leads not only to persistence of interdigital mesenchyme but also to cartilage differentiation giving digit-like structures (Hurle and Ganan, 1986). There is currently considerable interest in the mechanisms and the genetic basis of programmed cell death or apoptosis. From work in the nematode worm *Caenorhabditis elegans*, genes that control programmed death have been identified and mammalian homologues have also been found (Yuan et al, 1993); the significance of such genes for programmed cell death during limb development remains to be explored.

Skeletal dysplasias

There are a large number of abnormalities in which either the size or shape of parts of the limb are abnormal. It is now emerging that closely related members of the TGF-β family, including BMPs and growth/differentiation factors, play central roles in controlling skeletal form (reviewed by Erlebacher et al, 1995). Mutations in these genes are now known to underly some skeletal dysplasias. The *brachypodism* mouse mutation affects the *Gdf-5* gene, encoding a growth factor known as growth/differentiation factor-5. Transcripts of this gene are associated with developing skeletal elements in the limbs and the mutant phenotype is characterized by the limb skeleton being very reduced in length and the toes lacking the most distal elements (Storm et al, 1994). Mutations in the gene encoding another growth factor in the superfamily, BMP-5, lead to the *short ear* phenotype in which, in addition to external changes in size and shape of the ears, defects in sternum, ribs and vertebral processes are found (Kingsley et al, 1992). However, the limb skeleton in *short ear* is normal, raising the intriguing possibility that different but related growth factors are involved in modelling different parts of the skeleton.

Another family of growth factors has also been implicated in skeletal growth. **Achondroplasia**, in which the skeletal elements are very reduced in length, is now known to be due to a mutation in a gene encoding a receptor for FGFs (Rousseau et al, 1994; Shiang et al, 1994). It now appears that FGFs, as well as BMPs, are factors operating not only at the earliest stages in limb development (see earlier) but also in the control of skeletal form and growth at later stages too. In fact, mutations in FGFRs are now known to be the cause of a number of human syndromes involving limb abnormalities (Rutland et al, 1995; Wilkie et al, 1995).

AGENDA FOR THE FUTURE

Three main areas look set for an increase in understanding. One area is the further elucidation of signalling pathways that set up tissue patterns in the early limb bud. Most, if not all, of the steps that have so far been identified are probably indirect and it will be some time before the full details of the signalling pathways will be elucidated. A second area in which new insights are to be expected is the control of development of limbs in the context of the vertebrate body plan, and such knowledge will have important evolutionary implications. Finally, there will be the continuing elucidation of the genetic basis of human limb abnormalities. Here human clinical and molecular genetics will combine with experimental embryology in a potentially powerful and productive way.

Our progress in analysing the early pathways establishing tissue pattern has been rapid. However, there is a large conceptual gap between, say, the pattern of expression of a homeobox gene per se and the development of a recognizable skeletal element with its characteristic shape and growth, and so on. The morphogenesis of an individual element is a complex problem that is based on spatial control of cell behaviour. It will be a considerable challenge to understand how gene expression is translated into form.

REFERENCES

Abud, H.E., Skinner, J.A., McDonald, F.J. et al (1996) Ectopic expression of FGF-4 in chimaeric mouse embryos induces the expression of early markers of limb development in the lateral ridge. *Dev. Genet.* **19**, 51–65.

Akita, K. (1996) The effect of the ectoderm on the dorsoventral pattern of epidermis, muscles and joints in the developing chick leg: a new model. *Anat. Embryol.* **193**, 377–386.

Allen, F., Tickle, C. and Warner, A. (1990) The role of gap junctions in patterning of the chick limb bud. *Development* **108**, 623–634.

Basler, K. and Struhl, G. (1994) Compartment boundaries and the control of *Drosophila* limb pattern by hedgehog protein. *Nature* **368**, 208–214.

Beauchemin, M., Noiseux, N., Tremblay, M. and Savard, P. (1994) Expression of Hox A11 in the limb and the regeneration blastema of adult newt. *Int. J. Dev. Biol.* **38**, 641–649.

Boilly, B., Cavanaugh, K.P., Thomas, D. et al (1991) Acidic fibroblast growth factor is present in regenerating limb blastemas of axolotls and binds specifically to blastema tissues. *Dev. Biol.* **145**, 302–310.

Brockes, J.P. (1990) Retinoic acid and limb regeneration. *J. Cell Sci.* **13** (Suppl.), 191–198.

Brockes, J.P. (1994) New approaches to limb regeneration. *Trends Genet.* **10**, 169–173.

Brockes, J.P. and Kintner, C.R. (1986) Glial growth factor and nerve dependent proliferation in the regeneration blastema of urodele amphibians. *Cell* **45**, 301–306.

Brown, R. and Brockes, J.P. (1991) Identification and expression of a regeneration-specific homeobox gene in the newt limb blastema. *Development* **111**, 489–496.

Bryant, S.V. and Gardiner, D.M. (1992) Retinoic acid, local cell–cell interactions, and pattern formation in vertebrate limbs. *Dev. Biol.* **152**, 1–25.

Bulfone, A., Kim, H.J., Puelles, L. et al (1993) The mouse *Dlx-2 (Tes-1)* gene is expressed in spatially restricted domains of the forebrain, face and limbs in midgestation mouse embryos. *Mech. Dev.* **40**, 129–140.

Cameron, J.A., Hilgers, A.R. and Hinterberger, T.J. (1986) Evidence that reserve cells are a source of regenerated adult newt muscle *in vitro*. *Nature* **321**, 607–610.

Casimir, C.M., Gates, P.B., Ross-Macdonald, P.B. et al (1988) Structure and expression of a newt cardio-skeletal myosin gene: implications for the C value paradox. *J. Mol. Biol.* **202**, 287–296.

Chan, D.C., Wynshaw-Boris, A. and Leder, P. (1995) Formin isoforms are differentially expressed in the mouse embryo and are required for normal expression of *fgf-4* and *shh* in the limb bud. *Development* **121**, 3151–3162.

Chang, D.T., Lopéz, A., von Kessler, D.P. et al (1994) Products, genetic linkage and limb patterning activity of a murine *hedgehog* gene. *Development* **120**, 3339–3353.

Charité, J., de Graaff, W. and Deschamps, J. (1994) Ectopic expression of *Hoxb-8* causes duplication of the ZPA in the forelimb and homeotic transformation of axial structures. *Cell* **78**, 589–601.

Coelho, C.N., Upholt, W.B. and Kosher, R.A. (1992) Role of the chicken homeobox-containing genes Ghox-4.6 and Ghox-8 in the specification of positional identities during the development of normal and polydactylous chick limb buds. *Devl. Biol.* **115**, 629–637.

Cohn, M.J. and Tickle, C. (1996) Limbs: a model for pattern formation within the vertebrate body plan. *Trends Genet.* **12**, 253–257.

Cohn, M.J., Izpisúa-Belmonte, J.C., Abud, H., Heath, J. and Tickle, C. (1995) Fibroblast growth factors induce additional limb development from the flank of chick embryos. *Cell* **80**, 739–746.

Crossley, P.H. and Martin, G.M. (1995) The mouse *Fgf-8* gene encodes a family of polypeptides and is expressed in regions that direct outgrowth and patterning in the developing embryo. *Development* **121**, 439–451.

Crossley, P.H., Minowada, G., Macarthur, C.A. and Martin, G.R. (1996) Roles for FGF8 in the induction, initiation, and maintenance of chick limb development. *Cell* **84**, 127–136.

Davidson, D.R., Crawley, A., Hill, R.E. and Tickle, C. (1991) Position-dependent expression of two related homeobox genes in developing vertebrate limbs. *Nature* **352**, 429–431.

Davis, A.P. and Capecchi, M.R. (1994) Axial homeosis and appendicular skeleton defects in mice with a targeted disruption of *hoxd-11*. *Development* **120**, 2187–2198.

Davis, A.P., Witte, D.P., Hsieh-Li, H.M., Potter, S.S. and Capeccchi, M. (1995) Absence of radius and ulna in mice lacking *hoxa-11* and *hoxd-11*. *Nature* **375**, 791–795.

Dealy, C.N., Roth, A., Ferrari, D., Brown, A.M.C. and Kosher, R.A. (1993) *Wnt-5a* and *Wnt-7a* are expressed in the developing chick limb bud in a manner suggesting roles in pattern formation along the proximodistal and dorsoventral axes. *Mech. Dev.* **43**, 175–186.

Del Rio Tsonis, K., Washabaugh, C.H. and Tsonis, P.A. (1992) The mutant axolotl Short toes exhibits impaired limb regeneration and abnormal basement membrane formation. *Proc. Natl. Acad. Sci. USA* **89**, 5502–5506.

Dollé, P., Izpisúa-Belmonte, J.C., Falkenstein, H., Renucci, A. and Duboule, D. (1989) Coordinate expression of the murine *HOX-5* complex homeobox-containing genes during limb pattern formation. *Nature* **342**, 767–772.

Dollé, P., Izpisúa-Belmonte, J.C., Boncinelli, E. and Duboule, D. (1991) The *Hox-4.8* gene is localized at the 5' extremity of the *Hox-4* complex and is expressed in the most posterior parts of the body during development. *Mech. Dev.* **36**, 3–13.

Dollé, P., Price, M. and Duboule, D. (1992) Expression of the murine *Dlx-1* homeobox gene during facial, ocular and limb development. *Differentiation* **49**, 93–99.

Dollé, P., Dierich, A., LeMeur, M. et al (1993) Disruption of the *Hoxd-13* gene induces localized heterochrony leading to mice with neotenic limbs. *Cell* **75**, 431–441.

Dono, R. and Zeller, R. (1994) Cell-type specific nuclear translocation of fibroblast growth factor-2 isoforms during chicken kidney and limb morphogenesis. *Dev. Biol.* **163**, 316–330.

Dudley, A.T., Lyons, K.M. and Robertson, E.J. (1995) A requirement for bone morphogenetic protein-7 during development of the mammalian kidney and eye. *Gene Dev.* **9**, 2795–2807.

Duprez, D.M., Kostakopoulou, K., Francis-West, P.H., Tickle, C. and Brickell, P.M. (1996) Activation of *Fgf-4* and *HoxD* gene expression by BMP-2 expressing cells in the developing chick limb. *Development* **122**, 1821–1828.

Echelard, Y., Epstein, D., St-Jacques, B. et al (1993) Sonic hedgehog, a member of a family of putative signaling molecules, is implicated in the regulation of CNS polarity. *Cell* **75**, 1417–1430.

Erlebacher, A., Filvaroff, E.H., Gitelman, S.E. and Derynck, R. (1995) Toward a molecular understanding of skeletal development. *Cell* **80**, 371–378.

Fallon, J.F. and Crosby, G.M. (1977) Polarizing zone activity in limb buds of amniotes. In *Vertebrate Limb and Somite Morphogenesis* (Eds: D.A. Ede, J.R. Hinchliffe and M. Balls), pp. 55–69. Cambridge University Press: Cambridge.

Fallon, J.F., López, A., Ros, M.A. et al (1994) FGF-2: apical ectodermal ridge growth signal for chick limb development. *Science* **264**, 104–107.

Fekete, D.M. and Brockes, J.P. (1987) A monoclonal antibody detects a difference in the cellular composition of developing and regenerating limbs of newts. *Development* **99**, 589–602.

Ferretti, P. and Brockes, J.P. (1988) Culture of newt cells from different tissues and their expression of a regeneration-associated antigen. *J. Exp. Zool.* **247**, 77–91.

Ferretti, P. and Brockes, J.P. (1991) Cell origin and identity in limb regeneration and development. *Glia* **4**, 214–24.

Ferretti, P., Fekete, D.M., Patterson, M. and Lane, E.B. (1989) Transient expression of simple epithelial keratins by mesenchymal cells of regenerating newt limb. *Dev. Biol.* **133**, 415–424.

Ferretti, P., Brockes, J.P. and Brown, R. (1991) A newt type II keratin restricted to normal and regenerating limbs and tails is responsive to retinoic acid. *Development* **111**, 497–507.

Ferretti, P., Corcoran, J.P. and Ghosh, S. (1993) Expression and regulation of keratins in the wound epithelium and mesenchyme of the regenerating newt limb. *Prog. Clin. Biol. Res.* **383A**, 261–269.

Francis, P., Richardson, M., Brickell, P. and Tickle, C. (1994) Bone morphogenetic proteins and a signalling pathway that controls patterning in the developing chick limb. *Development* **120**, 209–218.

Francis-West, P.H., Robertson, K.E., Ede, D.A. et al (1995) Expression of genes encoding bone morphogenetic proteins and sonic hedgehog in talpid (ta(3)) limb buds: their relationships in the signaling cascade involved in limb patterning. *Dev. Dyn.* **203**, 187–197.

Gardiner, D.M., Blumberg, B., Komine, Y. and Bryant, S.V. (1995) Regulation of *HoxA* expression in developing and regenerating axolotl limbs. *Development* **121**, 1731–1741.

Géraudie, J. and Ferretti, P. (1997) Gene expression during amphibian limb regeneration. *Int. Rev. Cytol.* (in press).

Goodrich, L.V., Johnson, R.L., Milenkovic, L., McMahon, J.A. and Scott, M.P. (1996) Conservation of the *hedgehog/patched* signaling pathway from flies to mice: induction of a mouse *patched* gene by Hedgehog. *Genes Dev.* **10**, 301–312.

Green, C.R., Bowles, L., Crawley, A. and Tickle, C. (1994) Expression of the connexin 43 gap junctional protein in tissues at the tip of the chick limb bud is related to the epithelial–mesenchymal interactions that mediate morphogenesis. *Dev. Biol.* **161**, 12–21.

Hahn, H., Christiansen, J., Wicking, C. et al (1996a) A mammalian patched homolog is expressed in target tissues of sonic hedgehog and maps to a region associated with developmental abnormalities. *J. Biol. Chem.* **271**, 12125–12128.

Hahn, H., Wicking, C., Zaphiropoulos, P.G. et al (1996b) Mutations of the human homolog of Drosophila *patched* in the nevoid basal cell carcinoma syndrome. *Cell* **85**, 841–851.

Haramis, A.G. and Brown, Z.R. (1995) The *limb deformity* gene mutation disrupts the SHH/FGF-4 feedback loop and regulation of 5' *HoxD* genes during limb pattern formation. *Development* **121**, 4237–4245.

Hay, E.D. (1959) Electron microscopic observations of muscle dedifferentiation in regenerating Amblystoma limbs. *Dev. Biol.* **1**, 555–585.

Heikinheimo, K., Lawshe, A., Shackleford, G.M., Wilson, D.B. and McArthur, C.A. (1994) *Fgf-8* expression in the post-gastrulation mouse suggests roles in the development of the face, limbs and the central nervous system. *Mech. Dev.* **48**, 129–138.

Hill, R.E., Jones, P.F., Rees, A.R. et al (1989) A new family of mouse homeobox containing genes: molecular structure, chromosomal location and developmental expression of *Hox-7.1*. *Genes Dev.* **3**, 26–37.

Hinchliffe, J.R. and Ede, D.A. (1967) Limb development in the polydactylous talpid 3 mutant of the fowl. *J. Embryol. Exp. Morphol.* **17**, 385–404.

Hofmann, C. and Eichele, G. (1994) Retinoids in development. In *The Retinoids, Biology, Chemistry and Medicine* (Eds: M.B. Sporn, A.B. Roberts and D.S. Goodman), pp. 387–441. Raven Press: New York.

Honig, L. (1981) Positional signal transmission in the developing chick limb. *Nature* **291**, 72–73.

Hornbruch, A. and Wolpert, L. (1991) The spatial and temporal distribution of polarizing activity in the flank of the pre-limb-bud stages in the chick embryo. *Development* **111**, 725–731.

Hui, C.-C. and Joyner, A.L. (1993) A mouse model of Greig cephalopolysyndactyly syndrome: the *extra-toes* mutation contains an intragenic deletion of the *Gli3* gene. *Nature Genetics* **3**, 241–246.

Hurle, J.M. and Ganan, Y. (1986) Interdigital tissue chondrogenesis induced by surgical removal of the apical ectodermal ridge of the chick embryo leg bud in the stages previous to the onset of interdigital cell death. *Anat. Embryol.* **176**, 393–399.

Illingworth, C.M. and Barker, A.T. (1974) Trapped fingers and amputated finger tips in children. *J. Pediatr. Surg.* **9**, 853–858.

Izpisúa-Belmonte, J.C., Tickle, C., Dollé, P., Wolpert, L. and Duboule, D. (1991) Expression of the homeobox *Hox-4* genes and the specification of pattern in chick wing development. *Nature* **350**, 585–589.

Izpisúa-Belmonte, J.C., Brown, J.M., Duboule, D. and Tickle, C. (1992a) Expression of *hox-4* genes in the chick wing links pattern-formation to the epithelial mesenchymal interactions that mediate growth. *EMBO J.* **11**, 1451–1457.

Izpisúa-Belmonte, J.C., Ede, D.A., Tickle, C. and Duboule, D. (1992b) Misexpression of posterior *Hox-4* genes in *talpid* (ta³) mutant wings correlates with the absence of antero-posterior polarity. *Development* **114**, 959–963.

Jabs, E.W., Müller, U., Li, X. et al (1993) A mutation in the homeodomain of the human MSX2 gene in a family affected with autosomal dominant craniosynostosis. *Cell* **75**, 443–450.

Johnson, R.L., Rothman, A.L., Xie, J.W. et al (1996) Human homolog of *patched*, a candidate gene for the basal cell nevus syndrome. *Science* **272**, 1668–1671.

Kastner, P., Mark, M. and Chambon, P. (1995) Nonsteroid nuclear receptors: what are genetic studies telling us? *Cell* **83**, 859–869.

Kelley, R.O. and Fallon, J.F. (1978) Identification and distribution of gap junctions in the mesoderm of the developing chick limb bud. *J. Embryol. Exp. Morph.* **46**, 99–110.

Khrestchatisky, M., Djabali, M., Thouveny, Y. and Fontes, M. (1988) Expression of muscle actin genes in early differentiation stages of tail regeneration of the urodele amphibian *Pleurodeles waltlii*. *Cell Differ. Dev.* **25**, 203–212.

Kingsley, D.M., Bland, A.E., Grubber, J.M. et al (1992) The mouse short ear skeletal morphogenesis locus is associated with defects in a bone morphogenetic member of the TGF beta superfamily. *Cell* **71**, 399–410.

Kintner, C.R. and Brockes, J.P. (1984) Monoclonal antibodies identify blastemal cells derived from dedifferentiating muscle in newt limb regeneration. *Nature* **308**, 67–69.

Kintner, C.R. and Brockes, J.P. (1985) Monoclonal antibodies to the cells of a regenerating limb. *J. Embryol. Exp. Morphol.* **89**, 37–51.

Kochhar, D.M. (1977) Cellular basis of congenital limb deformity induced in mice by vitamin A. In *Morphogenesis and Malformation of the Limb* (Eds: D. Bergsma and W. Lenz). Birth Defects Original Article Series, vol. 13, pp. 111–154. Liss: New York.

Kostakopoulou, K., Vogel, A., Brickell, P. and Tickle, C. (1996) 'Regeneration' of wing bud stumps of chick embryos and reactivation of *Msx-1* and *Shh* expression in response to FGF-4 and ridge signals. *Mech. Dev.* **55**, 119–131.

Krauss, S., Concordet, J.P. and Ingham, P.W. (1993) A functionally conserved homolog of the Drosophila segment polarity gene *hh* is expressed in tissues with polarizing activity in zebrafish embryos. *Cell* **75**, 1431–1444.

Laufer, E., Nelson, C.E., Johnson, R.L., Morgan, B.A. and Tabin, C. (1994) Sonic hedgehog and FGF-4 act through a signaling cascade and feedback loop to integrate growth and patterning of the developing limb bud. *Cell* **79**, 993–1003.

Le Mouellic, H., Lallemand, Y. and Brûlet, P. (1992) Homeosis in the mouse induced by a null mutation in the *Hox 3.1* gene. *Cell* **69**, 251–264.

Lee, J. and Tickle, C. (1985) Retinoic acid and pattern formation in the developing chick wing: SEM and quantitative studies on the early effects on the apical ectodermal ridge and bud outgrowth. *J. Embryol. Exp. Morph.* **90**, 139–169.

Lo, D.C., Allen, F. and Brockes, J.P. (1993) Reversal of muscle differentiation during urodele limb regeneration. *Proc. Nat. Acad. Sci. USA* **90**, 7230–7234.

Lohnes, D., Mark, M., Mendelsohn, C. et al (1994) Function of the retinoic acid receptors (RARs) during development: craniofacial and skeletal abnormalities in RAR double mutants. *Development* **120**, 2723–2748.

Loomis, C.A., Harris, E., Michaud, J. et al (1996) The mouse *engrailed-1* gene and ventral limb patterning. *Nature* **382**, 360–363.

Lopez-Martinez, A., Chang, D.T., Chiang, C. et al (1995) Limb patterning activity and restricted posterior localization of the amino-terminal product of *sonic hedgehog* cleavage. *Curr. Biol.* **5**, 791–796.

Luo, G., Hofmann, C., Bronckers, A.L.J.J. et al (1995) BMP-7 is an inducer of nephro-genesis, and is also required for eye development and skeletal patterning. *Genes Dev.* **9**, 2808–2821.

Maas, R.L., Zeller, R., Woychik, R.P., Vogt, T.F. and Leder, P. (1990) Disruption of formin-encoding transcripts in two mutant limb deformity alleles. *Nature* **346**, 853–855.

Maas, R.L., Jepeal, L.I., Elfering, S.L. et al (1991) A human gene homologous to the formin gene residing at the murine limb deformity locus: chromosomal location and RFLPs. *Am. J. Hum. Genet.* **48**, 687–695.

MacCabe, J.A., Errick, J. and Saunders, J.W. (1974) Ectodermal control of the dorsoventral axis in the leg bud of the chick embryo. *Dev. Biol.* **39**, 69–82.

Maden, M. (1977) The role of Schwann cells in paradoxical regeneration in the axolotl. *J. Embryol. Exp. Morph.* **41**, 1–13.

Maden, M. (1982) Vitamin A and pattern formation in the regenerating limb. *Nature* **295**, 672–675.

Mangelsdorf, D.J., Umesono, K. and Evans, R.M. (1994) The retinoid receptors. In *The Retinoids, Biology, Chemistry and Medicine* (Eds: M.B. Sporn, A.B. Roberts and D.S. Goodman), pp. 319–349. Raven Press: New York.

Marigo, V., Scott, M.P., Johnson, R.L., Goodrich, L.V. and Tabin, C.J. (1996) Conservation in hedgehog signaling: induction of a chicken patched homolog by sonic hedgehog in the developing limb. *Development* **122**, 1225–1233.

Masuya, H., Sagai, T., Wakana, S., Moriwaki, K. and Shiroishi, T. (1995) A duplicated zone of polarizing activity in polydactylous mouse mutants. *Genes Dev.* **9**, 1645–1653.

Mizell, M. and Isaacs, J.J. (1970) Induced regeneration of hindlimbs in the newborn opossum. *Am. Zool.* **10**, 141–155.

Moore, K.L. (1988) *The Developing Human: Clinically Oriented Embryology*, 4th edn. W.B. Saunders: Philadelphia, PA.

Morgan, B.A., Izpisúa-Belmonte, J.C., Duboule, D. and Tabin, C.J. (1992) Targeted misexpression of *hox-4.6* in the avian limb bud causes apparent homeotic transformations. *Nature* **358**, 236–239.

Mortlock, D.P., Post, L.C. and Innis, J.W. (1996) The molecular basis of hypodactyly (*Hd*): a deletion in *Hoxal 3* leads to arrest of digital arch formation. *Nature Genetics* **13**, 284–289.

Muragaki, Y., Mundlos, S., Upton, J. and Olsen, B.R. (1996) Altered growth and branching patterns in synpolydactyly caused by mutations in HOXD 13. *Science* **272**, 548–551.

Neufeld, D.A. (1980) Partial blastema formation after amputation in adult mice. *J. Exp. Zool.* **212**, 31–36.

Niazi, I.A. and Saxena, S. (1978) Abnormal hindlimb regeneration in tadpoles of the toad, *Bufo andersoni*, exposed to excess vitamin A. *Folia Biol.* (Krakow) **26**, 3–11.

Niswander, L. and Martin, G.R. (1993) FGF-4 regulates expression of *Evx-1* in the developing mouse limb. *Development* **119**, 287–294.

Niswander, L., Tickle, C., Vogel, A., Booth, I. and Martin, G.R. (1993) FGF-4 replaces the apical ectodermal ridge and directs outgrowth and patterning of the limb. *Cell* **75**, 579–587.

Niswander, L., Jeffrey, S., Martin, G.R. and Tickle, C. (1994) A positive feedback loop coordinates growth and patterning in the vertebrate limb. *Nature* **371**, 609–612.

Nohno, T., Noji, S., Koyama, E. et al (1991) Involvement of the *chox-4* chicken homeobox genes in determination of anteroposterior axial polarity during limb development. *Cell* **64**, 1197–1205.

Ohuchi, H., Yoshioka, H., Tanaka, A. et al (1994) Involvement of androgen-induced growth factor (FGF-8) gene in mouse embryogenesis and morphogenesis. *Biochem. Biophys. Res. Comm.* **204**, 882–888.

Ohuchi, H.T.N., Yamauchi, T., Ohata, T. et al (1995) An additional limb can be induced from the flank of the chick embryo by FGF-4. *Biochem. Biophys. Res. Comm.* **209**, 809–816.

Olson, D.J., Christian, J.L. and Moon, R.T. (1991) Effect of Wnt-1 related proteins on gap junction communication in *Xenopus* embryos. *Science* **252**, 1173–1176.

Onda, H., Poulin, M.L., Tassava, R.A. and Chiu, I.M. (1991) Characterization of a newt tenascin cDNA and localization of tenascin mRNA during newt limb regeneration by in situ hybridization. *Dev. Biol.* **148**, 219–232.

Parr, B.A. and McMahon, A.P. (1995) Dorsalizing signal *Wnt-7a* required for normal polarity of D–V and A–P axes of mouse limb. *Nature* **374**, 350–353.

Parr, B.A., Shea, M.J., Vassileva, G. and McMahon, A.P. (1993) Mouse *Wnt* genes exhibit discrete domains of expression in the early embryonic CNS and limb buds. *Development* **119**, 247–261.

Patel, K., Nittenberg, R., Dsouza, D. et al (1996) Expression and regulation of *Cek-8*, a cell to cell signalling receptor in developing chick limb buds. *Development* **122**, 1147–1155.

Pecorino, L.T., Lo, C.D. and Brockes, J.P. (1994) Isoform-specific induction of a retinoid-responsive antigen after biolistic transfection of chimaeric retinoic acid/thyroid hormone receptors into a regenerating limb. *Development* **120**, 325–333.

Pecorino, L.T., Entwistle, A. and Brockes, J.P. (1996) Activation of a single retinoic acid receptor isoform mediates proximodistal respecification. *Curr. Biol.* **6**, 563–569.

Poswillo, D. (1975) Haemorrage in development of the face. *Birth Defects* **11**, 61–67.

Poulin, M.L. and Chiu, I.M. (1995) Re-programming of expression of the KGFR and *bek* variants of fibroblast growth factor receptor 2 during limb regeneration in newts (*Notophthalmus viridescens*). *Dev. Dyn.* **202**, 378–387.

Poulin, M.L., Patrie, K.M., Botelho, M.J., Tassava, R.A. and Chiu, I.M. (1993) Heterogeneity in the expression of fibroblast growth factor receptors during limb regeneration in newts (*Notophthalmus viridescens*). *Development* **119**, 353–361.

Ranson, M., Tickle, C., Mahon, K.A. and Mackem, S. (1995) *Gnot1*, a member of a new homeobox gene subfamily, is expressed in a dynamic, region-specific domain along the proximodistal axis of the developing limb. *Mech. Dev.* **51**, 17–30.

Reginelli, A.D., Wang, Y.Q., Sassoon, D. and Muneoka, K. (1995) Digit tip regeneration correlates with regions of *Msx1* (*Hox-7*) expression in fetal and newborn mice. *Development* **121**, 1065–1076.

Riddle, R., Johnson, R., Laufer, E. and Tabin, C. (1993) Sonic hedgehog mediates the polarizing activity of the ZPA. *Cell* **75**, 1401–1416.

Riddle, R.D., Ensini, M., Nelson, C. et al (1995) Induction of the limb homeobox gene *Lmx1* by WNT7a establishes dorsoventral pattern in the vertebrate limb. *Cell* **83**, 631–640.

Robert, B., Lyons, G., Simandl, B.K., Kuroiwa, A. and Buckingham, M. (1991) The apical ectodermal ridge regulates *Hox-7* and *Hox-8* gene expression in developing chick limb buds. *Genes Dev.* **5**, 2363–2374.

Rousseau, F., Bonaventure, J., Legeai-Mallet, L. et al (1994) Mutations in the gene encoding fibroblast growth factor receptor-3 in achondroplasia. *Nature* **371**, 252–254.

Rutland, P., Pulleyn, L.J., Reardon, W. et al (1995) Identical mutations in the *FGFR2* gene cause both Pfeiffer and Crouzon syndrome phenotypes. *Nature Genetics* **9**, 173–176.

Satokata, I. and Maas, R. (1994) *Msx1* deficient mice exhibit cleft-palate and abnormalities of craniofacial and tooth development. *Nature Genetics* **6**, 348–356.

Saunders, J.F. (1977) The experimental analysis of chick limb bud development. In *Vertebrate Limb and Somite Morphogenesis* (Eds: D.A. Ede, J.R. Hinchliffe and M. Balls), pp. 1–24. Cambridge University Press: Cambridge.

Saunders, J.F. and Errick, J. (1976) Inductive activity and enduring cellular constitution of a supernumerary apical ectodermal ridge grafted to the limb bud of the chick embryo. *Dev. Biol.* **50**, 16–25.

Saunders, J.F. and Gasseling, M.T. (1968) Ectodermal–mesodermal interactions in the origin of limb symmetry. In *Epithelial–Mesenchymal Interactions* (Eds: R. Fleischmajer and R.E. Billingham), pp. 78–97. Williams and Wilkins: Baltimore, MD.

Savage, M.P., Hart, C.E., Riley, B.B. et al (1993) Distribution of FGF-2 suggests it has a role in chick limb bud growth. *Dev. Dyn.* **198**, 159–170.

Savard, P. and Tremblay, M. (1995) Differential regulation of Hox C6 in the appendages of adult urodeles and anurans. *J. Mol. Biol.* **249**, 879–889.

Savard, P., Gates, P.B. and Brockes, J.P. (1988) Position dependent expression of a homeobox gene transcript in relation to amphibian limb regeneration. *EMBO J.* **7**, 4275–4282.

Shiang, R., Thompson, L.M., Zhu, Y.Z. et al (1994) Mutations in the transmembrane domain of FGFR3 cause the most common genetic form of dwarfism, achondroplasia. *Cell* **78**, 335–342.

Sicard, E.R. (1985) *Regulation of Vertebrate Limb Regeneration*. Oxford University Press: New York.

Simon, H.G. and Tabin, C.J. (1993) Analysis of *Hox-4.5* and *Hox-3.6* expression during newt limb regeneration: differential regulation of paralogous *Hox* genes suggest different roles for members of different *Hox* clusters. *Development* **117**, 1397–1407.

Singer, M. (1974) Neurotrophic control of limb regeneration in the newt. *Ann. NY Acad. Sci.* **228**, 308–322.

Small, K.M. and Potter, S.S. (1993) Homeotic transformations and limb defects in *Hox A11* mutant mice. *Genes Dev.* **7**, 2318–2328.

Song, K., Wang, Y. and Sassoon, D. (1992) Expression of *Hox-7.1* in myoblasts inhibits terminal differentiation and induces cell transformation. *Nature* **360**, 477–481.

Stevenson, R.E. and Meyer, L.C. (1993) The limbs. In *Human Malformations and Related Anomalies* (Eds: R.E. Stevenson, J.G. Hall and R.M. Goodman). Oxford Monographs on Medical Genetics vol. 27, pp. 699–804. Oxford University Press: Oxford.

Stocum, D. (1985) Role of the skin in urodele limb regeneration. In *Regulation of Vertebrate Limb Regeneration* (Ed.: R.E. Sicard). Oxford University Press: New York.

Stocum, D.L. (1991) Retinoic acid and limb regeneration. *Semin. Dev. Biol.* **2**, 199–210.

Storm, E.E., Huynh, T.V., Copeland, N.G. et al (1994) Limb alterations in brachypodism mice due to mutations in a new member of the TGF beta-superfamily. *Nature* **368**, 639–643.

Summerbell, D. (1974) A quantitative analysis of the effect of excision of the AER from the chick limb bud. *J. Embryol. Exp. Morphol.* **35**, 241–260.

Summerbell, D., Lewis, J. and Wolpert, L. (1973) Positional information in chick limb morphogenesis. *Nature* **244**, 492–496.

Taylor, G.P., Anderson, R., Reginelli, A.D. and Muneoka, K. (1994) FGF-2 induces regeneration of the chick limb bud. *Dev. Biol.* **163**, 282–284.

Thaller, C. and Eichele, G. (1987) Identification and spatial distribution of retinoids in the developing chick limb bud. *Nature* **327**, 625–628.

Thornton, C.S. (1968) Amphibian limb regeneration. *Adv. Morphogen.* **7**, 205–249.

Tickle, C. (1981) The number of polarizing region cells required to specify additional digits in the developing chick wing. *Nature* **289**, 295–298.

Tickle, C. and Eichele, G. (1994) Vertebrate limb development. *Annu. Rev. Cell Biol.* **10**, 121–152.

Tickle, C., Alberts, B.M., Wolpert, L. and Lee, J. (1982) Local application of retinoic acid to the limb bud mimics the action of the polarizing region. *Nature* **296**, 564–565.

Tickle, C., Lee, J. and Eichele, G. (1985) A quantitative analysis of the effect of all-trans-retinoic acid on the pattern of chick wing development. *Dev. Biol.* **109**, 82–95.

Vogel, A. and Tickle, C. (1993) FGF-4 maintains polarizing activity of posterior limb bud cells in vivo and in vitro. *Development* **119**, 199–206.

Vogel, A., Roberts-Clarke, D. and Niswander, L. (1995a) Effect of FGF on gene expression in chick limb bud cells *in vivo* and *in vitro*. *Dev. Biol.* **171**, 507–520.

Vogel, A., Rodriguez, C., Warnken, W. and Belmonte, J. (1995b) Dorsal cell fate specified by chick *Lmx-1* during vertebrate limb development. *Nature* **378**, 716–720.

Vortkamp, A., Gessler, M. and Grzeschik, K.-H. (1991) *GLI-3* zinc-finger gene interrupted by translocation in Greig syndrome families. *Nature* **352**, 539–540.

Wallace, H. (1981) *Vertebrate Limb Regeneration*. Wiley: Chichester.

Wilkie, O.M., Slaney, S.F., Oldridge, M. et al (1995) Apert syndrome (craniosynostosis/syndactyly) results from localised mutations of *FGFR2* and is allelic with Crouzon syndrome. *Nature Genetics* **9**, 165–172.

Williams, C.J., Considine, E.L., Knowlton, R.G. et al (1993) Spondyloepiphyseal dysplasia and precocious osteoarthritis in a family with an Arg75-Cys mutation in the procollagen type II gene. *Hum. Genet.* **92**, 499–505.

Winter, R.M., Schoroer, R.J. and Meyer, L.C. (1993) Hands and feet. In *Human Malformations and Related Anomalies* (Eds: R.E. Stevenson, J.G. Hall and R.M. Goodman). Oxford Monographs on Medical Genetics, vol. 27, pp. 805–843. Oxford University Press: Oxford.

Wolpert, L., Tickle, C. and Sampford, M. (1979) The effect of cell killing by X-irradiation on pattern formation in the chick limb. *J. Embryol. Exp. Morphol.* **50**, 175–198.

Woychik, R.P., Maas, R.L., Zeller, R., Vogt, T.F. and Leder, P. (1990) 'Formins': proteins deduced from the alternative transcripts of the *limb deformity* gene. *Nature* **346**, 850–853.

Wozney, J.M., Capparella, J. and Rosen, V. (1993) The bone morphogenetic proteins in cartilage and bone development. In *Molecular Basis of Morphogenesis* (Ed.: M. Bernfield), pp. 221–230. Wiley-Liss: New York.

Yang, Y. and Niswander, L. (1995) Interaction between the signaling molecules WNT7 and SHH during vertebrate limb development: dorsal signals regulate anteroposterior patterning. *Cell* **80**, 939–947.

Yokouchi, Y., Sasaki, H. and Kuriowa, A. (1991) Homeobox gene expression correlated with the bifurcation process of limb cartilage development. *Nature* **353**, 443–445.

Yuan, J., Shaham, S., Ledoux, S., Ellis, H.M. and Horvitz, H.R. (1993) The *C. elegans* cell death gene *ced-3* encodes a protein similar to mammalian Interleukin-1-beta converting enzyme. *Cell* **75**, 641–652.

Zeller, R., Jackson-Grusby, L. and Leder, P. (1989) The limb deformity gene is required for apical ectodermal ridge differentiation and antero-posterior limb pattern formation. *Genes Dev.* **3**, 1481–1492.

Zhao, W.G. and Neufeld, D.A. (1995) Bone regrowth in young mice stimulated by nail organ. *J. Exp. Zool.* **271**, 155–159.

Zou, H. and Niswander, L. (1996) Requirement for BMP signaling in interdigital apoptosis and scale formation. *Science* **272**, 738–741.

8 The Neural Tube

ANDREW J. COPP

Neural Development Unit, Institute of Child Health, London, UK

There can be few parts of the mammalian embryo that play such a pivotal role in development as the neural tube. This dorsal midline structure runs the entire length of the embryo giving rise to all of the neurones and most of the glia of the central nervous system. Moreover, its derivative, the neural crest, contributes to the peripheral nervous system and to a variety of other organ and body systems including the craniofacial skeleton, thymus, thyroid, parathyroid and important cardiac structures. In addition to these cellular contributions, the neural tube is critically important as an inducer of the formation of other organ systems, for instance, the mesodermally derived vertebrae and the ectodermally derived inner-ear primordium (the otic vesicle).

Defects of the central nervous system arise when the processes of neural tube development become disturbed, particularly during the embryonic and fetal periods. The abnormalities may be structural, as when the neural tube fails to close during the third and fourth weeks of human development, leading to the malformations anencephaly and myelomeningocele (see later). These defects are of major clinical importance, both as a cause of death around birth (perinatal mortality) and as a source of disability in children and adults. They affect between 1 in 300 and 1 in 5000 liveborn babies, depending on geographical location. Disturbance of later nervous system development yields functional rather than gross structural deficits, leading for instance, to epilepsy, mental retardation or behavioural disturbance. Up to 4% of children are affected by functional defects of this type, probably the commonest and most challenging type of disability that is faced by society today (Office of Population and Surveys, 1989).

In order to diagnose, effectively manage and ultimately prevent congenital nervous system defects, it is essential that we understand the genetic, molecular and cellular mechanisms of nervous system development and the ways in which these processes can be disturbed. This chapter will review the main events of nervous system development and the main types of congenital defect, and will then consider how modern molecular developmental biology is providing insight into the processes of nervous system development, both normal and abnormal.

Embryos, Genes and Birth Defects. Edited by P. Thorogood.
© 1997 John Wiley & Sons Ltd.

OVERVIEW OF NERVOUS SYSTEM DEVELOPMENT

The first event in the development of the nervous system is **neural induction**, in which the neural plate, the immediate precursor of the neural tube, forms as a result of a cellular interaction between the ectoderm and mesoderm of the gastrula-stage embryo. Neural induction probably begins as soon as the ectoderm and mesoderm come into contact, at the start of gastrulation (Sharpe and Gurdon, 1990). Concurrent with its induction, the neural plate becomes **regionally patterned** along each of its axes: craniocaudal, dorsoventral and mediolateral. This patterning represents a latent potential for differentiation that can be visualized at this early stage only as patterns of differential gene expression (Figure 8.1a). The patterning foreshadows the later development of morphological and functional subdivisions of the neural tube, for example, the distinct regions of the brain and the regionalization of neurones in the spinal cord. While regional patterning is under way, the neural plate also undergoes **morphogenesis**: folds arise at its lateral edges, approach one other in the dorsal midline and fuse (Figure 8.1b). Once neural fold fusion is complete, the inner aspect of the neural folds forms a continuous layer across the midline, comprising the roof plate of the neural tube. Similarly, the outer aspects of the neural folds fuse to form the continuous mid-dorsal surface ectoderm. In this way, the neural tube takes up its internal, dorsal, midline position in the embryo.

The early events of nervous system development, described above, are collectively referred to as **neurulation**. A complicating factor in the development of higher vertebrates, including birds and mammals, is that neurulation does not occur simultaneously at all levels of the craniocaudal axis, in contrast to lower vertebrates, as exemplified by the amphibian *Xenopus laevis*. In mammals, neural induction initially defines a region of neural plate whose developmental fate is confined to forming the brain and upper spinal regions of the future nervous system. Lower spinal regions form progressively (thoracic, lumbar, sacral and caudal) by the emergence of cells from the primitive streak as it regresses towards the caudal end of the embryo.

Neural crest migration is closely correlated in time with closure of the neural tube. In all mammals and birds studied, the cranial neural crest cells migrate from the tips of the neural folds, just prior to closure of the neural tube. In contrast, neural crest cells in the spinal region emerge from the roof of the neural tube just **after** its closure. Newly emerged spinal neural crest cells follow one of two migration routes (Serbedzija et al, 1990), either beneath the surface ectoderm (dorsolateral route) or between the neural tube and somite (ventrolateral route). Cranial neural crest cells appear to migrate entirely along the dorsolateral route. Neural crest cells subsequently give rise to differentiated derivatives in the peripheral nervous system and in several organs and body structures (see Chapters 9, 10, 11 and 15).

The neural tube is complete by the end of the fourth week of human embryonic development (equivalent to 10.5 days of gestation in the mouse). The period immediately following this is marked by **differentiation of the neuronal and glial cell lineages** from the wall of the neural tube, which at this stage

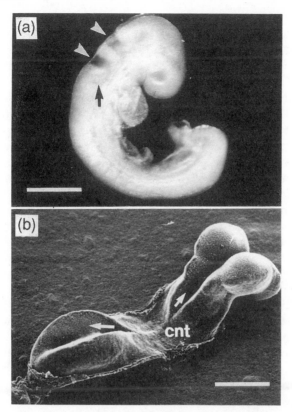

Figure 8.1 Early development and regional specification of the nervous system in the mouse embryo. (a) Whole-mount in-situ hybridization of *Krox-20* expression in the 9.5-day mouse embryo. Coincident with closure of the neural tube in the hindbrain region, this pattern-specifying gene is expressed specifically within rhombomeres 3 (weaker expression, more rostral arrowhead) and 5 (stronger expression, more caudal arrowhead). Black arrow indicates position of the developing otocyst which is located opposite rhombomeres 5 and 6. Scale bar: 0.5 mm. (b) Scanning electron micrograph of 8.5-day mouse embryo showing the early stages in closure of the neural tube. Closure has been initiated in the future cervical region (cnt) and is now progressing rostrally (to the right) and caudally (to the left) as shown by the arrows. Scale bar: 0.25 mm. (Part (b) from Copp et al, 1990)

comprises an actively proliferating, pseudostratified **neuroepithelium**. An important principle is that the neuroepithelial cells at any particular craniocaudal level of the neural tube differentiate into only those cell types that will characterize the mature nervous system at that level. Thus, the anterior hindbrain neural tube uniquely contains cells destined to form the cerebellar Purkinje neurones whereas the forebrain neuroepithelium contains cells destined to develop as pyramidal neurones. Transplantation studies in the chick show that, soon after neural tube closure, cells of the future cerebellar region are already irreversibly committed to particular pathways of differentiation (Alvarado-Mallart et al,

1990), presumably as a result of intracellular events that occurred during the phase of regional patterning.

Cell proliferation is a prominent feature of the primitive neuroepithelial cells of the neural tube, with rapid cell cycle times (e.g. 8–10 h at 10.5 days of mouse development). The onset of differentiation towards neuronal and glial lineages coincides with the loss of contact of neuroepithelial cells with the lumen of the neural tube, and their cessation of proliferation. The only exceptions to this rule are the ependyma, a population of glial cells that differentiates in situ at the luminal border of the neural tube, and cells of the subventricular zone of the cerebral hemispheres, which continue to proliferate for a time after migrating away from the neural tube lumen. However, these cells also cease proliferation before they migrate to the cortical plate.

Cell migration is an integral feature of the early development of the neural tube. In the spinal cord, post-mitotic neuronal and glial precursors move only short distances to take up a position in the intermediate and outer, marginal, layers, where they differentiate. At the other extreme, neuronal precursors migrate considerable distances during development of the layered structure of the cerebral cortex. The post-mitotic neuroblasts migrate in a series of waves across the intermediate zone to form the cortical plate. Cells that arrive first populate deep layers of the cortical plate whereas later-arriving cells populate progressively more superficial layers. The cortical plate thus expands as development proceeds, giving rise to the adult cortex. The mode of migration of neurones to the cortical plate involves guidance by cellular processes of the **radial glia**, which are oriented perpendicularly to the pial surface of the developing cortex. Neurones are intimately apposed to the surface of the radial glial cells and it is thought that cell–cell interactions are important in promoting correct migration of the cortical neurones.

Somewhat surprisingly, at this time of intensive growth and differentiation, there is also considerable **programmed cell death** or **apoptosis** in the early nervous system. This is regionally restricted, for instance characterizing the cortical subplate (Allendoerfer and Shatz, 1994) and spinal motor neurones (Oppenheim, 1991). The function of such cell death is not clear: it may be responsible for removal of entire structures that play a temporally limited role in nervous system development. Additionally, cell death could play a role in removing cells with persistent multipotentiality after differentiative decisions have been made in the majority of cells.

We have seen that formation of the neural tube begins in the third week of human development. **Nervous system function** can be first detected from about 6 weeks in the human embryo (de Vries, 1992), correlating with the onset of peptide neurotransmitter production, which can be detected in neuroblasts during development of the cerebral cortical plate (Allendoerfer and Shatz, 1994). The nervous system continues to develop rapidly throughout the remaining weeks of fetal development, and into postnatal life. During this later developmental period, **synaptic connections** are formed linking the different parts of the central nervous system with each other, and with the periphery. Upon these connections depend the majority of body functions and all of our mental activities.

DEFECTS OF NERVOUS SYSTEM DEVELOPMENT

Defective nervous system development results in a diverse group of diseases ranging from major malformations that are incompatible with postnatal life to disabilities that only slightly affect the physical or mental function of the individual. For the purpose of the present discussion, these disorders will be categorized according to the type of developmental event that appears to be disturbed (Table 8.1).

Global defects of neural induction are expected to arrest development at an early stage. Indeed, several mouse mutations cause embryonic death, early in the post-implantation period without formation of neural structures, although no specific evidence currently exists to implicate neural induction in the pathogenesis of these malformations. In humans, global defects of neural induction are unlikely to come to the attention of the clinician, except as cases of early pregnancy loss, and so are not distinguished as a clinical entity. A localized defect of neural induction has been invoked to account for the complex malformation **holoprosencephaly**, in which subdivision of the forebrain to form the telencephalic vesicles (containing the future lateral ventricles) is defective, yielding a single poorly developed forebrain structure. This malformation can be associated with fusion of the optic vesicles and eye primordia, yielding the birth defect **cyclopia**, with lack of olfactory bulb development, yielding the defect **arrhinencephaly**, and with lack of other midline structures, as in **agenesis of the corpus callosum**. There is no indication that forebrain neuroepithelial differentiation is defective per se in holoprosencephaly, as would be expected if a defect of the neural induction process itself were responsible. Rather, it has been suggested that holoprosencephaly is an example of a 'developmental field defect' in which the domain of neural induction in the forebrain is narrower than normal, providing insufficient breadth for subsequent development of the paired telencephalic vesicles. Alternatively, holoprosencephaly could represent a disturbance of the co-ordinated growth that underlies morphogenesis of the early neural plate following induction, so that the development of distinct bilateral telencephalic vesicles is not realized and the forebrain remains a single midline structure. Resolution of this issue will require analysis of the early development of holoprosencephaly in an experimental model system (see note added in proof).

Defects of neural patterning are expected to yield misplacements, deletions or duplications of major subdivisions of the nervous system. Experimentally, it has been shown that regional specification of the midbrain and hindbrain in the mouse is dependent on the co-ordinated expression of several embryonic genes. Thus, *Wnt-1* is required for development of the midbrain and rostral hindbrain (McMahon and Bradley, 1990). Embryos homozygous for a null mutation in this gene exhibit agenesis of the midbrain and cerebellum (Figure 8.2). Likewise, the gene *Krox-20* is needed for correct development of the cranial nerves originating in the hindbrain (Swiatek and Gridley, 1993). Nervous system patterning can also be disturbed by exogenous factors such as excess retinoic acid, which results in duplication of the facial nerve (cranial nerve VII) when administered to

Table 8.1 The main embryonic processes of nervous system development and the defects that result from their disruption in human and mouse

Event or processes	Developmental function	Type of anomaly expected from disturbance of the process	Candidate abnormalities in human	Candidate abnormalities in mouse
Neural induction	Formation of neural plate from ectoderm due to the influence of underlying mesodermal derivatives	General defect: absence of neuroepithelial differentiation Local defect: inadequate area of neural plate formed for normal subsequent development	General defects probably produce early embryonic lethality, leading to first trimester abortion. Local deficit of forebrain induction is implicated in holoprosencephaly	Possible neural induction defects in pre-neurulation lethal mutations in which neural tissue is not formed, for example in the mutations *Ve*, *Bld*
Nervous system patterning	Specification of regional identity in craniocaudal and dorsoventral axes within the early nervous system	Absence of duplication of regional elements of the nervous system. Homeotic transformations (i.e. misplacement of region elements)	Cerebellar agenesis, Dandy–Walker syndrome (?)	*Wnt-1* gene null mutations, resulting in lack of midbrain and cerebellar structures. Duplication of the VIIth nerve resulting from retinoic acid treatment
Neural tube morphogenesis	Elevation, apposition and fusion of the neural folds to form the neural tube. Canalization of the caudal (secondary) neural tube	Open malformations of the brain and/or spinal cord. Herniation of central nervous system structures through incomplete formation of skull vault and vertebral neural arches	Open neural tube defects: craniorachischisis, anencephaly, myelomeningocele. Closed 'neural tube defects': encephalocele, meningocele	Neural tube defects resulting from action of several mutant genes (e.g. *curly tail*, *loop tail*, *Splotch*) and numerous teratogenic exogenous agents (e.g. valproic acid, retinoic acid)

Neural crest development	Migration and differentiation of neural crest cells	Absence or maldevelopment of neural crest-derived structures	Craniofacial defects, skin hypopigmentation, hearing loss (pigmentation in the stria vascularis), aplasia of thymus, thyroid and parathyroid, conotruncal heart defects, aganglionosis of the terminal bowel (Hirschsprung's disease)	Defects as in human resulting from genes including *Sp, Ph, ls, W, Sl* and many teratogenic exogenous agents (e.g. retinoic acid)
Neuronal proliferation and programmed cell death	Proliferation of mitotic neuroepithelial cells in the ventricular zone of the neural tube. Programmed death of neurones at particular sites within the nervous system, e.g. cortical subplate, motor neurones	Abnormal neuronal numbers in specific regions of the nervous system	Microencephaly in which brain mass is reduced. Megalencephaly could result from failure of programmed cell death	Micrencephaly resulting from the action of many teratogenic agents
Neuronal migration	Migration of post-mitotic neuroblasts from the ventricular zone of the neural tube to their final destinations in the brain and spinal cord	Misplacement of groups of neurones within the nervous system	'Neuronal migration disorders' including heterotopic neurones and disorders of cerebral gyral formation, including lissencephaly, pachygyria and polymicrogyria	Generalized disruption of neuronal migration as seen in the *reeler* mutant. More limited neuronal heterotopies seen in the *dreher* mutant and as a result of irradiation and puncture wounds in neonates
Neuronal/glial differentiation	Divergence and differentiation of the neuronal and glial lineages appropriate to each level of the neuraxis	Regionally restricted absence or malfunction of specific cell types	Granule cell aplasia in the cerebellum	Several mutants disturb differentiation or survival of specific cell types in the cerebellum e.g *pcd*, Purkinje cell degeneration; *we*, granule cell loss

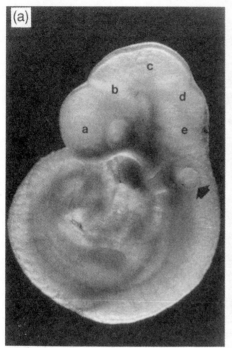
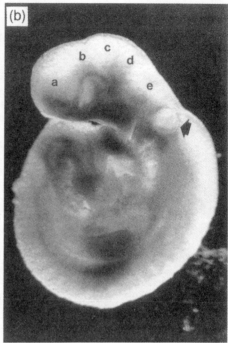

Figure 8.2 Targeted mutation of the *Wnt-1* gene in the mouse. Mouse embryos at 10.5 days of gestation (27-somite stage) from a mating between *Wnt-1*$^{+/-}$ heterozygotes. The regions of the developing brain are indicated: a, telencephalon; b, diencephalon; c, mesencephalon; d, metencephalon; e, myelencephalon. (a) *Wnt-1*$^{+/-}$ embryo with normal appearance; (b) *Wnt-1*$^{+/-}$ mutant embryo showing hypoplasia of midbrain and metencephalic region of the hindbrain. Magnification: approx. × 20. (Reproduced by permission of McMahon and Bradley, 1990)

mouse embryos at a specific stage of development (Marshall et al, 1992; and see Chapter 5). In humans, malformations such as **cerebellar agenesis** may result from defects of neural patterning, where an element in the craniocaudal neural axis is seemingly missing from an early developmental stage. It has been suggested that the related **Dandy–Walker syndrome**, in which hindbrain development is disturbed leading to absence of the cerebellar vermis and cystic dilatation of the fourth ventricle, may also be an anomaly of neural patterning.

Defects of neural tube morphogenesis include the major category of **open neural tube defects**, namely **anencephaly**, in which the cranial neural tube fails to close, **myelomeningocele**, in which the lower spinal neural tube remains open, and **craniorachischisis,** where there is a failure of neural tube closure over the entire body axis. There are close parallels between these malformations in experimental animals and in humans. In the mouse, at least 10 different genes cause non-closure of the neural tube, with different mutations affecting specific craniocaudal levels of the body axis, thereby mimicking the human situation. Study of the mouse models shows that the initial defect is almost always non-closure of the neural tube and that, with subsequent development, there is erosion of the exposed neuroepithelium so that, later in gestation, severe damage to the affected nervous system is present. **Closed neural tube defects** also occur in humans: **encephaloceles** and **meningoceles** may affect any level of the brain and spinal cord respectively and comprise herniation of neural tissue and/or meninges through openings in the skull or the neural arches of the vertebral column. It seems likely that these are primarily defects of mesodermal development during skeletogenesis, and so perhaps should not be classified developmentally as 'neural tube defects' as such. However, given the important role of the neural tube in inducing skeletal tissue development, it is possible that an underlying abnormality of skeletal induction by the neural tube may be involved in the genesis of these malformations.

An important group of defects of nervous system development are the so-called 'neuronal migration disorders' (Rorke, 1994). In their most extreme form, these disorders can comprise apparent duplication of the cerebral cortex, giving the appearance of a 'double cortex' (Figure 8.3). These lesions are classified pathologically as **laminar heterotopias** (i.e. plate-like groups of misplaced neurones). Normally, a broad layer of white matter (axonal processes) separates the grey matter (neuronal cell bodies) from the ventricular wall of the fully developed cerebral hemisphere. In the laminar heterotopias, an additional layer of grey matter lies beneath the cortex, separated from it and from the ventricular wall by white matter. Although rare, laminar heterotopias are especially found in females with problematic epilepsy. **Nodular heterotopias** are commoner

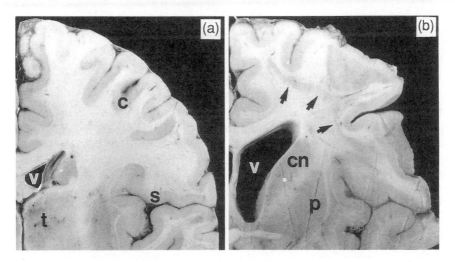

Figure 8.3 Neuronal migration defect, the 'double cortex' malformation, in coronal sections of human brain. (a) Normal brain showing the single, uniform layer of cerebral cortical grey matter overlying the white matter. (b) Abnormal brain with an additional layer of grey matter (arrows) within the white matter, underlying the cortical ribbon. Sections are taken from non-identical levels of the brain, hence the difference in size of the lateral ventricles. c, cerebral cortical ribbon; cn, caudate nucleus; p, putamen; s, sylvian fissure; t, thalamus; v, lateral ventricle. Magnification: actual size

malformations, comprising restricted groups of neurones situated in abnormal positions, particularly within the cerebral hemispheres, hippocampus and cerebellar cortex. They can comprise relatively discrete islands containing small numbers of nerve cells which may be asymptomatic or can be associated with epileptic foci: surgical specimens of excised brain tissue from individuals with intractable seizure disorders often contain heterotopic neurones. Heterotopias may also be associated with complex maldevelopments of the cerebral cortex such as **polymicrogyria**, in which the cortex exhibits increased numbers of poorly formed folds (gyri), and **pachygyria**, in which the gyri are fewer than normal or even completely absent (**lissencephaly**). All of these conditions are frequently accompanied by epilepsy and mental retardation.

It is not clear whether clinical malformations result from a deficiency of programmed cell death in the developing nervous system. However, the rare condition **megalencephaly**, in which the entire brain is of massive size, may result from a reduction in programmed cell death. Fundamental studies of the embryonic and fetal development of heterotopias are required before definite conclusions can be drawn about the possible role of disturbances to normal levels of programmed cell death.

Cell proliferation is clearly an integral component of nervous system development and may be implicated in the genesis of many defects of the central nervous system in which the neuronal mass is reduced. For instance, in **microcephaly** there is reduced mass of the brain (strictly called 'micrencephaly'). This finding is a frequent accompaniment to mental retardation. Some cases of micrencephaly have been suggested to result from a reduction in the number of cell divisions undergone by the germinal layer of the neural tube. Thus, fewer neuroblasts are generated, and the ependyma is formed prematurely.

It was stated earlier that the early development of the nervous system is a period of differentiation of the various cell types that are appropriate for each level of the body axis. In some disorders of nervous system development there is **aplasia of specific neuronal and glial cell types**, which is indicative of malfunction of a particular cell lineage. This is seen in some rare cerebellar syndromes in humans and has been described in a number of mouse genetic mutations affecting the cerebellum. For instance, cerebellar Purkinje cells are defective or degenerate in the *lurcher* and *purkinje cell degeneration* mutants while the cerebellar granule cells are defective in the *staggerer* and *weaver* mutants.

RECENT PROGRESS IN UNDERSTANDING CENTRAL NERVOUS SYSTEM DEVELOPMENT

GENE EXPRESSION IN THE NERVOUS SYSTEM

In recent years, we have come to appreciate the tremendous diversity and complexity of gene expression in the developing vertebrate nervous system. The discovery of these genes has resulted mainly from screening for homologues of genes that are expressed in other related contexts (see Chapter 1), for instance, during *Drosophila* development or during neoplastic transformation. Alternative approaches, which do not rely on homology to known genes, are now being developed: for instance, it is possible to use transgenic technology to 'trap' genes by inserting a reporter sequence into, or adjacent to, an expressed gene (Joyner, 1991; and see Chapter 4). Expression of the trapped gene is revealed by co-expression of the reporter, and the inserted sequence provides a means of cloning the endogenous gene.

As might be expected, particular cellular functions such as synaptic activity have proven to be associated with specific patterns of gene expression (Burden, 1993). Perhaps more significant for the early development of the nervous system has been the discovery that specific classes of genes, particularly transcription factors such as those containing homeobox, helix-loop-helix and leucine zipper DNA-sequence motifs, are expressed early in development. The protein products of these genes bind to specific DNA target sequences in the regulatory regions of downstream genes and so co-ordinate cascades of gene activity during development. Moreover, these genes are regionally expressed: for instance, the developing forebrain and hindbrain differ radically in their patterns of expression of homeobox-containing genes, with *Hox* and *Krox* genes expressed in the hindbrain and a different set of homeobox-containing genes, including *Otx*, *Emx* and *Dlx*, expressed in the forebrain (Wilkinson, 1993; Finkelstein and Boncinelli, 1994; and see Chapter 10).

NEURAL INDUCTION

A great deal of effort, mainly using amphibians and birds, has been aimed at identifying the molecular mechanisms of neural induction (reviewed by Kelly and Melton, 1995). A dramatic demonstration of neural induction is the capacity of the amphibian 'organizer', a region of the embryo situated at the dorsal lip of the blastopore, to induce a secondary body axis when transplanted to a non-midline region of a host embryo. The chick and mouse equivalents of the organizer (named 'Hensen's node' and the 'embryonic node' respectively) are situated at the cranial end of the primitive streak, and have similar inducing properties. A graft of organizer/Hensen's node tissue contributes mesodermal cells to the secondary axis, but induces the neural component of the new axis from host tissue that would not normally have differentiated along this pathway (reviewed by Guthrie, 1991). A molecular component of the neural-inducing mechanism appears to be diffusible, since induction can occur through a filter interposed between mesoderm and ectoderm (Toivonen et al, 1976). However, it has also been shown that inducing signals can pass along the plane of the neural tissue, rather than directly from mesoderm to adjacent ectoderm (Guthrie, 1991). Many candidates have been suggested for the neural-inducing molecules, and recent molecular studies have identified several gene products that are present in the organizer and which can induce neural tissue in amphibian ectoderm (Green, 1994). The activins appear to have neural-inducing properties but this can probably be explained by their ability to induce mesoderm, which itself has neural-inducing activity. Two genes, *noggin* and *follistatin*, have no mesoderm-inducing ability and yet can induce neural tissue. However, a further possibility has arisen as a result of experiments in which a dominant-negative mutant form of the activin receptor has been expressed in amphibian embryos. Mesoderm induction is blocked, but neural induction occurs suggesting that the neural state may be a default pathway of differentiation that is prevented by certain concentrations of activin. Further advances in our understanding of neural induction can be expected in the near future.

CRANIOCAUDAL PATTERNING OF THE NERVOUS SYSTEM

During neural induction, the specific regional character of the neuroepithelium along the craniocaudal axis is induced by an interaction between mesoderm and overlying ectoderm. In both amphibia and mice, anterior mesoderm can induce the expression of genes characterizing anterior neuroepithelium when co-cultured with posterior ectoderm that would not normally express these genes (Sharpe and Gurdon, 1990; Ang and Rossant, 1993). The difference between lower and higher vertebrates is that neural induction is complete in amphibia before the onset of neural folding whereas in mammals it is a long drawn-out process that continues from gastrulation to the end of the neurulation period. The reason for this difference is that neurulation occurs simultaneously along the entire body axis of the amphibian whereas, as noted earlier, in mammals the process occurs progressively in a craniocaudal sequence.

Regional specification has been studied in detail in the mouse hindbrain where, just prior to neural tube closure, neuroepithelial cells begin to express genes belonging to the Hox family of homeobox-containing genes. In general, Hox genes are expressed along much of the body axis but they have differing rostral boundaries of expression, with the boundary situated in some cases within the hindbrain (see Chapter 10). The hindbrain consists of six segments or rhombomeres and each expresses a different combination of Hox genes. This has led to the suggestion that regional specification within the hindbrain may be determined by a 'Hox code' (Hunt and Krumlauf, 1992). Experimental evidence is accumulating to support this idea. For instance, treatment of gastrulation-stage mouse embryos with retinoic acid alters the pattern of Hox-gene expression causing cells of rhombomeres 2 and 3 to express *Hoxb-1*, which is normally expressed only by cells of rhombomeres 4 and 5. The regional character of rhombomeres 2 and 3 is altered so that they now give rise to a nerve resembling cranial nerve VII (facial) rather than cranial nerve V (trigeminal) as would normally occur. Thus, the facial nerve is duplicated in the embryos treated with retinoic acid (Marshall et al, 1992). Further evidence for a Hox code comes from studies in which Hox genes are inactivated in transgenic mice. The most prominent abnormalities in these mice affect the neural crest and skeletal derivatives (see Chapter 10), but nervous system defects, particularly involving the cranial nerves, have also been described in mutations of those Hox genes whose anterior expression boundary is located within the hindbrain (reviewed by Wilkinson, 1993).

DORSOVENTRAL PATTERNING OF THE NERVOUS SYSTEM

Concurrent with patterning in the craniocaudal axis, the nervous system also develops regional specialization in the dorsoventral axis. This has been studied in detail in the spinal cord where, from dorsal to ventral, the following cell types differentiate soon after closure of the neural tube: roof-plate cells, neural crest, dorsal sensory relay neurones, motor neurones and floor-plate cells (Figure 8.4a). Domains of gene expression, particularly involving homeobox-containing Pax genes that are restricted in the dorsoventral axis (Figure 8.4b), precede the differentiation of these neural cell types and may be implicated in their specification, in an analogous way to the proposed Hox code. Interactions between the notochord and the neural tube appear to be instrumental in setting up the pattern of dorsoventral gene expression. The notochord is closely apposed to the ventral surface of the neural plate and tube, and manipulations such as ultraviolet irradiation of the amphibian embryo, or extirpation of Hensen's node in the chick, prevent the notochord from developing and lead to failure of the floor plate to differentiate (Clarke et al, 1991). It has been shown that an interaction between notochord and neuroepithelium, requiring cell contact, is necessary for the formation of floor-plate cells in vitro (Placzek et al, 1990). In addition, signals from the notochord and floor plate are capable of

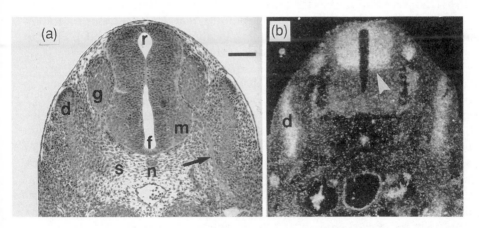

Figure 8.4 Regionalization of morphology and gene expression in the mouse neural tube. (a) Transverse section through the lumbar region of 11.5-day embryo showing differentiation of, from dorsal to ventral, the roof plate (r), dorsal root ganglia (g), motor neurones (m) and floor plate (f). Arrow indicates a motor nerve root. The somite has differentiated into dermamyotome (d), a lateral, epithelial derivative, and sclerotome (s), which comprises mesenchymal cells migrating ventromedially to surround the notochord (n). Bright field, haematoxylin and eosin. Scale bar: 0.1 mm. (b) Similar transverse section to (a), viewed under dark-field illumination after in-situ hybridization for *Pax-3* gene expression. White grains indicate sites of mRNA localization. Note the sharp boundary (arrowhead) between the dorsal neural tube that expresses *Pax-3* and the ventral neural tube that is negative. Dermamyotome (d) is also positive for *Pax-3*, as are the dorsal root ganglia. Scale bar: 0.15 mm

inducing the differentiation of motor neurones in fragments of neuroepithelium that would normally form other cell types (Yamada et al, 1993). Thus, it appears that signals from the notochord are responsible for specifying ventral aspects of the neural tube pattern. Recently, mammalian homologues of two *Drosophila* developmental genes have been found to play a role in the interaction between the notochord and neural tube. *Sonic hedgehog* (*Shh*) and *hepatocyte nuclear factor-3β* (*HNF-3β*) are both expressed in the notochord and later in the floor plate. Moreover, ectopic expression of *Shh* induces the expression of genes characteristic of the floor plate (Echelard et al, 1993). Since *HNF-3β* is expressed before *Shh*, it seems possible that *HNF-3β* may serve to regulate *shh* during development (see note added in proof).

The formation of dorsal cell types, for instance the neural crest, appears to be independent of the notochord (Artinger and Bronner-Fraser, 1992). It is possible that differentiation of dorsal cell types is a 'default pathway' in neural tube development. Alternatively, other signals may be active in inducing dorsal pattern formation. For instance, *dorsalin-1*, a member of the family of transforming growth factors (TGFs), has the ability to induce the formation of neural crest cells (Basler et al, 1993). This finding points to the existence of specific inducing signals for dorsal cell types within the neural tube. Significantly, it has recently been demonstrated that hindbrain neuroepithelium can regenerate neural crest if the original crest is ablated (Scherson et al, 1993). Furthermore, the regeneration of crest from cells within the lateral aspects of the neural tube, and which would have otherwise contributed to the brain, indicates that dorsoventral specification is relatively labile until well after the specification of cell fate and positional identity along the anteroposterior axis of the neural tube (Hunt et al, 1995).

NEURAL TUBE MORPHOGENESIS

Morphogenesis of the neural tube occurs concurrently with regional specification of the nervous system, and yet the molecular regulation of the two processes appears to be quite distinct. For instance, inactivation of Hox genes has not been found to yield neural tube defects, making it unlikely that Hox genes play a major role in neural tube closure. On the other hand, transcription factors such as those encoded by the homeobox gene *Pax-3* and the zinc-finger gene *Gli-3* are certainly involved in neural tube closure. These genes are disrupted in the *Splotch* and *Extra toes* mutations respectively, and the mutant phenotypes include neural tube defects (Copp and Bernfield, 1994). *Pax-3* mRNA is expressed with the neural cell adhesion molecule (N-CAM) in the neural folds during neurulation and the latter is misregulated in *Splotch* embryos suggesting that *Pax-3* may regulate N-CAM. However, recent evidence indicates that the N-CAM abnormality in *Splotch* embryos involves premature addition of sialic acid residues, a post-translational modification of the protein that is probably only indirectly related to *Pax-3* function (Neale and Trasler, 1994). *Gli-3* is expressed in the dorsal parts of the neural folds and in the mesoderm at the stage of neural tube closure, but it is not yet clear how *Gli-3* participates in neural tube closure.

The frequent occurrence of neural tube defects in human and experimental animals suggests that closure of the neural tube may be a relatively poorly 'buffered' developmental event, in comparison with neural patterning in the craniocaudal axis, which appears to be protected against disturbance by overlap of function among members of the paralogous groups of Hox genes (see Chapter 10). One reason for this lack of buffering may be the complex nature of the embryonic requirements for successful neural tube closure. Neural patterning appears to be essentially a process of assignment of positional values to cells, which guides their future pathway of differentiation. Neural tube closure similarly involves specific gene expression but, in addition, requires a co-ordinated series of mechanical changes, derived from changes in cell and tissue shape. Indeed, it has been demonstrated that spinal neural tube defects in the *curly tail* mouse mutant result from a mechanical defect in which non-neural tissues, the notochord and hindgut endoderm, proliferate abnormally slowly causing ventral curvature of the body axis (Copp et al, 1990). Experimental production of ventral curvature of the body axis in normal mouse and chick embryos also inhibits neural tube closure (Van Straaten et al, 1993). Thus, both molecular and mechanical influences can disturb the closure of the neural tube. Conversely, a growing list of factors can prevent faulty closure in genetically predisposed embryos. For instance, low doses of retinoic acid prevent the spinal neural tube defects in *curly tail* embryos (Chen et al, 1994) and recent studies indicate that this effect may be mediated via up-regulation of the expression of retinoic acid receptors, which may participate in the control of growth in the hindgut endoderm (Chen et al, 1995). Folic acid has similarly been found to prevent some cases of human neural tube defects (Wald et al, 1991), but the developmental basis of this effect remains to be determined.

DIFFERENTIATION AND MIGRATION OF NEURONAL AND GLIAL CELL LINEAGES

Much research effort has gone into defining the process of divergence of the neuronal and glial lineages in the developing cerebral cortex and cerebellum. Single neuroepithelial cells can be labelled by transfection with a replication-defective retroviral vector that contains a reporter gene such as bacterial β-galactosidase (*LacZ*). The subsequent development of the labelled cell and its clonal descendants can then be correlated with the pattern of differentiation as discerned by staining with antibodies specific for different neuronal and glial subsets. Studies of this type have shown that labelled clones most often contain only a single neuronal or glial cell type, suggesting that lineage specification occurs prior to the final mitotic division of neuroepithelial stem cells (Grove et al, 1993). A question that crucially affects the interpretation of studies of this type is whether spatially related cells labelled with the reporter gene are clonally related or derived from more than one infected cell. Recently, this problem has been solved by using the polymerase chain reaction to identify individual retroviruses (i.e. single integration events) after infection with a library of such constructs (Walsh and Cepko, 1993).

Labelling of early neuroepithelial cells has also provided evidence on the mode of migration of neuroblasts from the ventricular zone towards the cerebral cortex. The prevailing view is that neuroblasts migrate radially from the ventricular zone towards the cortex along processes of radial glial cells. This view is supported by the finding that, in the *reeler* mutant mouse where neuronal migration is disturbed in both the cerebral and cerebellar regions, processes of the radial glia lack their regular distribution and are haphazardly oriented (Pinto-Lord et al, 1982; Yuasa et al, 1993). However, clones of retrovirally labelled cells are sometimes found to be dispersed tangentially rather than radially organized (Tan and Breen, 1993; Walsh and Cepko, 1993). It appears that two mechanisms may operate: radial migration based on guidance by radial glia and tangential dispersion based on an unknown mechanism.

As mentioned earlier, several mouse mutations have been described in which particular neuronal cell types develop abnormally in the cerebellum. These defects characteristically produce an ataxic gait, a phenotype that is readily identified in mice. Although microscopic analysis can reveal the cell types affected by these defects, an experimental approach is necessary in order to identify the cell type in which the mutant gene acts to produce the observed defect. Mouse **chimeras**, individuals in which cells of two distinct phenotypes are combined as a result of experimental intervention, have been used extensively to investigate mechanisms of cerebellar neuronal defects. Chimeric individuals express genes from both donor and host strains, but in different cells, in contrast to hybrid animals which co-express genes from both donor and host strain in every cell. Chimeras are created to contain both mutant and wild-type cells, with the additional use of a marker that can distinguish between cells of the two genotypes in histological sections. The cerebellum of chimeras is then assessed to determine whether the cellular abnormality is corrected in genetically mutant cells (indicating an environment-dependent defect) or whether mutant cells persist in developing abnormally in chimeras (indicating a cell-autonomous defect). Studies of this sort have been successful in identifying a cell-autonomous defect of Purkinje cells in the *purkinje cell degeneration* (*pcd*) mutation, whereas aberrant migration of Purkinje cells in the *reeler* homozygotes can be rescued in chimeras, suggesting a non-autonomous defect involving trophic support from neighbouring cells (Mullen and Herrup, 1979). It is interesting to note that the *reeler* gene product has recently been identified as a secreted protein with homology to adhesion molecules (D'Arcangelo et al, 1995), consistent with the findings from the chimeric analysis.

NEURONAL PROGRAMMED CELL DEATH

A great deal of information has emerged in recent years on the mechanisms of cell death during normal embryonic and fetal development. 'Programmed' or 'physiological' cell death is usually equated with the morphological process of **apoptosis**, in which cells die by nuclear condensation and fragmentation into membrane-bound bodies without release of cytoplasmic contents. This contrasts

with necrosis, a pathological process, in which cells rupture and cytoplasmic contents are released. Programmed cell death requires new gene expression and should probably be considered as a state of terminal differentiation. There is evidence from the nematode worm *Caenorhabditis elegans* that a series of genes is required to specify which cells are destined to die or to survive during development (Ellis and Horvitz, 1986). Although no such pathway has yet been implicated in the control of mammalian programmed cell death, several genes have been found to participate in its regulation. For instance, the *bcl-2* gene encodes an inner mitochondrial membrane protein that acts to prevent programmed cell death, probably by inhibiting the generation of damaging oxygen free radicals (Hockenbery et al, 1993). When over-expressed, *bcl-2* can prevent the degeneration of neurones in response to deprivation of neurotrophic factors in vitro (Allsopp et al, 1993) or cutting their axons in vivo (Dubois-Dauphin et al, 1994). A related gene, *bcl-x*, may also play an important role in protecting neurones from programmed cell death in vivo (Boise et al, 1993). Thus, although details are emerging of the intracellular regulation of programmed neuronal cell death (reviewed by Davies, 1995), it is still unclear how neuronal loss is regulated during development and whether disturbance of this process can yield central nervous system defects.

AGENDA FOR THE FUTURE

There is hardly a single topic in the development of nervous system malformations that does not require further in-depth study. In the case of malformations such as holoprosencephaly, we do not even understand which embryonic event is primarily affected (see note added in proof). Is there a defect of forebrain induction or in morphogenesis of the forebrain following induction? Other defects, such as neuronal heterotopias, have not been well studied in terms of the cellular processes that are responsible. Are they solely defects of neuronal migration, or is disturbance of cell proliferation and programmed cell death also involved? In each of these examples, the current lack of experimentally tractable model systems is an impediment to progress. By contrast, in other areas such as neural tube defects there are excellent mouse models available; here the need is for detailed studies of the cell and molecular biology of defective embryos as the malformations develop. The advent of gene expression studies in the developing nervous system, together with refinement of the techniques of gene targeting and transgenic mouse production, seems likely to herald a period of rapid advance in our understanding of the embryonic events underlying nervous system malformations.

ACKNOWLEDGEMENTS

I am most grateful to Dr Andrew McMahon for allowing me to reproduce Figure 8.2, and to Mr Nick Greene, Dr Brian Harding and Dr Simon Conway for providing unpublished material for Figures 8.1a, 8.3 and 8.4b respectively.

150 EMBRYOS, GENES AND BIRTH DEFECTS

REFERENCES

Allendoerfer, K.L. and Shatz, C.J. (1994) The subplate, a transient neocortical structure: its role in the development of connections between thalamus and cortex. *Annu. Rev. Neurosci.* **17**, 185–218.

Allsopp, T.E., Wyatt, S., Paterson, H.F. and Davies, A.M. (1993) The proto-oncogene *bcl-2* can selectively rescue neurotrophic factor-dependent neurons from apoptosis. *Cell* **73**, 295–307.

Alvarado-Mallart, R.-M., Martinez, S. and Lance-Jones, C.C. (1990) Pluripotentiality of the 2-day-old avian germinative neuroepithelium. *Dev. Biol.* **139**, 75–88.

Ang, S.-L. and Rossant, J. (1993) Anterior mesendoderm induces mouse *Engrailed* genes in explant cultures. *Development* **118**, 139–149.

Artinger, K.B. and Bronner-Fraser, M. (1992) Notochord grafts do not suppress formation of neural crest cells or commissural neurons. *Development* **116**, 877–886.

Basler, K., Edlund, T., Jessell, T.M. and Yamada, T. (1993) Control of cell pattern in the neural tube: regulation of cell differentiation by *dorsalin-1*, a novel TGFβ family member. *Cell* **73**, 687–702.

Boise, L.H., González-Garcia, M., Postema, C.E. et al (1993) *bcl-x*, a *bcl-2*-related gene that functions as a dominant regulator of apoptotic cell death. *Cell* **74**, 597–608.

Burden, S.J. (1993) Synapse-specific gene expression. *Trends in Genetics* **9**, 12–16.

Chen, W., Morriss-Kay, G.M. and Copp, A.J. (1994) Prevention of spinal neural tube defects in the curly tail mouse mutant by a specific effect of retinoic acid. *Dev. Dyn.* **199**, 93–102.

Chen, W., Morriss-Kay, G.M. and Copp, A.J. (1995) Genesis and prevention of spinal neural tube defects in the *curly tail* mutant mouse: involvement of retinoic acid and its nuclear receptors RAR-beta and RAR-gamma. *Development* **121**, 681–691.

Clarke, J.D.W., Holder, N., Soffe, S.R. and Storm-Mathisen, J. (1991) Neuroanatomical and functional analysis of neural tube formation in notochordless *Xenopus* embryos: laterality of the ventral spinal cord is lost. *Development* **112**, 499–516.

Copp, A.J. and Bernfield, M. (1994) Etiology and pathogenesis of human neural tube defects: insights from mouse models. *Curr. Opin. Pediatr.* **6**, 624–631.

Copp, A.J., Brook, F.A., Estibeiro, J.P., Shum, A.S.W. and Cockroft, D.L. (1990) The embryonic development of mammalian neural tube defects. *Prog. Neurobiol.* **35**, 363–403.

D'Arcangelo, G., Miao, G.G., Chen, S.-C. et al (1995) A protein related to extracellular matrix proteins deleted in the mouse mutant *reeler*. *Nature* **374**, 719–723.

Davies, A.M. (1995) The bcl-2 family of proteins and the regulation of neuronal survival. *Trends Neurosci.* **18**, 355–358.

de Vries, J.I.P. (1992) The first trimester. In *Fetal Behaviour: Developmental and Perinatal Aspects.* (Ed.: J.E. Nijhuis), pp. 3–16. Oxford University Press: Oxford.

Dubois-Dauphin, M., Frankowski, H., Tsujimoto, Y., Huarte, J. and Martinou, J.-C. (1994) Neonatal motorneurons overexpressing the *bcl-2* protooncogene in transgenic mice are protected from axotomy-induced cell death. *Proc. Natl. Acad. Sci. USA* **91**, 3309–3313.

Echelard, Y., Epstein, D.J., St-Jacques, B. et al (1993) Sonic hedgehog, a member of a family of putative signaling molecules, is implicated in the regulation of CNS polarity. *Cell* **75**, 1417–1430.

Ellis, H.M. and Horvitz, H.R. (1986) Genetic control of programmed cell death in the nematode C. elegans. *Cell* **44**, 817–829.

Finkelstein, R. and Boncinelli, E. (1994) From fly head to mammalian forebrain: the story of *otd* and *Otx*. *Trends Genet.* **10**, 310–315.

Green, J.B.A. (1994) Roads to neuralness: embryonic neural induction as derepression of a default state. *Cell* **77**, 317–320.

Grove, E.A., Williams, B.P., Li, D.-Q. et al (1993) Multiple restricted lineages in the embryonic rat cerebral cortex. *Development* **117**, 553–561.

Guthrie, S. (1991) Horizontal and vertical pathways in neural induction. *Trends Neurosci.* **14**, 123–126.

Hockenbery, D.M., Oltvai, Z.N., Yin, X.-M., Milliman, C.L. and Korsmeyer, S.J. (1993) *Bcl-2* functions in an antioxidant pathway to prevent apoptosis. *Cell* **75**, 241–251.

Hunt, P. and Krumlauf, R. (1992) *Hox* codes and positional specification in vertebrate embryonic axes. *Annu. Rev. Cell Biol.* **8**, 227–256.

Hunt, P., Ferretti, P., Krumlauf, R. and Thorogood, P. (1995) Restoration of normal *Hox* code and branchial arch morphogenesis after extensive deletion of hindbrain neural crest. *Dev. Biol.* **168**, 584–597.

Joyner, A.L. (1991) Gene targeting and gene trap screens using embryonic stem cells: new approaches to mammalian development. *BioEssays* **13**, 649–656.

Kelly, O.G. and Melton, D.A. (1995) Induction and patterning of the vertebrate nervous system. *Trends Genet.* **11**, 273–278.

Marshall, H., Nonchev, S., Sham, M.H. et al (1992) Retinoic acid alters hindbrain *Hox* code and induces transformation of rhombomeres 2/3 into a 4/5 identity. *Nature* **360**, 737–741.

McMahon, A.P. and Bradley, A. (1990) The *Wnt-1* (*int-1*) proto-oncogene is required for development of a large region of the mouse brain. *Cell* **62**, 1073–1085.

Mullen, R.J. and Herrup, K. (1979) Chimeric analysis of mouse cerebellar mutants. In *Neurogenetics: Genetic Approaches to the Nervous System* (Ed.: X.O. Breakfield), pp. 173–196. Elsevier: New York.

Neale, S.A. and Trasler, D.G. (1994) Early sialylation on N-CAM in splotch neural tube defect mouse embryos. *Teratology* **50**, 118–124.

Office of Population Censuses and Surveys (1989) *The Prevalence of Disability Among Children.* Her Majesty's Stationery Office: London.

Oppenheim, R.W. (1991) Cell death during development of the nervous system. *Annu. Rev. Neurosci.* **14**, 453–501.

Pinto-Lord, M.C., Evrard, P. and Caviness, V.S., Jr (1982) Obstructed neuronal migration along radial glial fibers in the neocortex of the reeler mouse: a Golgi-EM analysis. *Dev. Brain Res.* **4**, 379–393.

Placzek, M., Tessier-Lavigne, M., Yamada, T., Jessell, T. and Dodd, J. (1990) Mesodermal control of neural cell identity: floor plate induction by the notochord. *Science* **250**, 985–988.

Rorke, L.B. (1994) The role of disordered genetic control of neurogenesis in the pathogenesis of migration disorders. *J. Neuropathol. Exp. Neurol.* **53**, 105–117.

Scherson, T., Serbedzija, G., Fraser, S. and Bronner-Fraser, M. (1993) Regulative capacity of the cranial neural tube to form neural crest. *Development* **118**, 1049–1061.

Serbedzija, G.N., Fraser, S. and Bronner-Fraser, M. (1990) Pathways of trunk neural crest cell migration in the mouse embryo as revealed by vital dye labelling. *Development* **108**, 605–612.

Sharpe, C.R. and Gurdon, J.B. (1990) The induction of anterior and posterior neural genes in Xenopus laevis. *Development* **109**, 765–774.

Swiatek, P.J. and Gridley, T. (1993) Perinatal lethality and defects in hindbrain development in mice homozygous for a targeted mutation of the zinc finger gene *Krox20*. *Genes Dev.* **7**, 2071–2084.

Tan, S.-S. and Breen, S. (1993) Radial mosaicism and tangential cell dispersion both contribute to mouse neocortical development. *Nature* **362**, 638–640.

Toivonen, S., Tarin, D. and Saxen, L. (1976) The transmission of morphogenetic signals from amphibian mesoderm to ectoderm in primary induction. *Differentiation* **5**, 49–55.

Van Straaten, H.W.M., Hekking, J.W.M., Consten, C. and Copp, A.J. (1993) Intrinsic and extrinsic factors in the mechanism of neurulation: effect of curvature of the body axis on closure of the posterior neuropore. *Development* **117**, 1163–1172.

Wald, N., Sneddon, J., Densem, J., Frost, C., Stone, R. and MRC Vitamin Study Research Group (1991) Prevention of neural tube defects: results of the Medical Research Council Vitamin Study. *Lancet* **338**, 131–137.

Walsh, C. and Cepko, C.L. (1993) Clonal dispersion in proliferative layers of developing cerebral cortex. *Nature* **362**, 632–635.

Wilkinson, D.G. (1993) Molecular mechanisms of segmental patterning in the vertebrate hindbrain and neural crest. *BioEssays* **15**, 499–505.

Yamada, T., Pfaff, S.L., Edlund, T. and Jessell, T.M. (1993) Control of cell pattern in the neural tube: motor neuron induction by diffusible factors from notochord and floor plate. *Cell* **73**, 673–686.

Yuasa, S., Kitoh, J., Oda, S. and Kawamura, K. (1993) Obstructed migration of Purkinje cells in the developing cerebellum of the reeler mutant mouse. *Anat. Embryol.* **188**, 317–329.

NOTE IN PROOF

Recently it was reported that *Sonic hedgehog* is a strong candidate for holoprosencephaly. The gene maps close to *HPE3* locus on chromosome 7q36 and harbours mutations in patients with autosomal dominant holoprosencephaly (Belloni et al 1996, *Nature Genet.* **14**, 353–356; Roessler et al 1996, *Nature Genet.* **14**, 357–360). Moreover, inactivation of *Sonic hedgehog* by gene targeting in the mouse causes a holoprosencephaly-like phenotype (Chiang et al 1996, *Nature* **383**, 407–413). Thus, a known inducer of neural patterning appears to be critically involved in forebrain induction.

9 The Gut and Enteric Nervous System

MICHÈLE KEDINGER[1] and DON NEWGREEN[2]

[1]INSERM unité 381, Strasbourg, France and [2]The Murdoch Institute, Royal Children's Hospital, Melbourne, Australia

The morphological and functional steady-state of the gut results from a complex interplay among various cell components. At the centre of this integrative system, epithelial and mesenchymal cells form the prime interactive unit, which is further regulated by hormonal, immune and neural inputs. In the light of this complexity, it is not surprising that the development of the gut is correspondingly complex, with contributions from all three germ layers. Thus, the endoderm, splanchnic mesoderm and ectoderm supply the epithelial cells of the mucosa, mesenchymal cell types and neural components respectively.

Due to its permanent and rapid epithelial cell renewal, the gut represents a fascinating model of dynamic cell biology, in which the involvement of cell communications has to be considered not only during development but also in the adult organ. This chapter focuses on the main features of gut morphogenesis and innervation as well as proliferation, migration and phenotypic differentiation in the mature epithelium. These events are fundamental in normal mucosal physiology and are the main targets in many pathological states. Emphasis will be directed successively on (1) the formation of the endodermal–mesenchymal cell assemblages necessary to generate form and cytodifferentiation, and (2) the establishment of the intrinsic nervous system of the gut by cell migration and differentiation. Both of these are mediated by adhesive and other interactions between the cells and the extracellular microenvironment.

The extracellular milieu consists of a dynamic and developmentally regulated assemblage of a variety of interacting molecules. Some of them are located at the interface between epithelial and mesenchymal-derived cells and are capable of directing specific cell behaviour; their regulation plays a key role in the maintenance of the steady-state of the main morphological and functional properties of the gut. Others form the ground substance of the connective tissue and are implicated in the morphogenetic steps and in the migration, homing and differentiation of the neural cells. This provides an introduction to a discussion of the major developmental defect of the enteric nervous system (ENS), Hirschsprung's disease, in humans and phenotypically similar regional intestinal aganglionoses of developmental origin in animals. How will current knowledge on cell interactions and on extracellular matrix molecules in the developing gut

Embryos, Genes and Birth Defects. Edited by P. Thorogood.
© 1997 John Wiley & Sons Ltd.

help the understanding of pathological states affecting this organ? This question will be approached by illustrating more particular examples.

MAIN CHARACTERISTICS OF THE ADULT GUT

THE INTESTINAL WALL

The mucosa

The functional element of the small intestinal mucosa consists of the **crypt–villus unit** (Figure 9.1) lined by a simple epithelium that is in direct contact with the luminal content. The structural support of the villi is provided by a connective tissue layer, the **lamina propria**. The variety of elements present in the lamina propria (blood and lymph vessels, nerve fibres, smooth muscle cells and fibroblasts) reflects its involvement in numerous important functions. The intestinal epithelium is separated from the lamina propria by a continuous basement membrane.

The small intestinal epithelium is a highly differentiated structure whose constituent cells display complex morphological specialization suitable for the large range of specific intestinal functions (Figure 9.1). It contains four principal terminally differentiated cell types: **absorptive**, **goblet**, **endocrine** and **Paneth cells**. Absorptive cells or enterocytes represent the main cell type of the intestinal epithelium (90%). They are characterized by the presence at their luminal surface of a microvillous brush border, possessing integral membrane digestive hydrolases and transporters which are involved in the final phases of nutrient digestion and absorption. They are sustained by a sophisticated cytoskeletal core. The folding of the apical membrane enhances dramatically the apical surface directly involved in active absorption. The goblet cells (c. 6%) are filled with mucus granules in the apical cytoplasm and are supposed to play a protective role in the epithelium. Various endocrine cells are characterized by basally located secretory granules containing neurohormonal peptides. Owing to their dual localization to both endocrine cells and the ENS, these neuropeptides may display important functions in regulating intestinal absorption and secretion, blood flow and motility. Paneth cells, located at the base of the crypts, contain large supranuclear granules. The presence in the granules of lyzozyme, of immunoglobulins and of defensin-related gene products indicates that this cell type may be involved in the regulation of the intestinal microflora.

In contrast to the small intestine, the colon exhibits deep crypts and a luminal surface devoid of villi (Figure 9.1). Furthermore, goblet cells represent the predominant cell type of the colonic crypt epithelium, absorptive cells being essentially located in the flat surface epithelium. These colonocytes do not express the digestive brush border molecules characteristic of the small intestinal absorptive cells, but are responsible for colonic water and electrolyte transport.

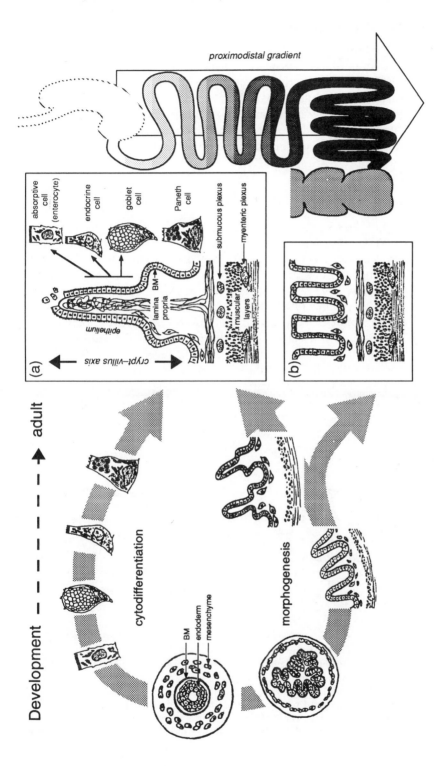

Figure 9.1 Main cytodifferentiative and morphogenetic events leading to maturation of the small intestine and colon. (a) Epithelial cytodifferentiation occurring during development, and along the crypt–villus axis in the adult small intestine. (b) Colon. The morphological and functional proximodistal gradient of the small intestine and colon is shown. BM, basement membrane

The submucosa and muscle layers

Along the small intestine as well as along the colon, a thin strip of smooth muscle cells, the muscularis mucosae, separates the mucosa from the submucosa, which is a loose connective tissue layer. The most external tissue layer of the gut consists of a continuous peripheral smooth muscle coat that extends over the whole length of the small and large bowel. It is composed of inner circular and outer longitudinal muscle layers which are mainly responsible for gastrointestinal peristalsis. They are also involved in the maintenance of the processes of digestion.

The ENS: structure and function

The ENS is by far the largest and most complex division of the autonomic nervous system (ANS) (Furness and Bornstein, 1995) and shows great autonomy from the central nervous system (CNS). This is due to a complete reflex circuitry, comprising sensory and intermediary as well as motor neurones (Wood, 1987), with few ENS neurones receiving any direct input from the CNS (Kirchgessner and Gershon, 1989). The ENS is laid out as numerous small interconnected ganglia in the **myenteric** (or Auerbach's) **plexus**, between the circular and longitudinal muscle coats of the gut and in the **submucous** (or Meissner's) **plexus**, internal to the circular muscle layer (Figure 9.2a). Many neurone types occur in the ENS, and these are not clustered but are mixed with other neurone types. The ENS supporting cells are also specialized and resemble the glia of the CNS rather than supporting cells elsewhere in the ANS (Gershon and Rothman, 1991). Regional differences in the ENS occur, with the number of

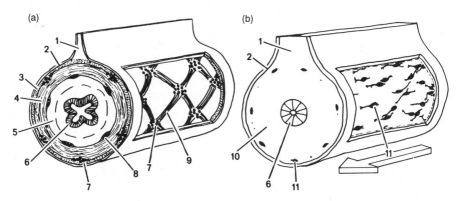

Figure 9.2 (a) The gut, shown at the end of organogenesis, is attached dorsally by the mesentery (1) and is covered by the serosal epithelium (2). Tissues arranged concentrically are longitudinal (3) and circular (4) smooth muscle, submucosa and lamina propria (5) and mucosal epithelium (6). The enteric nervous system (ENS) consists of the myenteric (7) and submucosal (8) ganglia, with interganglionic nerve fibres (9). (b) At early developmental stages the gut mesenchyme (10) is a relatively uniform layer. Neural crest (NC) derived ENS precursor cells (11) migrating in the arrowed direction occur close to the serosa (2). The vanguard NC cells are often single but the trailing cells quickly form a crude network

cells in the ganglia, the relative size of the myenteric and submucous plexus ganglia and the proportion of neurone types varying along the intestine.

EPITHELIAL CRYPT–VILLUS COMPARTMENTALIZATION AND THE CONCEPT OF INTESTINAL STEM CELLS

The adult tissue is endowed with an enormous capacity for proliferation and differentiation. Cell division is confined to the crypts; this proliferative zone derives from a resident stem cell population located near the base of the crypts. Several lines of evidence demonstrate that in the adult organ, the four main differentiated epithelial cell lineages derive from a common pluripotent crypt stem cell. Cell differentiation is bidirectional: while most phenotypes arise from cell migration and differentiation towards the apex of the villi, Paneth cells differentiate towards the bottom of the crypts. Each villus is surrounded by several crypts, and is composed of cells migrating out of these crypts. Ultrastructurally the differentiating cells can be visualized by the presence of intermediate cell phenotypes. Their functional maturation is characterized either by a progressive increase in the level of specific molecules, or by the turning on of specific genes which takes place at the crypt–villus junction. Additionally, a sequential expression of enteroendocrine products has been demonstrated in a population of upwardly migrating enteroendocrine cells. At the villus tip, the epithelial cells exfoliate into the intestinal lumen. The process of proliferation–migration and exfoliation takes 2–3 days in rodents, 5–6 days in humans. In contrast, Paneth cells are renewed at a significantly slower rate (c. 25 days). In the small intestine, there is a small percentage of crypts that do not appear to export cells to villi. These crypts may contain a population of facultative stem cells that may contribute to gut epithelium regeneration after injury.

Several techniques have led to significant advances during the last decade: namely, production of mouse chimeras by the aggregation of four- to eight-cell embryos from inbred strains varying in the expression of specific gut markers (Ponder et al, 1985; Schmidt et al, 1988), analysis of spontaneous or ethylnitrosourea-induced somatic mutations in such heterozygous mice (Winton and Ponder, 1990) and the creation of transgenic mice in which the transgene consists of the promoter regions of several fatty-acid binding proteins linked to a reporter gene (Cohn et al, 1991). (See reviews by Potten and Loeffler, 1990; Gordon et al, 1992; Kedinger 1994.)

THE ANTEROPOSTERIOR MORPHOLOGICAL AND FUNCTIONAL GRADIENT

The small intestine is not segmented but can be subdivided into three portions: the **duodenum**, which is the most proximal portion of the small intestine; the **jejunum**; and the **ileum**, which is terminated at the ileocaecal junction. Although the crypt–villus structures are found over the whole length of the small intestine, the villi exhibit a decreasing gradient in height and their shape is somewhat different at the various anteroposterior levels. The colon also consists of three anatomically and morphologically distinct portions, but the crypt architecture is maintained throughout its length.

Several cytodifferentiative features are worth noting:

(1)   One cell type is unique to the most proximal part of the duodenum; these cells are organized as small submucosal glands, the **Brünner's glands**, which originate as tubular downgrowth from the crypts and express a protein from the trefoil peptide family (Otto and Wright, 1994).

(2)   The number of goblet cells increases with the distal progression along the small intestine.

(3)   To date, as many as 16 types of endocrine cells have been identified in the human gastrointestinal tract, each with a specific regional distribution along the tract.

(4)   Specialized clusters of lymphoid aggregates, or **Peyer's patches**, are more prominent in the ileum. The associated epithelium overlying these aggregates is composed of M cells, specialized epithelial cells that transport luminal antigens, allowing access to immunocompetent cells.

(5)   Paneth cells are absent from the colon except from its most proximal part.

In addition to this morphological and cytological proximodistal gradient, there is a functional gradient that is paralleled by region-specific variations in the level or type of gene expression: digestive enzymes, or transporters of sugars, amino acids and vitamins, or intracellular molecules specific for the corresponding cell metabolisms. The genetic control of the anteroposterior gradient of differentiation in the gut is beginning to be explored. In this respect, it is important to note that several homeogenes exhibit peculiar proximodistal gradients of expression in the intestinal tract including the colon: *Cdx-1* presents a regular increasing gradient from the duodenum to the colon and *Hoxa-7* is expressed exclusively in the colon (James and Kazenwadel, 1991; Freund et al, 1992). Interestingly, an over-expression of *Hoxa-4* leads to developmental alterations of the colon (Tennyson et al, 1993; see later). These observations strongly suggest that the products of these genes function in cell fate specification in the developing gut. Furthermore, experiments conducted on fatty-acid binding proteins and sucrase-isomaltase gene promoters have already shown that multiple, nuclear, transacting factors believed to recognize various regions of the promoters may be involved in defining the spatial and temporal patterns of gene transcription (Gordon et al, 1992; Traber, 1994).

GUT MORPHOGENESIS AND CYTODIFFERENTIATION

INTESTINAL MORPHOGENESIS

The intestinal tube derives from the association of the embryonic endoderm with the splanchnic mesoderm. Although the overall processes involved in the ontogenic maturation of the gastrointestinal tract are closely similar in almost all animal species, the temporal patterns vary between them. In humans, the endoderm appears around the eighth day of gestation and rapidly forms the epithelial border of the digestive tract. It is surrounded at 15 days by the splanchnic mesoderm that will give rise to the connective tissue, muscle and serosal layers. The primitive gut is formed at 3 weeks; it is initially closed at both cranial and caudal regions, which open respectively at 4 and 9 weeks. Three distinct gut anlagen, the fore-, mid- and hindgut, will develop respectively into the duodenum, the major part of the small intestine and colon, and the distal colon. In rats, intestinal tube formation is initiated at 9 days of gestation.

At 8–10 weeks in the human fetus and 14–15 days in the rat, the intestinal tube is composed of an inner stratified endoderm comprising undifferentiated cells characterized by large nuclei and few cytoplasmic organelles. At the tiny lumen border, intercellular junctional complexes as well as rare irregular apical microvilli are obvious. At its basal surface, the deepest epithelial cell layer is delineated by a regular basement membrane which represents the endodermal–mesenchymal interface. The underlying mesenchymal cells are elongated and parallel to the basement membrane (Figure 9.1). From that stage onwards, a high level of cellular proliferative activity and an active tissue remodelling lead to the formation of villi and later of crypts. Villus outgrowth results from two distinct events that occur simultaneously: in the stratified epithelium, secondary lumens are formed which progressively fuse together and with the main lumen (Chen and Kataoka, 1991), and in the underlying mesenchyme, cuboidal cells accumulate at sites of presumptive protruding villus buds (Colony and Conforti, 1993). During fold formation, the presence at the surface of both epithelial and mesenchymal cells of numerous cytoplasmic processes extending towards the basement membrane emphasizes the role of epithelial–mesenchymal interactions in the morphogenesis and cellular differentiation of the developing gastrointestinal tract (see later). In the rat, differentiation of the circular and, with a slight delay, of the longitudinal muscle layers proceeds until the end of gestation. The muscularis mucosae can be seen only after birth and smooth muscle α-actin-expressing pericryptal fibroblasts become visible when the crypts are formed (Kedinger et al, 1990).

Between the newly formed villi, the formation of crypts results from an epithelial downgrowth into the mesenchyme, associated with a progressive restriction of the proliferative cells to the inter-villus regions. Crypt formation is achieved once villus morphogenesis is complete at around 15 weeks of gestation in humans and around birth in rodents. Before this stage, mitoses are distributed randomly within the stratified and subsequent simple epithelium (see Klein, 1989). It has been established (Schmidt et al, 1988; Winton and Ponder, 1990; Gordon et al, 1992) that the nascent crypts have a polyclonal origin; they become monoclonal by a mechanism of cell selection that is still not well understood. In addition, patches of adjacent crypts in the adult tissue derive from a common embryonic intestinal stem cell. Thus, progenitor cells that are present in the embryonic gut (at 7 days in mice) produce descendants that form the pluripotent stem cell population of adult crypts. The number of such progenitors increases during gut development whereas their proliferative potential becomes more restricted.

CYTODIFFERENTIATION IN THE DEVELOPING INTESTINE

The conversion of stratified into simple epithelium involves the formation of tight junctions which delineate two distinct membrane domains, assessed by the differential expression of molecules involved in the digestive function (i.e. enzymes and transporter proteins) at the luminal/apical side of the differentiating absorptive cells (Louvard et al, 1992). Concomitantly, different cell types emerge from the immature primitive cells that will differentiate chronologically (Figure 9.1): absorptive, goblet and endocrine cells. Following crypt formation, endocrine cells diversify and Paneth cells appear (Kedinger, 1994). Despite temporal differences between species, a clear parallelism between morphological and enzymatic differentiation has been regularly demonstrated. For instance, in the developing human small intestine, the first outgrowth of villi coincides with the appearance of detectable disaccharidase and peptidase activities. The progressive enhancement of the **apical brush borders** is accompanied by a concomitant increase in most enzyme activities up to 14 weeks. Most of the enzymatic changes that are seen during fetal life in humans occur postnatally in rodents. Drastic changes take place at weaning when the animals adapt from milk to solid food (Dauça et al, 1990; Henning et al, 1994). Indeed lactase, needed to hydrolyse lactose found in milk, is detectable in the rat intestine on day 18 of gestation, has its maximal activity at birth and then declines, reaching low levels after weaning. Among the digestive enzymes that are involved in digestion of solid food, some are increased and others begin to be expressed (sucrase-isomaltase) at weaning, when adult modes of digestion become fully operative.

The onset of morphological and functional maturation occurs in a proximodistal sequential pattern. The emergence of a functional regionalization along the small intestine is exemplified by the expression pattern of lactase. Lactase mRNA is expressed regularly over the whole length of the rat small intestine during the suckling period. Although it is still expressed in the jejunum after weaning, it disappears from the distal ileum (Duluc et al, 1993). In addition, lactase expression in the proximal region of the gut is patchy: it is expressed in a restricted number of cell islets interspersed among non-expressing cells (Maiuri et al, 1992). The establishment of the proximodistal gradient during development results from an intrinsic programme for differentiation. Indeed, transplantation of fetal intestinal segments into chick embryos or nude mice shows that fetal rodent intestines taken after (Rubin et al, 1992), or even prior to, cytodifferentiation (Duluc et al, 1994) develop the appropriate jejuno-ileal gradient of villus height/crypt depth and express characteristic cell lineage specific markers. These intrinsic developmental properties do not preclude an additional functional regulation by hormones, nutrients, growth factors and neuropeptides (reviewed by Henning et al, 1994).

The morphological steps of colon development are closely similar to those described for the small intestine (Figure 9.1). However, it should be noted that, although the mature colon is characterized by deep glands and a flat surface epithelium, it exhibits a transient villus-phase during development. This phase is obvious during fetal life in humans (at 14–30 weeks), and during the first postnatal week in rodents. These villi are covered by polarized cells that express small intestinal-type enzymes like sucrase-isomaltase in the human fetal colon and lactase in the postnatal rat colon (Lacroix et al, 1984; Menard and Pothier, 1987; Foltzer-Jourdainne et al, 1989). Concomitant with the onset of the adult colonic structure and function, the expression of these enzymes is turned off.

INFLUENCE OF EPITHELIAL–MESENCHYMAL INTERACTIONS

Close contacts between endodermal and mesenchymal cells in the fetal intestine, and between crypt epithelial cells and myofibroblastic cells in the adult organ, have been reported. These observations point to the potential role of such heterologous cell communications in (1) directing morphogenesis and associated cytodifferentiation, and (2) the maintenance of the steady-state of the adult crypt stem cells (Valentich and Powell, 1994).

The role of epithelial–mesenchymal cell interactions in such processes has been studied using various types of interspecies or heterotopic embryonic tissue associations (Figure 9.3). The main conclusions of such experiments have been reviewed by Haffen et al (1989) and Yasugi (1993); several conclusions relating to the gut can be drawn:

(1) Each of the intestinal endodermal and mesenchymal tissue components exerts permissive effects on the development of its associated counterpart. Interspecies chick/rodent epithelial–mesenchymal associations have been established experimentally. Their development as intracoelomic grafts leads to chimeric intestines which exhibit a morphogenetic pattern similar to that of the species from which the mesenchyme was taken, and an epithelial functional cytodifferentiation which is that of the species from which the endoderm was derived (Kedinger et al, 1981). Also, in xenograft experiments using tissue recombinants composed of endodermal and mesodermal segments originating from different positions along the anteroposterior axis of rat fetal small intestine, the endoderm of the chimeric intestines develops its own functional cytodifferentiation characteristics (Duluc et al, 1994).

(2) Endodermal–mesenchymal contacts are required to allow the expression of their reciprocal permissive interactions. Most experiments demonstrate that intestinal epithelial or mesenchymal anlagen are unable to differentiate in vitro or in vivo unless heterologous cellular contacts are achieved (Kedinger et al, 1987; Takiguchi-Hayashi and Yasugi, 1990). However, it has recently been reported that late fetal intestinal cells immortalized with the thermolabile SV40 T-antigen gene exhibit some differentiation characteristics when they are under non-permissive growth temperature conditions (Paul et al, 1993).

(3) Morphological integrity of the endoderm or mesenchyme is not required for morphogenesis (in vivo grafts) and/or differentiation (in vivo/in vitro) of both cell components. This is exemplified in vitro by the ability of

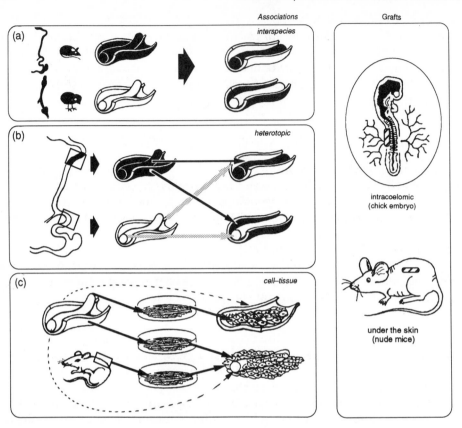

Figure 9.3 Experimental strategies used to analyse both the nature and properties of epithelial–mesenchymal interactions in the gut and the establishment of the subepithelial basement membrane. (a) *Interspecies associations*: the endoderm is dissociated mechanically from the mesenchyme after a 1-hour collagenase treatment of intestinal anlagen taken from E14-rat (or E12-mouse) fetuses or 5-day chick embryos. (b) *Heterotopic associations* are composed of cross-associations of the dissociated endoderm and mesenchyme from the proximal jejunum, the distal ileum and the colon (not indicated). (c) *Cell–tissue associations* comprise either an intact mesenchyme or an intact endoderm combined to the complementary tissue anlage as a cultured cell sheet. Skin fibroblastic cells were also analysed. The various associations are cultured overnight on a gel enriched in 10% chick embryonic extract, to ensure cohesion of the tissues, before grafting either into the coelomic cavity of 3-day chick embryos, or under the skin of nude mice, depending on the subsequent use. The two hosts offer a different hormonal environment and a different time-period for the development of the grafts (10–13 days in chick embryos, up to 8 weeks in nude mice)

layered-mesenchymal and endodermal co-cultures to express respectively smooth-muscle actin and apically located digestive enzymes (Figure 9.4). The development, as intracoelomic grafts, of endoderms associated with sheets of cultured mesenchymal cells, or conversely of cultured endodermal cells with intact mesenchymes, leads to well-organized and functionally active intestinal structures (Kedinger et al, 1986, 1990).

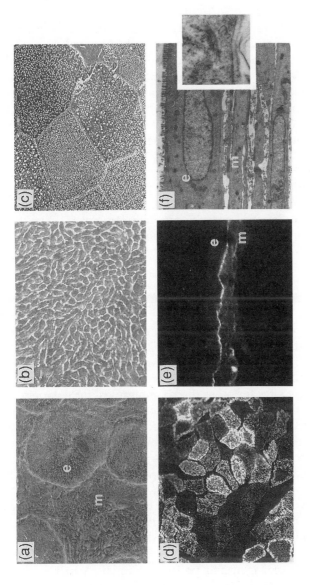

Figure 9.4 Co-cultures of 14-day fetal rat intestinal endodermal microexplants on top of a confluent layer of mesenchymal cells (Kedinger et al, 1987). (a), (b) Living cells photographed after 24 h and 4 days in culture. (c)–(f) illustrate various aspects of the co-cultures after 4 days. (c) Scanning electron micrograph of the apical surface of polarized epithelial cells. (d) Apical immunocytochemical localization of lactase. (e) Immunocytochemical localization of laminin at the epithelial/mesenchymal interface on a transverse cryosection of the co-culture. (f) Ultrastructural aspect of the co-culture and higher magnification (inset) of the basement membrane underneath the epithelial cell layer. e, epithelial cells; m, mesenchymal cells

(4)   Inductive interactions have also been demonstrated in various types of tissue association developed after transplantation; they concern: (a) the ability of the jejunal or ileal mesenchyme to induce fetal rat colonic endoderm to turn on a small intestinal-type enzymatic differentiation (Foltzer-Jourdainne et al, 1989; Duluc et al, 1994). This observation is of particular importance given the peculiar expression of small intestinal-like phenotypes in colonic cancer cells; (b) the same inductive action of gut mesenchyme on avian gizzard endoderm, which changes its morphological and cytodifferentiation pattern (Haffen et al, 1989); (c) an inductive potency of the intestinal endoderm towards the surrounding mesenchymally derived cell layer, which is demonstrated by its ability to induce skin fibroblastic cells to form subnormal peripheral muscle and inner lamina propria-like layers (Kedinger et al, 1990).

(5)   Functional epithelial–mesenchymal cell interactions are maintained in the mature gut. Indeed postnatal primary crypt cell cultures and, to a lesser extent, crypt cell lines can be induced by fetal mesenchyme to achieve complete cytodifferentiation together with villous morphogenesis (Kedinger et al, 1986). On the other hand, cell cultures established from postnatal intestinal lamina propria are able to direct (like the fetal mesenchyme) an intestine-like differentiation of avian gizzard endoderm (Haffen et al, 1983).

THE EXTRACELLULAR MATRIX: A POTENTIAL MEDIATOR OF EPITHELIAL–MESENCHYMAL INTERACTIONS

The basal pole of the intestinal endoderm or epithelium is in contact with specialized extracellular matrix (ECM) molecules assembled to form the basement membrane (BM), at the epithelial–mesenchymal interface. ECM molecules (over fifty different proteins) are composed of many domains and each has multiple binding sites for other matrix molecules, for a variety of other molecules such as growth factors and, most importantly, for cells. In the last 15 years, increasing attention has been directed towards the composition, deposition and role of the ECM in various organs; ECM molecules are considered as dynamic effectors in morphogenesis and in the generation and maintenance of epithelial cell polarity (e.g. Howlett and Bissell, 1993; Ingber, 1993). This exoskeleton interacts with cell surface receptors such as integrins, which transduce information from the cell environment to the intracellular compartment (Hynes, 1992; Sastry and Horwitz, 1993).

The **intestinal subepithelial BM** has been shown to contain the major ubiquitous components found in BM of various other tissues: laminin-1, entactin/nidogen, type IV collagen and perlecan (Simon-Assmann et al, 1986, 1989, 1995; Beaulieu et al, 1991). The properties of these molecules as well as their potential assembly have been reported by Timpl (1989) and Paulsson (1992). In addition, the ground substance of the intestinal stroma comprises mainly fibrillar collagens (types I and III), fibronectin and tenascin. Proteoglycans, composed of protein cores appended to which are various types of sulphated glycosaminoglycans (GAGs), and the unsulphated GAG, hyaluronan, have also been identified (Simon-Assmann et al, 1995).

In parallel to the observation that isolated intestinal endodermal cells (or, more generally, non-transformed intestinal epithelial cells) are unable to differentiate in vitro unless they are in close contact with mesenchymally derived cells, it is worth noting that an organized deposition of BM molecules is achieved only in co-culture conditions (Figure 9.4). Immunocytochemical data, using double-labelling of BM molecules and of epithelial differentiation markers, point to the potential importance of the BM molecular organization at the epithelial–mesenchymal interface for differentiation processes, according to a precise chronology: (1) heterologous cell contacts; (2) polarized BM molecule deposition at the epithelial–mesenchymal interface; (3) epithelial cell polarization and differentiation (Simon-Assmann et al, 1988; Kedinger et al, 1989).

Concerning the two first steps, the construction of interspecies (rodent/avian) hybrid intestines, in which the origin of BM molecules can be traced with species-specific antibodies, confirms the importance of heterologous cell contacts in the elaboration of the BM. Indeed, the subepithelial BM has been shown to be composed of molecules deposited either by the epithelial or by the mesenchymal cells, or by both, according to the constituent (Figure 9.5). Furthermore, interesting changes in their cellular origin can be observed as a function of the development of the hybrids; for example: (1) **type IV collagen** is mostly produced by the mesenchyme, except at the earliest stages of development of the hybrids, when epithelial cells also contribute to its deposition; (2) the constituent **laminin α1** chain is mostly deposited by the epithelial cells, but also by mesenchyme at the later stages of development of the hybrid intestines (Simon-Assmann et al, 1990b; Simon-Assmann and Kedinger, 1993).

The involvement of BM molecules in epithelial differentiation has been demonstrated by the fact that expression of apical hydrolases can be blocked by adding anti-laminin antibodies to the co-culture medium (Simo et al, 1992). Similarly, by using monoclonal antibodies directed against various epitopes of laminin chains, it has been shown that the COOH-terminal end (E3 fragment) of the α1 chain directs epithelial cell polarization during kidney organogenesis (Klein et al, 1988). In current experiments, De Arcangelis et al (1996) have blocked expression of the laminin α1 chain in the colonic cancer cell line Caco2 by stable transfection of an antisense cDNA. The α1-deficient clones exhibit altered differentiation properties and do not allow the establishment of a normal BM in co-cultures.

The physiological expression of the α1 chain of laminin in the developing and mature human intestine is also of interest: (1) at the earliest embryonic stages studied it is found exclusively at the endodermal–mesenchymal interface; (2) this restricted localization is maintained during the phase of villus protrusion; (3) in the mature intestine a gradient of expression is obvious: laminin α1 chain is present at the BM level along the villi but is absent from the crypts. Even more interesting is the fact that an isoform of laminin, in which the α1 chain is replaced by the α2 chain (merosin or laminin-2), displays a complementary expression pattern, with a restricted localization in the crypt BM (Beaulieu and

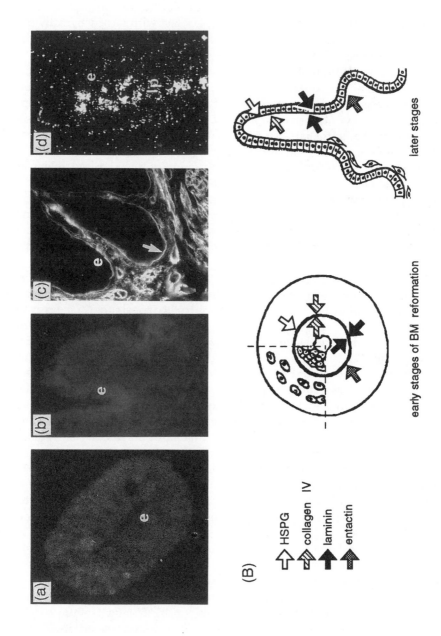

Vachon, 1994; Simon-Assmann et al, 1994). In addition, first expression of laminin-2 occurs only when crypts develop: at 15–17 weeks of gestation in human small intestine and around birth in mouse (Simon-Assmann et al, 1994).

These observations, as far as the $\alpha 1$ chain is concerned, fit with a role for this molecule in epithelial cell polarization. The potential role of the $\alpha 2$ chain in the maintenance of an extracellular microenvironment specific to the crypt stem cell niche or proliferative cells was analysed in a mutant $\alpha 2$-deficient (dy/dy) mouse. The fact that dy mice, mainly characterized by a severe muscular dystrophy (Xu et al, 1994), die prematurely could be linked to intestinal abnormalities. However, this assumption has not been confirmed since these mutants have an apparently normal intestine as far as the gross morphology, and cytodifferentiation are concerned (Simon-Assmann et al, 1994). This observation means either that the $\alpha 2$ laminin chain does not act on the maintenance of the crypt steady-state, or that replacement pathways can occur. This might be the case in the dy/dy mouse intestine in which, in contrast to the human organ, the $\alpha 1$ laminin chain is also found in the crypt BM.

Finally, two other ECM molecules, **hyaluronan** and **tenascin**, are of relevance. Changes have been reported in the amount of hyaluronan expressed and in the localization of tenascin along the crypt–villus axis during development; moreover, both molecules have been reported to be abnormal in pathological situations (see later). Hyaluronan is a large, polyanionic, unsulphated GAG produced at a high rate by the intestinal tissue during fetal development. In parallel, the sulphated GAGs are found to be under- or un-sulphated. After birth, these processes are reversed: there is a drastic decrease in the production of hyaluronan and an increase in the degree of sulphation of the other GAGs (Bouziges et al, 1991). In physiological terms, the fetal hyaluronan-rich extracellular environment could allow plasticity, cell movements and tissue remodelling. This fits with the finding that hyaluronan receptors are present at the basolateral surface of dividing epithelial cells (Alho and Underhill, 1989). Furthermore, the huge size of hyaluronan molecules could prevent the accessibility to the cell of other ECM molecules involved in cell

---

Figure 9.5 Cellular origin of basement membrane (BM) molecules. (A) Origin of type IV collagen: the experimental design consists of the construction of interspecies hybrid intestines (see Figure 9.3), composed in this case of chick mesenchyme and rat endoderm. (a)–(c) Immunodetection of type IV collagen with antibodies directed against rodent antigens (a, b) or against chick antigens (c). (a) Rat endoderm separated from the mesenchyme after collagenase treatment: there are no residual collagen molecules. (b), (c) Hybrid intestine developed in the coelom of a chick embryo for 13 days: only the antibodies that cross-react with the species from which the mesenchyme is derived (chick) decorate the BM (c; arrow). (d) The mesenchymal origin of this molecule is also confirmed by in situ hybridization: the transcripts are confined to the mesenchymally derived lamina propria (Simon-Assmann et al, 1990a). e, endoderm or epithelium; lp, lamina propria. (B) Cellular origin of several BM molecules determined using the strategy of interspecies chimeric intestines: early stages of BM reformation (4 days) and during villus outgrowth (13 days after grafting). HSPG, heparan sulphate proteoglycan. Arrows indicate the epithelial and/or mesenchymal origin of the BM molecules found at the epithelial/mesenchymal interface

polarization/differentiation (Gallagher, 1989). Tenascin, a hexameric glycoprotein, is found to be expressed in the mature intestine, with an increasing gradient from the base to the tip of the villi. Although tenascin is a connective tissue ECM molecule, it is concentrated just beneath the epithelial cells. This peculiar expression gradient, together with the fact that tenascin disturbs the adhesion of epithelial cells to their ECM substrate in vitro, suggests that this molecule plays a physiological role in the shedding of epithelial cells from the villus tip (Probstmeier et al, 1990).

DEVELOPMENT OF THE ENTERIC NERVOUS SYSTEM

EMBRYONIC ORIGIN OF THE ENS: THE NEURAL CREST

The neural crest (NC) arises on the dorsal midline of the neural tube (Figure 9.6b), and gives rise to pigment cells and cranio-facial connective tissues as well as nervous tissues (reviewed by Newgreen, 1992). The origin of the ENS was linked to the NC in a series of in-ovo microsurgical ablations of the dorsal neural primordium (i.e. NC plus immediately adjacent neural tube) of chicken embryos (Yntema and Hammond, 1954). After allowing time for the enteric neurones to become normally recognizable histologically (the only means available at the time), the ENS in NC-ablated embryos failed to develop in gut that was otherwise normal. This provided strong, but not totally compelling, evidence that the avian ENS, like the rest of the ANS, is of NC origin. Using *Xenopus*, transplantation of the neural folds (i.e. NC with only slight inclusion of neural tube) between two related species has resulted in development in host embryos of an ENS whose cells are of the fold-donor species (Epperlein et al, 1990). Thus, the entire ENS in all vertebrates stems from NC cells, which migrate to the gut in a remarkably conservative development programme (Newgreen, 1992). The NC, however, stretches along the entire body axis; identifying the precise regions that give rise to the ENS has proven remarkably difficult, and has generated controversy which has impacted on ideas about the aetiology of Hirschsprung's disease.

Unitary origin of the ENS: the vagal NC

Yntema and Hammond (1954) noted a total loss of the enteric neurones when a hindbrain NC region termed the vagal level, between the otocyst and somite 8, was ablated, whereas ablations outside this region (Yntema and Hammond, 1955) left the ENS undisturbed (see Figure 9.6a). These studies indicated that enteric neuronogenic potential is normally confined to the vagal level, and that consequently vagal NC cells must populate the viscera in a unidirectional rostrocaudal wave (Yntema and Hammond, 1954). Recently, smaller scale ablations (Peters-van der Sanden et al, 1993a) and cell labelling (Epstein et al, 1994) have suggested that the NC between somites 3 and 6 has particular importance for ENS development.

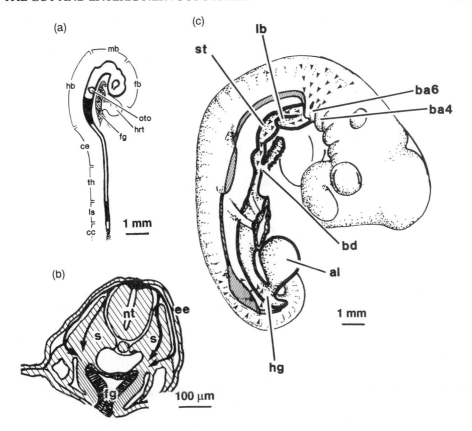

Figure 9.6 (a) Axial levels of the vertebrate neural tube (heavily outlined structure) of a 2-day chicken embryo. fb, forebrain; mb, midbrain; hb, hindbrain; ce, cervical; th, thoracic; ls, lumbosacral; cc, coccygeal. The enteric nervous system is derived from the vagal neural crest (NC) from the hindbrain caudal to the ear vesicle or otocyst (oto), from the immediate post-vagal NC and from the lumbosacral NC. These levels are indicated by solid black. Note the relatively rostral position of the foregut (fg) and heart (hrt) at these stages. (b) Pathways of NC cell migration (arrows) from the dorsal neural tube (nt) to the foregut (fg) mesenchyme (double-hatched) are shown at the vagal level (somite 5) of a 1.75-day chicken embryo. A ventral pathway leads through the somitic mesenchyme (s), and a dorsolateral pathway follows the cell-free space between the epidermal ectoderm (ee) and the somite. (c) Chicken embryo at about 4 days incubation, with the body wall removed to show the gut (heavily outlined structure). Migrating NC cells (arrowheads) from the vagal region moving through branchial arches 4 and 6 (ba4, ba6) and the post-branchial region have populated the lung bud (lb), oesophagus, stomach (st) and duodenum to the bile ducts (bd). Lumbosacral NC cells have just entered the hindgut (hg) near the stalk of the allantois (al)

The rostrocaudal sequence of colonization of the chicken intestine by neurone precursors has been deduced from gut segments grown in isolation by grafting to the chorioallantoic membrane of a host embryo, followed by histological assessment for the presence or absence of ENS neurones (Allan and Newgreen, 1980). The results indicated a sole rostral source of ENS neurone precursors, consistent with a vagal origin. Further evidence for a rostrocaudal wave of immigration was provided by transecting the intestine of chicken embryos in ovo (Meijers et al, 1989), after which the gut caudal to the transect failed to develop ENS ganglia. A single rostrocaudal order of appearance of ENS neuroblasts has also been deduced, using the growth-in-isolation technique, by grafting to the kidney capsule in mice (Southwell, 1982; Nishijima et al, 1990; Kapur et al, 1992) as well as in rats (Cass et al, 1992).

Many studies on the sequence of appearance of endogenous markers for NC cells or neurones have indicated a unidirectional rostrocaudal progression. In principle, the most reliable, from the viewpoint of origin and progress of precursor cells, would be those that focus on stem NC characters rather than on differentiation markers. Such studies have been reported in Aves (Tucker et al, 1986) and rats (Newgreen and Hartley, 1995) using the HNK-1 (or identical NC-1) monoclonal antibody, which with certain caveats labels migrating NC cells. These studies describe a single rostrocaudal sequence, but a methodologically identical study by Pomeranz and Gershon (1990) detected an additional caudorostral wave (see below).

Unidirectional appearance of differentiation markers in humans, mice and chickens (e.g. Okamoto and Ueda, 1967; Webster, 1973; Allan and Newgreen, 1980; Kapur et al, 1992; Fairman et al, 1995) must be interpreted cautiously, since at best they give an outside limit for the NC migration sequence and timetable in the gut simply because terminal differentiation need not follow precursor immigration by any consistent time lag. Even with the HNK-1 antibody, detailed comparison shows that the timetable in bird embryos is delayed relative to the results of the growth-in-isolation experiments of Allan and Newgreen (1980) and, the further caudal in the gut, the greater the delay.

Dual origin of the ENS: the vagal and lumbosacral NC

Cell labelling is, in principle, the most exact means of tracing the origins of the ENS. It has been accomplished by transplanting equivalent regions of the neural primordium (neural tube plus NC) between chicken and quail embryos (Le Douarin and Teillet, 1973), since the cells of the two species are histologically distinguishable but developmentally compatible. This confirmed the vagal origin of ENS cells throughout the intestine and gave a rostrocaudal migration timetable matched exactly by that of Allan and Newgreen (1980). Likewise, the cervicothoracic NC (i.e. caudal to the vagal level) was reported as not contributing to the ENS (but see below). However, the lumbosacral level (in birds, caudal to somite 28) also gave labelled cells in the ENS caudal to the umbilicus (Figure 9.6a). This showed that the rostral gut has a single vagal source for its ENS; the caudal gut, a dual source; and implied that there are rostrocaudal and caudorostral waves of colonization (Figure 9.6c). This has been confirmed using microinjection of cell marker dyes and viral probes in chicken and mouse embryos (Pomeranz et al, 1991a; Serbedzija et al, 1991). The initial number of lumbosacral cells was, however, small in comparison with the vagal invasion (Serbedzija et al, 1991), and the time of initial colonization was earlier than originally reported by Le Douarin and Teillet (1973).

Growth-in-isolation of mouse embryonic hindgut in organ culture has indicated the presence of neurone precursors as early as embryonic day 9 (E9), before the presumed immigration of the vagal cells, thus implying a closer source, the sacral NC (Rothman and Gershon, 1982). This conflicts with the kidney capsule growth-in-isolation experiments (see above) of Southwell (1982), Nishijima et al (1990), Cass et al (1992) and Kapur et al (1992). Nishijima et al (1990), who detected no neuronal differentiation in hindgut isolated at E9, found the growth and differentiation of the grafted intestine approached normal only with the kidney capsule technique and suggested that the organ culture method allowed NC cells to develop neuronal characteristics that would normally be suppressed. Artefactual expression of a neuronal phenotype in gut-related tissues in vitro has been described elsewhere (Teitelman, 1990). Alternatively, since Serbedzija et al (1991) report that lumbosacral NC cells enter the hindgut at about E10, it is possible that the neurones in these E9 grafts represent contamination with juxta-intestinal pelvic plexus neuroblasts.

Several studies on the sequence of appearance of endogenous markers for ENS cells have reported bidirectional waves. The most significant of these is the HNK-1 immunolabelling of chicken embryos (Pomeranz and Gershon, 1990). Here a very large number of labelled cells extended rostrally from the cloaca, to meet the caudally moving, vagal-derived cells. Interestingly, these cells contrasted with the vagal ENS precursors in that they did not co-express neuronal markers. Since the specificity of HNK-1 for NC cells is not absolute (Newgreen et al, 1990), at least some of these labelled cells may be gut mesenchyme cells (Meijers et al, 1989), especially given the numerical disparity compared with the few cells revealed by labelling studies (Serbedzija et al, 1991). It is not clear why these cells were undetected by Tucker et al (1986), who used the same antibody and specimen preparation techniques.

Triple origin of the ENS: the vagal, lumbosacral and post-vagal neural crest

The ENS in the oesophagus differentiates surprisingly late (Fairman et al, 1995) in Aves, and involves few vagal NC-derived cells (Epstein et al, 1994) despite the proximity of the foregut to the vagal level of the NC. In addition ablation of the entire vagal NC in Aves (Peters-van der Sanden et al, 1993a) left a residual ENS in the foregut. Likewise in the mouse, genetic knockouts of the gene for the cell surface receptor, *ret* (see later), which predominantly affects vagal derivatives, resulted in the loss of the ENS except in the foregut (Durbec et al, 1996). Cell labelling in mice gave confirming evidence that a trunk-level (i.e. non-vagal) region of the NC contributes some of the foregut ENS, but not the ENS elsewhere (Durbec et al, 1996). This additional source is in the NC immediately caudal to the vagal level, but neither its quantitative importance nor its qualitative role as to types of neurones provided is settled.

Origin of the ENS: conclusion

The most economical explanation of the conflicting opinions on the origin of the ENS hinges on techniques. In general, the proponents of the vagal-only view used methods that revealed neurones, while those proposing other origins used techniques that revealed crest cells of any differentiation pathway. Thus, the vagal NC gives rise to, and is the most important source of, ENS neurones and support cells throughout the gut in mammals, birds and amphibians. Early studies ruled out a contribution to the ENS by NC between the vagal and lumbosacral levels, but recently more detailed studies have revealed that this level of the NC provides some of the ENS, including neurones, but only in the foregut. The lumbosacral NC gives rise to ENS support cells in the post-umbilical intestine, but its contribution to neurones is probably slight and/or delayed. Nevertheless, the contributions of all these sources in terms of cell types and numbers need to be established in detail. The idea that although there are two sources for ENS cells in the caudal gut, yet only the rostral (i.e. vagal) source is obligatory, simplifies interpretation of the causes of Hirschsprung's disease (see later).

ENS PRECURSOR CELL MIGRATION

In the region of the vagal-level somites, two pathways from the NC to the gut potentially exist: a dorsolateral route in cell-free ECM between the epidermis and the somites, and a ventral route percolating through the sclerotomal mesenchyme of the somites (Figure 9.6b). In birds, NC cells are found in both, but most migrate through the somites (Kuritani and Kirby, 1991). Most NC cells in birds reach the foregut just caudal to the branchial arches, with some passing through branchial arches 6 and 4 (Tucker et al 1986; Phillips et al, 1987; Lumsden et al, 1991; and see Figure 9.6c). Once near the foregut, NC cells form left and right strands which foreshadow the route of vagal axons (Tucker et al, 1986), but do not immediately invade nearby foregut mesenchyme. The foregut gives rise to the gut down to the duodenum and, given the compressed scale of the gut compared to the neural axis at these early developmental stages (Figure 9.6a), vagal NC cells require virtually no longitudinal movement to reach the gut down to the level of the bile ducts. Caudal to the developing duodenum, vagal NC cells migrate longitudinally within the gut mesenchyme itself, typically favouring the region close to the serosal surface (Figure 9.2b), the vanguard advancing at a rate of 40 µm/h (Allan and Newgreen, 1980). The NC cells behind this vanguard are found immediately outside the presumptive circular muscle layer (Tucker et al, 1986), i.e. already in position to form the myenteric plexus. Cells are not seen at the submucous plexus site until later and it is not clear whether they derive, by a secondary migration, from local myenteric cells, or are a separate immigrant wave. Sacral NC cells migrate ventrally through the adjacent sclerotome before entering the hindgut at the cloaca, near the stalk of the allantois (Figure 9.6c), and migrating rostral in the gut mesenchyme layer (Pomeranz and Gershon, 1990).

   The timetable of rostrocaudal migration of vagal NC cells is substantially as indicated by Le Douarin and Teillet (1973) and Allan and Newgreen (1980) in chickens, and by Southwell (1982) in mice. The timetable of caudorostral migration by lumbosacral NC cells is as described by Pomeranz et al (1991a) and

Serbedzija et al (1991) for chicken and mouse embryos. In humans, the vagal timetable must be in advance of the histological observations of Okamoto and Ueda (1967), and the presumed sacral input timetable is unknown (Figure 9.7).

Role of microenvironmental properties in ENS precursor cell migration

NC cell distribution is, in general, strongly influenced by contacts with the microenvironment (Figure 9.8), which structurally consists of other cells (both mesenchyme and NC) and the ECM, the latter being the focus of most research (Newgreen, 1992). The ECM molecules fibronectin, laminin-1, tenascin and chondroitin sulphate proteoglycan occur near migrating NC cells in the intestine, but their distribution is far wider than that of NC cells (Tucker et al, 1986; Newgreen and Hartley, 1995), suggesting alternative or additional molecular controls are necessary to define migration pathways. Additional indicators of a role for ECM arise from *lethal spotting* (*ls*) mice, which have intestinal aganglionosis similar to Hirschsprung's disease (see later). Here a microenvironmental defect (Kapur et al, 1993; Rothman et al, 1993) curtails NC migration in the distal colon, which is associated with localized over-expression of ECM (Payette et al, 1988; Tennyson et al, 1990). If this abnormality prevents NC cell migration, the normal role of these ECM molecules may be to limit and refine crest migration pathways.

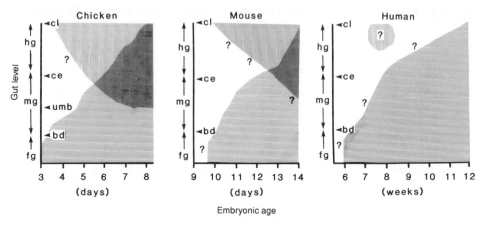

Figure 9.7 Timetables of entry of vagal (horizontal hatching) and lumbosacral (vertical hatching) neural crest (NC) cells into the foregut (fg), midgut (mg) and hindgut (hg) of chicken, mouse and human embryos. The unhatched region is aneural. Positional markers include the bile ducts (bd), umbilicus (umb), caeca (ce) and cloaca (cl). The vagal timetable in the human is imprecise, being based on histological identification of neurones of the enteric nervous system (ENS): a timetable of arrival of ENS precursors would be shifted slightly to the left of that presented. The slope of the lumbosacral timetable is imprecise in the chicken and mouse, and completely unknown in the human. The length of gut (*y*-axis), corrected for time of NC cell entry, is about 5–7 mm in all cases, suggesting that the rate of cell movement is very much slower in humans than in chickens and mice

The stage of gut development is also important for NC cell colonization, for two reasons. First, the gut tube at these stages is growing rapidly, especially in length. Any delay in the longitudinal spread of NC cells could be amplifed disproportionately, in terms of gut still to be populated, by this growth. Such an asynchrony has been suggested as being important in generating colonic aganglionosis in *piebald lethal* (s[l]) mice (Webster, 1973; and see later), a defect similar to Hirschsprung's disease in humans. Nevertheless, a detailed comparison of gut growth parameters with NC cell migration has not been made in human, rodent or bird embryos. Secondly, avian NC cell immigration is impaired, but not entirely prevented, when the recipient gut tissue is considerably older and more differentiated than normal (Meijers et al, 1989). Stage-dependent changes in gut tube morphology, cell differentiation and ECM deposition occur and in birds and rats this histodifferentiation proceeds rostrocaudally, to be met in the hindgut by a caudorostral wave of maturation (Allan and Newgreen, 1980; Newgreen and Hartley, 1995). This means that vagal NC cells in the small intestine migrate in a uniform mesenchyme, while further caudally they enter gut that is progressively more mature. Any delay in NC cell migration along normally differentiating gut could be exacerbated by the requirement to move through tissue more mature than normally encountered, as well as by the growth asynchrony discussed above.

Role of NC properties in ENS precursor cell migration

Intrinsic properties of NC cells are also important for migration (Newgreen, 1992), and there is some degree of regional NC specialization even prior to migration. Vagal NC cells in Aves can migrate to the gut even when grafted to an atypical location, unlike non-vagal NC cells (Le Douarin and Teillet, 1974), although the latter can reach the gut when grafted into the vagal NC site. This implies that, although microenvironmental pathways to the foregut occur at the vagal level, vagal NC cells have additional intrinsic mechanisms enabling them to reach their normal target from elsewhere. Chemotactic receptors for gut-derived attractor molecules have been proposed to exist on vagal NC cells by Le Douarin and Teillet (1974). Once in the gut, however, NC cells of all levels of origin can migrate to sites appropriate for ENS development (Le Douarin and Teillet, 1974; Smith et al, 1977; Newgreen et al, 1980), although they may not necessarily develop into appropriate cell types.

The size of the vagal NC population is also important, since gross reduction in cell numbers leads to a normal ENS in the rostral levels of the gut and a complete absence at caudal levels in chicken embryos (Yntema and Hammond, 1954), thus microsurgically mimicking Hirschsprung's disease in humans and aganglionosis in rodents. Since great increases in ENS precursor cell numbers occur during the colonization of the gut (Meijers et al, 1987), a similar outcome could be expected if cell numbers were subnormal during, as well as prior to, immigration. In other regions the first NC cells to migrate distribute themselves furthest (Serbedzija et al, 1991), so it is likely that this also occurs in the gut. This mode of distribution has been interpreted as being driven by NC population pressure via contact inhibition of locomotion, whereby contact between cells induces movement away from contact (Newgreen, 1992). This would also explain the negative effects of pre-existing ENS cells on the ability of exogenous ENS precursor cells to invade avian gut (Meijers et al, 1989). The ability of NC-derived cells in the avian gut to populate regions lacking such cells declines with developmental age, as shown by heterochronic tissue recombinations, but considerably later than the stage of normal cessation of migration (Meijers et al, 1989). This suggests that for a considerable time the ENS harbours cells sufficiently immature to be able to recapitulate early migration and differentiation events.

These studies, drawn from many models, suggest that Hirschsprung's disease could be generated by defects during and even prior to the NC migratory stage, and these could directly affect the NC cells themselves, or the milieu in which they migrate.

GROWTH AND DIFFERENTIATION OF ENS CELLS

ENS growth and differentiation before, during and after NC migration

The NC precursors show a gradual restriction of potentialities from an initial state in which, while heterogeneous in proliferative and differentiative potential, many cells are pluripotent. Even before migration, there is a pronounced bias in ENS-forming ability since avian vagal premigratory NC populations provided over 50 times as many neurones in co-cultured colon as did cervicothoracic and lumbosacral levels (Newgreen et al, 1980; Peters-van der Sanden et al, 1993b). This difference is probably due to superior growth and differentiation ability rather than immigration within the colon, since the last two levels provide NC cells to the position of the ENS where they differentiate mostly into ectopic melanocytes (Smith et al, 1977; Newgreen et al, 1980). This specialization of the vagal region may be related to the spatially restricted differential expression of various Hox genes along the hindbrain. This so-called Hox code is thought to specify different segment identities along the neural axis, involving both the CNS and the NC (Graham, 1992).

Migratory NC cells in the branchial arches have lost the potentiality to form melanocytes and dorsal root ganglion-type sensory neurones, a potential that is present in premigratory NC Cells (Ciment and Weston, 1985; Ito and Sieber-Blum, 1993). Equivalent restrictive changes in the differentiation potential of vagal NC cells can be expected en route prior to reaching the gut. Later still, cells localized in the stomach and intestine become progressively even more restricted, losing adrenergic neurone potentiality (Sextier-Sainte-Claire Deville et al, 1994). In contrast, the ability to produce SMP, a marker of non-ENS support cells, is not irrevocably lost: suppression of the synthesis of this protein seems to require constant inhibitory modulation within the normal ENS (Dulac and Le Douarin, 1993). The number of ENS support cells may also be modulated since contact with enteric neurones suppresses growth (Eccleston et al, 1989). Thus the number and cell types of enteric glia may be matched to those of the neurones, by a continuous interaction.

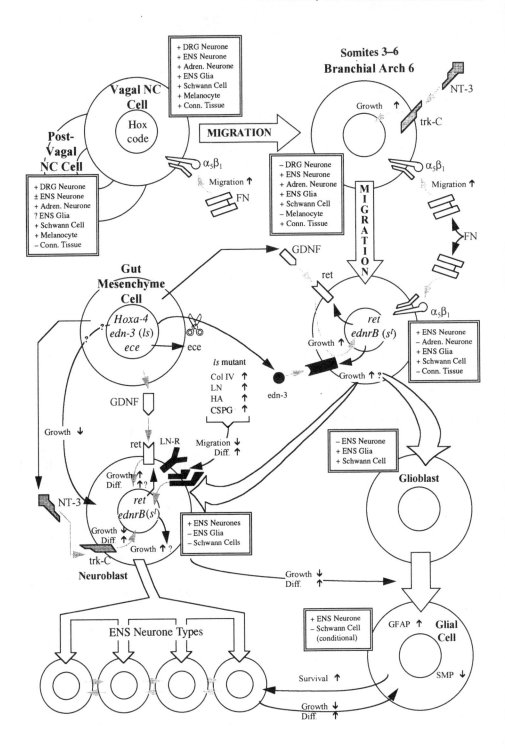

Role of the microenvironment in growth and differentiation of the ENS

The ENS population increases dramatically in size, during and after the migratory phase (Meijers et al, 1987) and this is controlled by the local gut environment as shown by tissue recombination grafts in birds (Smith et al, 1977; Newgreen et al, 1980). The pattern of ENS differentiation also seems to be linked to the local microenvironment, as tissue recombination experiments also show (Smith et al, 1977). Differentiation of the NC cells at any point in the gut into various classes of ENS neurones and support cells occurs in a distinct but overlapping sequence (Pham et al, 1991). Superimposed on this is a graded sequence along the length of the gut, some differentiation markers showing a unidirectional sequence, but others showing a bidirectional wave. In addition, different levels of the gut vary dramatically in their ability to induce or support ENS differentiation. Cervicothoracic NC, for example, can form ENS in the foregut (Le Douarin and Teillet, 1974; Durbec et al, 1996), but not the hindgut (Newgreen et al, 1980).

Figure 9.8 Summary of major events thought to be involved in the migration, growth and differentiation of vagal neural crest (NC) cells into the enteric nervous system (ENS). The development of the ENS exhibits a multitude of cell interactions to regulate growth, migration and differentiation of the neural cells in relation to their mesenchymal surroundings. Migration may be controlled in part by interaction of cell surface receptors (e.g. $\alpha 5\beta 1$ integrin) with extracellular matrix (ECM) molecules (e.g. fibronectin, FN). Other ECM molecules like laminin (LN), collagen IV (Col IV), hyaluronan (HA) and chondroitin sulphate proteoglycan (CSPG) may also be involved in ENS cell migration or differentiation; these molecules and the ENS are co-ordinately disturbed when the *edn-3* gene is mutated. An identical ENS failure results from mutation in the gene for the receptor for edn-3, *ednrB*. Which cells synthesize edn-3 and its receptor is uncertain, but the receptor is likely to be found at least on the NC cells and the ligand produced at least by the mesenchyme. A necessary correlate to edn-3/ednrB is the *ece* gene whose product cleaves edn-3 to give the active form. The ret tyrosine kinase on the NC cells is the receptor for glial cell line-derived neurotrophic factor (GDNF), a growth factor probably produced by the mesenchyme cells. Absence of activity of either of these grossly impairs growth, survival and differentiation of ENS cells. Another growth factor, neurotrophin NT-3, acts via the cell surface tyrosine kinase receptor trk-C. At early stages this may act to stimulate cell division and at later stages may promote differentiation. The *Hoxa-4* gene also acts in the gut mesenchyme and regional over-expression leads to subnormal ENS development. Even prior to migration the vagal level NC is subtly different from other levels, and this may be derived from the level-specific code of active Hox genes. A progressive restriction of differentiative potential (listed in boxes) occurs as the cells migrate from the vagal NC through the branchial arch/somites to the gut. Terminal neuronal differentiation may be controlled by a range of growth factors (e.g. NT-3) which act to match the differentiation of the neurones with their intestinal surroundings (which include other neurones). ENS glia differentiate, as indicated by the expression of glial fibrillary acidic protein (GFAP), also in response to their surroundings, but unlike neurones require continuous contact with ENS neurones to avoid reverting to an inappropriate Schwann cell type, marked by the expression of Schwann cell myelin protein (SMP). DRG, dorsal root ganglion

Several types of ENS cells are absent in clonal cultures yet occur in mass cultures of rat gut. This also indicates that interactions between ENS precursors and their surroundings, including mesenchyme cells, other NC cells, and their secreted products, must also occur to ensure correct differentiation. The role of interactions mediated by direct cell contact in ENS development has not been studied, but preliminary and interesting data concern the effects of secreted products, neurotrophins and ECM (Figure 9.8).

Neural growth, survival and differentiation can be influenced by cytokines including **neurotrophins** (Sieber-Blum, 1991; Birren et al, 1993) and their receptors (Barbacid, 1993). ENS precursor cells isolated from rat gut respond to neurotrophin NT-3, probably derived normally from the mesenchyme (Hohn et al, 1990), by differentiation and survival of neurones and glial cells, but not by increased mitosis (Chalazonitis et al, 1994). This is presumably mediated by the receptor tyrosine kinase, trk-C. In contrast, NT-3 is mitogenic for avian NC cells at a younger stage (Kalcheim et al, 1992). Ignoring possible technical or species differences, this suggests that a switch in the type of response to the same neurotrophin occurs during ENS cell differentiation. Other neurotrophins (nerve growth factor, NGF; brain-derived neurotrophic factor, BDNF; NT-4/5) had no effect on the rat ENS precursor cells, but the failure of many cell types to differentiate at all (Chalazonitis et al, 1994) suggests that additional, multiple factors are necessary, as in other NC systems (Birren et al, 1993). A candidate, as yet not functionally tested, is ciliary neurotrophic factor (CNTF), since its mRNA, along with that of the CNTF α-receptor, is reportedly expressed in mouse gut mesenchyme (Rothman et al, 1994). Additional factors have been indicated by mutant and gene knockout mice; these include Glial cell line-derived neurotrophic factor (GDNF) and endothelin-3 (EDN-3). These are discussed later, because of their direct relevance to Hirschsprung's disease. The interplay between neurotrophins and their receptors in ENS development is likely to be very complex, with many as yet unidentified molecules playing a part.

ECM provides important signals for neural cell development (Lander and Calof, 1993). Recent tissue culture experiments show that laminin promotes rat ENS neuronal and glial differentiation (Pomeranz et al, 1993). In vitro and in vivo this basal lamina-associated molecule is correlated with a specific NC cell surface laminin-binding protein at the time of neural differentiation in the ENS (Pomeranz et al, 1991b). Over-expression of laminin also parallels aganglionosis in *ls* mice (see later), with the suggestion that it inhibits NC cell migration by promoting terminal differentiation (Payette et al, 1988). The role of ECM in promoting or permitting various differentiational programmes is only beginning to be explored in the ENS, but given the large body of background knowledge on ECM and its roles, rapid advances can be expected.

Although a coherent picture has not emerged, it is obvious that the development of the ENS after migration is dependent on numerous released molecules and ECM derived from the gut environment and from the NC cells themselves. These control the survival, growth and differentiation of the NC cells: obviously disturbance to these could result in Hirschsprung's disease.

MAIN CLASSES OF DEFECT AFFECTING THE GUT: THE CONTRIBUTION OF CURRENT KNOWLEDGE ON NORMAL DEVELOPMENT

This section will be subdivided into two parts: one concerning pathologies affecting the mucosa, and another dealing with innervation defects; selection has been made for those pathologies in which data from developmental studies have provided some insight into aetiology.

DISEASES AFFECTING THE GUT MUCOSA

Specific malabsorption syndromes

Briefly, the first group covers specific congenital deficiencies affecting individual **brush-border membrane proteins** (either digestive enzymes or transporters), without morphological alterations. Two of these deficiencies are of particular interest – sucrase-isomaltase and lactase deficiencies – because their study at the cellular level has brought invaluable information on the elucidation of normal cell function, mainly in terms of intracellular protein traffic. At least six different phenotypes of congenital sucrase-isomaltase deficiency in humans have been characterized by the combined use of immunoelectron microscopy and immunochemical analysis of the protein. Each reflects an abnormality in a specific step from protein synthesis (transcription–translational steps) to brush-border membrane integration (post-translational events). These observations, together with a concomitant study of the biosynthetic steps in a differentiated colonic cancer cell line, have provided important clues as to the normal protein traffic in polarized cells (see Louvard et al, 1992). On the other hand, adult lactase deficiency has to be considered separately from **congenital lactase disease**; it is linked to the developmental turn-off of intestinal lactase activity described earlier in rodents, and which is obvious in most mammals (except for 30% of adult humans who may retain high lactase activity). In adult humans this deficiency results in lactose intolerance. In lactase-deficient intestinal mucosa, there is a residual low level of lactase activity. The immunocytochemical localization of the protein shows that small patches of positive cells are scattered among the mostly negative villi (Maiuri et al, 1991). This observation cannot be related to a coherent population of special absorptive cells arising from a crypt stem cell: in this case, the positive areas would appear as vertical ribbons along the villus, emerging from some crypts (Ponder et al, 1985; and see earlier). The expression pattern of the residual enzyme in adult lactose-intolerant patients rather resembles the mottled pattern found in the chimeric intestine (Schmidt et al, 1988) before crypt formation, and which corresponds to clones of cells differentiating from various individual cells. This observation remains an intriguing feature which cannot be explained by the current knowledge about adult stem cells but will perhaps help to its further understanding.

Enterocolitis

Enterocolitis can be due to various pathogens or to unknown factors (crypto-genetic diseases). Among these disorders special attention has been directed during this last decade to the chronic **inflammatory bowel diseases** (IBDs), **Crohn's disease** and **ulcerative colitis**. There is an increasing prevalence of this type of disorder for which the first onset occurs in young patients. The pathophysiological symptoms of IBD are subsequent to morphological lesions of the small intestinal or colonic mucosa, with crypt distortion and loss of villus architecture leading to superficial ulceration often surrounded by regenerating polypoid-like areas. In the case of Crohn's disease, the lamina propria displays mononuclear and plasma cell infiltration, with the formation of granulomas; in addition a fibrotic transmural reaction often results in obstructions that necessitate intestinal resection (Schumacher, 1993). Furthermore, chronic IBD predisposes towards the development of carcinomas.

Although IBDs are not developmental diseases, they have been chosen for consideration here because the destruction of the overall mucosal morphological steady-state could be due to alterations of cell interactions and ECM organization, and because some of these changes recapitulate some developmental features. As in other inflammatory states, intestinal inflammation is characterized by increased concentrations of cytokines (Sartor, 1994). The latter are known to modulate cell synthesis and/or degradation of ECM molecules and their integrin receptors (Nathan and Sporn, 1991; Postlethwaite and Kang, 1992). Thus, by analogy with the proliferative and remodelling phases described in inflammation, one can speculate that enhanced release of cytokines in the mucosal connective tissue in IBD patients may alter, on the one hand, proliferation of the fibroblasts and, on the other, production of ECM molecules by these cells. In turn, ECM conformational changes may alter the equilibrium between epithelial proliferation and differentiation.

The following three examples illustrate the possible involvement of changes in the extracellular microenvironment in the morphological disruption that characterizes IBD.

(1)   In intestinal biopsies taken from patients with active Crohn's disease, an increased immunostaining of hyaluronan in the distended lamina propria has been observed together with an increased luminal release which has been interpreted as being the reflection of a high villous vulnerability (Ahrenstedt et al, 1992). It is tempting to correlate these observations with the synthesis of high levels of hyaluronan by the fetal intestine (see earlier), when morphogenetic remodelling occurs.

(2)   A substantial loss of sulphated GAGs from the subepithelial BM is described in IBD and in particular in Crohn's disease, which can be associated with tumour necrosis factor-α (TNF-α) producing macrophages (Murch et al, 1993). TNF-α could inhibit the synthesis of sulphated GAGs and thus disrupt the continuity of the BM. On the other hand, TNF-α is known to induce apoptosis in target cells (Iwanaga et al, 1994).

(3)   The third example illustrating changes in the ECM patterning concerns tenascin. Riedl et al (1992) describe that, while tenascin content at the BM

level is restricted to the mucosal surface in normal tissue, it is heavily increased in the inflamed mucosa and extends towards the bottom of the crypts. The over-expression of this molecule outside the areas of normal desquamation might cause an overall decreased adherence of the epithelium in inflamed mucosa.

Conversely, increased levels of **transforming growth factor-β** (TGF-β) in inflammatory diseases could favour re-epithelialization of the wounded mucosa. Indeed, TGF-β has been shown to induce intestinal epithelial cell migration in vitro (Ciacci et al, 1993) and to stimulate the expression of β1 integrins and adhesion to collagen (Hafez et al, 1992). Related to this, it is of interest that there is an increased expression of β1 integrins on crypt and villus epithelial cells of inflamed human intestine (MacDonald et al, 1990). Furthermore, TGF-β significantly increases the production of fibrillar collagens (mainly type III collagen) by fibroblastic cells present in the lamina propria in active Crohn's disease (Stallmach et al, 1992). Again, this effect can be considered as a significant factor in intestinal repair processes. However, the chronic stimulation of such events may lead to an over-production of fibrotic molecules (Raghow, 1994) and finally to the obstructions seen in IBD.

Another noteworthy observation made in IBD-involved mucosa concerns the emergence of a peculiar cell lineage that is normally not expressed in the gut. This lineage consists of cells secreting **epidermal growth factor** (EGF) and a protein from the trefoil factor family, PS2; cells appear initially from the base of the crypts adjacent to the lesion, grow as a tubule and emerge on to the mucosal surface (Wright et al, 1990; Rio et al, 1991). This cell lineage which could be involved in proliferation/regeneration and ulcer healing, could arise from a spontaneous deviation of the pluripotent stem cells in pathological situations.

Colonic tumours

Colonic tumours as well as colonic cancer cell lines have been often shown to express small intestinal differentiation markers, brush-border digestive enzymes or transporters (Zweibaum et al, 1991). Linked to the observations made in the developing human and rodent colon, in which transient villus morphogenesis and expression of small intestinal markers have been reported (see earlier), it is tempting to ascribe this behaviour of cancer cells to a resurgence of fetal characteristics. This raises the possibility of a mixed population of stem cells in the colon for which the normal predominance of the 'colon type' could be developmentally regulated, and de-regulated in metaplasia. The finding that clonal populations – isolated from a monoclonal cell line derived from human colon carcinoma HT29 cells – are able to differentiate as absorptive, secretory or mucus cells, allows this cell line to be considered as a potent model of intestinal stem cells (Huet et al, 1987; Zweibaum et al, 1993). However, it is important to remember that colonic endodermal differentiation can be modulated by a heterologous mesenchymal environment (see earlier).

DEVELOPMENTAL ABNORMALITIES AFFECTING THE ENS: INTESTINAL AGANGLIONOSIS IN HUMANS AND ANIMALS

The inability of the gut to transmit a peristaltic wave, with proximal faecal accumulation (**megacolon**) is a common human birth defect. Overwhelmingly this is due to a regional absence or reduction of ENS ganglia, a condition termed **Hirschsprung's disease**, which occurs in around 1 in 5000 live births, with over-representation in males (reviewed by Cass, 1986). Similar conditions occur in animal models, such as *lethal spotting* (*ls*), *piebald lethal* (*s^l*) (Lane, 1966) and *Dominant megacolon* (*Dom*) (Lane and Liu, 1984) in mice, *spotting lethal* (*sl*) in rats (Ikadai et al, 1979) and lethal white foal syndrome in horses (McCabe et al, 1990). Intestinal aganglionosis (Schuchardt et al, 1994; Pichel et al, 1996) and hypoganglionosis (Wolgemuth et al, 1989) have been produced in mice by knockout of the *ret* and *GDNF* gene and over-expression of the *Hoxa-4* gene, respectively. Aganglionosis has also been produced by partial vagal NC ablation in chickens (Yntema and Hammond, 1954; Peters-van der Sanden et al, 1993a).

Regional distribution of intestinal aganglionosis

The outstanding unifying feature of all these enteric aganglionoses is that the affected region involves the caudal-most gut. Thus, in *ls* neonatal mice, the aganglionosis involves only the caudal few millimetres of the colon; in *s^l* mice, about half the colon; in *Dom* mice, a variable extent at the distal colon; in *sl* rats, the entire colon plus a variable extent of the ileocaecal region; while the *ret* and *GDNF* knockout mice show almost total absence of the ENS with the exception of the foregut. In humans, short-segment and long-segment forms of Hirsch-sprung disease (HD) have been identified in the distal bowel and were until recently thought to represent separate clinical entities (Badner et al, 1990).

The striking rostrocaudal pattern of intestinal aganglionosis points to disturbance in a rostrocaudal pattern of normal early development in the ENS. Given the interactive nature of NC development, defects could arise in the NC cells themselves or in their local environment, either at the site of origin at the dorsal neural tube, in the migration pathways before reaching the gut, in the gut in general or in the gut localized to the aganglionic zone. Mutations could affect the ability of NC-derived cells to migrate, divide, survive or differentiate (see Figure 9.8).

Hirschsprung's disease in humans and animals

The RET/GDNF system

Short- and long-segment forms of Hirschsprung's disease have been localized to defects in chromosome 10q11.2 (Lyonnet et al, 1993) and specified to the RET gene (Edery et al, 1994a; Romeo et al, 1994). It is likely that most familial and some sporadic cases of Hirschsprung's disease arise from mutations in RET (Pelet et al, 1994). In developing mice, the homologous gene *ret* is expressed in, but not confined to, migratory and post-migratory NC cells of the entire ANS including the ENS (Pachnis et al, 1993), and RET protein is found in the human ENS (Martucciello et al, 1995). The simplest conclusion, therefore, is that this is an inherent NC defect that affects cells migrating, multiplying or differentiating in the gut. Interestingly, in *ret* knockout mice, the foregut ENS not derived from the vagal NC is preserved while the non-ENS derivative of the vagal NC, the sympathetic superior cervical ganglion, regresses (Durbec et al, 1996). Thus a companion requirement is that *ret* function, while NC-wide, is vital only for derivatives of the vagal NC. A slim possibility remains, however, that this defect is also in the microenvironment of the NC cells, since *ret* is also expressed in mice in the posterior branchial arch epithelia at a stage when vagal NC cells, not yet *ret*-positive, bound for the gut, are migrating nearby (Pachnis et al, 1993). Fate-restricting decisions are likely to be made in this region by migrating NC cells (Ciment and Weston, 1985; Ito and Sieber-Blum, 1993), which hypothetically could require interaction with *ret*-expressing epithelia.

The *RET* gene codes for a putative cell surface tyrosine kinase receptor. The mutations that cause HD, premature stop codons and deletions in the kinase domain, would be expected to inactivate RET protein. The phenotype is, however, quite variable in that identical *RET* mutation can result in long-segment HD, short-segment HD or a functionally normal ENS (Romeo et al, 1994; Edery et al, 1994b). Mice with one *ret* gene knocked-out have an apparently normal ENS, but homozygeous *ret* knockout mice show total absence of the ENS. This suggests that normal ENS development is quantitatively dependent on the *RET* gene product, with humans teetering on the edge of sufficiency with one functional *RET* gene, while for mice this is more than sufficient. This may be a case of simple haploid insufficiency, but given the dimerisation often seen with receptor tyrosine kinases (Barbacid, 1993), it may reflect a dominant-negative effect. A non-mutually exclusive alternative for this variability is the activity of modifier genes.

The ligand for RET has recently been shown to be **GDNF**; this growth factor acts through cell surface RET plus an obligatory co-receptor, GDNF receptor-α (GDNF-Rα; Treanor et al, 1996). GDNF itself is a distant member of the TGF-β family of dimeric growth factors. Gene knockout of *GDNF* in mice creates a phenotype very similar to *Ret* knockout, including almost complete absence of the ENS (Pichel et al, 1996). The cellular source of GDNF in the early developing gut is not entirely clear, but is probably the enteric mesenchyme cells, thus giving a paracrine relationship between the NC cells and their microenvironment. However, self-production of GDNF by the NC cells is an additional possibility. The GDNF-Rα is a cell-surface linked molecule so is presumed to originate in the RET-possessing cells (i.e. the NC cells). However, Treanor et al (1996) have shown that this co-receptor is also effective when released: it could also be produced by the mesenchyme cells of the gut and still be effective. The requirement for GDNF and GDNF-Rα revealed by these research studies obviously places their genes as candidates for additional genes implicated in Hirschsprung's disease.

Other mutations in *RET*, expected to result in a constitutively active receptor, do not cause Hirschsprung's disease but instead result in **familial medullary thyroid carcinoma** and **multiple endocrine neoplasias 2A and 2B**. Since these originate as hyperplasias, it is therefore logical to assume that Hirschsprung's disease-type inactivating mutations cause hypoplasia. This conveniently ties in with the production of a Hirschsprung's disease-like condition in birds simply by reducing the number of vagal NC cells (Yntema and Hammond, 1954; Peters-van der Sanden et al, 1993a). Together, these suggest that numerical insufficiency of vagal NC cells during the migratory phase inside the gut, as a result of a relative lack of a RET-mediated interaction with GDNF, results in diminished migratory drive and consequent failure to fully populate the most distant gut. It must be assumed that lumbosacral NC cells, thought to be already resident in the hindgut (see earlier), are unable to form an ENS in the absence of the vagal cells (Newgreen et al, 1980).

Attractive as this simple scenario is, it is not yet possible to rule out survival, proliferative or differentiational abnormalities subsequent to normal migration in RET-mutation Hirschsprung's disease. These alternatives to an effect at the migratory stage are compatible with several lines of evidence. First, GDNF in tissue culture induces post-migratory events such as neuronal differentiation and survival of a variety of peripheral neurones (Buj-Bello et al, 1995; Ebendal et al, 1995). Secondly, transfection of the RET gene into neuroblastoma cells confers the ability to differentiate as neurones (D'Alessio et al, 1995). Thirdly, in ret knockout mice the vagal NC-derived superior cervical sympathetic ganglion is absent not because cells fail to migrate to form it but because it regresses after formation (Durbec et al, 1996).

Thus, further detailed studies on RET and its ligand GDNF, and on their origin and distribution, are still required in normal and in ret and GDNF knockout mice, as well as in humans.

The EDNRB/EDN-3 system

In a recent study of an inbred Mennonite kindred, Puffenberger et al (1994) identified a point mutation in the gene for the **endothelin-B receptor** (EDNRB) at chromosome 13q22. About one-fifth of heterozygotes for this mutation showed Hirschsprung's disease but about a quarter of homozygotes failed to develop the clinical condition. As with RET, this could reflect a normal stochastic process in ENS formation which is near a threshold for production of Hirschsprung's disease. Additionally, this could point to specific co-effector elements whose functional status could ameliorate or intensify the risk of Hirschsprung's disease. In this light, the same group has also shown the presence of a further risk gene for Hirsch-sprung's disease at chromosome 21q22.3. Mutation of the EDNRB gene accounts for the report of an association of Hirschsprung's disease with Waardenburg syndrome (both affect hindbrain NC derivatives), where neither RET nor PAX3, the gene associated with typical Waardenburg type I, was found to be involved (Hofstra et al, 1996).

The s^l/s^l mutant of mice is caused by mutation in the same gene, ednrB, as that of the Mennonite cases of Hirschsprung's disease and the mutation in the sl/sl rat is also in this gene (Hosoda et al, 1994; Ceccherini et al, 1995). Unlike in humans, in the rodents all homozygotes are affected whereas all heterozygotes are normal. This difference no doubt results from a combination of complete loss of receptor function in the rodents versus residual function in humans, plus the variability in function of other risk genes for Hirschsprung's disease in humans. This mutation in the *ednrB* gene (Hosoda et al, 1994) seems to cause a retardation of ENS appearance, beginning far rostral to the zone that finally remains aganglionic (Webster, 1973; Cass et al, 1992; Newgreen and Hartley, 1995), pointing (as in *ls*) to a widespread early defect which results in a localized abnormality later. Tissue combination experiments assaying the defects in NC-derived pigmentation in the *piebald* (*s*) allele suggest the gene is expressed in NC cells (Mayer, 1977). Avian NC cells in tissue culture respond to edn-3 by cell division (Lahav et al, 1996). This could mean that the s^l defect, like *ret*, involves the ENS precursor cells rather than their microenvironment. However, production of chimeric mice with both normal and s^l/s^l cells indicates that the latter could be rescued (as shown by s^l/s^l cells in the colonic ENS) by the normal cells (Kapur et al, 1995). This result is difficult to explain if the s^l/s^l cells intrinsically lack a vital cell surface receptor: they should be incapable of reacting to any 'rescue factor'.

The ligand for EDNRB is **EDN-3**, coded for in mice by the *ls* gene. This lies in a region of mouse chromosome 2, potentially subject to parental imprinting (Le Tissier et al, 1993), and in a region syntenic with human chromosome 20q. This recessive condition arises as a point mutation of the *edn-3* gene, which prevents proteolytic processing of the precursor protein into the active form. An identical phenotype is produced by targeted disruption of the gene (Baynash et al, 1994). The endothelins are a family of 21-amino acid diffusible peptides that act through a number of G-protein coupled receptors, the EDN-3 receptor being EDNRB.

As yet, the cellular processes in the ENS controlled by the EDN-3/EDNRB system are not yet known. However, cell growth and locomotion are candidate effects because Lahav et al. (1996) report that edn-3 is a potent cell growth stimulator for avian NC cells in tissue culture. Similarly, cell proliferation was induced by edn-1 in transformed NC-derived cells, but the same factor also increased cell migration by increased directed locomotion (Yohn et al, 1994). Similar effects on cell movement could also occur with **edn-3** with NC cells that form the ENS. Understanding the function of this system is hampered because the spatiotemporal pattern of gene expression in development has not yet been elucidated. Apparently, however, in *ls/edn-3* mutant mice the defect lies not in the NC cells but in their microenvironment (unlike *ret*; see earlier), as shown by a variety of combination experiments (Kapur et al, 1993; Rothman et al, 1993), although Baynash et al (1994) consider that the site of gene action may be in the NC cells. A major abnormality in the microenvironment does occur in *ls/ls* mice: an early expressed local superabundance of mesenchymal ECM, including laminin, collagen type IV, hyaluronan and chondroitin sulphate proteoglycan, which was suggested to terminate NC cell migration by inducing precocious neuronal differentiation (Payette et al, 1988; Tennyson et al, 1990). However, these molecules could have a more direct effect on NC cell migration, since they modulate the cell-substrate adhesions on which migration depends (see Newgreen, 1992). The nexus between the *ls/edn-3* gene mutation and the ECM accumulation is unclear, but the idea that there is a direct link fits uneasily with the observation that 20% or less of normal mesenchyme cells in chimeric gut can rescue the *ls* phenotype (Kapur et al, 1993).

The ECM abnormalities were originally described as co-localizing with the region of ENS abnormality, the distal colon (Payette et al, 1988). However, studies on the appearance of the ENS in *ls/ls* mice using several techniques describe a gradual slowing of migration that begins well rostral to the final affected region (Cass et al, 1992; Kapur et al, 1992; Coventry et al, 1994). This suggests either that ENS or ECM abnormalities are more widely distributed than first reported, or that the ECM alterations are not causally related to the ENS defect. However, they probably are not simply a result of aganglionosis, since abnormal over-expression of ECM has not been reported consistently in Hirschsprung's disease in humans (compare Parikh et al, 1992 with Clavel et al, 1988), and seems to be less obvious in s^l/s^l mice and *sl/sl* rats (Newgreen and Hartley, 1995), although both have more extensive aganglionosis than the *ls* mice (Cass et al, 1992).

This model suggests that loss of edn-3 increases ECM accumulation in the gut mesenchyme and that this in turn causes the ENS abnormalities. In the light of the mutation in the cognate receptor gene *ednrB* in s^l mice, another possibility is that the *ls* mutation acts on the ENS precursor cells, denying them edn-3. The less extensive aganglionosis in *ls/edn-3* mutants compared to $s^l/ednrB$ mutants may be due to low levels of diffusible edn-1 and -2 in the former which can also be recognized by the ednrB receptor. Although not yet found, mutations in the human *EDN3* gene should be considered as candidates for causing Hirschsprung's disease. Likewise, defects in endothelin-converting enzyme (ECE), which activates EDN-3, could also potentially result in Hirschsprung's disease.

Other Hirschsprung's disease systems

Even less is known about the *Dom* mice (gene on chromosome 6, syntenic with human chromosome 8q), which show dominant but variable aganglionosis of the colon. Defects in the early development of the ENS of *Dom* mice extend over a longer region than ultimately remains aganglionic (Kapur et al, 1996), just as in *ls* and s^l mouse mutants. Analysis of chimeric mice that possess both normal and *Dom/Dom* cells indicates that, as with *ls* mice, the *Dom* mutation affects microenvironmental signals necessary to generate the ENS of the caudal gut (Kapur et al, 1996). The human homologue of *Dom* is an obvious candidate for a Hirschsprung's disease gene. The hypoganglionosis produced by over-expression of the *Hoxa-4* gene (Wolgemuth et al, 1989) probably acts on the ENS cells via the gut mesenchyme cells where *Hoxa-4* is normally expressed (Tennyson et al, 1993). The Hox genes are transcription factors and their target genes whose products impact upon ENS development are at present unknown.

The *piebald* trait in humans, which shows a high incidence of Hirschsprung's disease-like features, has been ascribed to mutations in c-*kit* (Fleischman et al, 1991; Spritz et al, 1991). Like RET, c-kit is a receptor tyrosine kinase, but it is not expressed in ENS cells but in gut mesenchyme-derived interstitial cells of Cajal

(Lecoin et al, 1996; Young et al, 1996). The c-kit ligand, stem cell factor, is present in gut mesenchyme (Keshet et al, 1991).

Thus several genes other than *RET* and *EDNRB* can give Hirschsprung's disease-like phenotypes. Identifying these will help unravel the network of interactions that govern ENS development. The overall importance of these other genes is great, especially since for more than 80% of cases of Hirschsprung's disease a cause has not yet been established.

The availability of so many animal models of Hirschsprung's disease, with mutations in several different genes, is a resource of extraordinary value since they provide the potential to identify those genes, which participate in ENS development. This will not only specify several steps in the cascade of events that generates a normally functional ENS, but also pinpoint genes at risk in the causation of Hirschsprung's disease.

AGENDA FOR THE FUTURE

New molecular and genetic approaches together with sophisticated experimental strategies have allowed dramatic progress in the knowledge of gut development and differentiation during the last two decades. Nevertheless, several important issues remain to be elucidated. As an example, although the concept of the intestinal stem cell is widely accepted, attempts to define markers of this cell population, specific stem cell growth factors, or other environmental factors allowing their isolation and culture remain unsuccessful. This is ironic given the need to understand, in particular, why the colon, but not the small intestine, develops tumours. Another crucial aspect that remains to be elucidated, linked to the stem cell populations, concerns the proximodistal control of epithelial cell differentiation and its related function. Indeed, there are a number of pathological situations (either genetic or subsequent to massive small intestinal resections leading to important malabsorptions), that would be improved by the transdifferentiation of colonic stem cells into small intestinal ones, or by the transplantation of small intestinal stem cells into the colon (Tait et al, 1994). Such developments may be helped by the ongoing studies on homeotic genes, and by the rapid progress in the functional analysis of the promoters (and nuclear trans-acting factors) of several human and animal intestinal genes, which will allow us in the near future to get further insight into the control of tissue-, proximodistal- and temporal-specific gene expression.

Based on the observations and data reported herein we propose that epithelial and mesenchymal cells, together with the ECM, act as crucial regulators during intestinal development and adult cell renewal. In addition to the mechanical role of ECM in maintaining the structural integrity of the tissues, the constituent molecules play a key role in cellular migration, proliferation and differentiation. It is of interest that in Hirschsprung's-like disease developed in *lethal spotting* mice, as well as in IBD and colonic tumours, structural and functional alterations of the tissue can be correlated with extracellular compositional changes.

The most important issue in the near future will be to know how tissue- or cell-specific gene expression is regulated by the extracellular microenvironment, and how gene expression of matrix molecules, of matrix receptors or of degradation enzymes is controlled in a given developmental or physio (patho)logical state. A promising way to analyse the involvement of these extracellular molecules in gut physiology would be to inhibit their expression using either antisense sequences associated with promoters of tissue-specific genes turned on at precise developmental stages, or targeted mutations of tissue-specific regulatory sequences. Further clarification will come from the study of transcriptional activation or inhibition of extracellular molecules in response to individual cytokines and also by the molecular analysis of pathological states in which some processes recapitulate basic phenomena observed during gut development. Related to these regulatory processes, the characterization of mesenchymal cell populations which are under hormonal, immune and neural control, and which may modulate information transfer between the mucosal connective tissue and the epithelium (Valentich and Powell 1994), remains an important open field. Finally, studies of the link between growth factors and homeobox gene expression, which could mediate signalling implicated in epithelial–mesenchymal interactions, would be of particular potential interest in terms of intestinal proximodistal regulation, and of pathology.

The development of the vertebrate ENS results in the formation of a complex nervous system broadly comparable to the CNS, and shows similar neurogenetic events, such as controlled cell growth, cell migration and differentiation, involving interactions with other cells, with ECM and with cytokines. Nevertheless, it is far simpler in terms of number of components, and its development actually facilitates isolation of these components spatially or temporally, for purposes of analysis. Understanding the development of the ENS will therefore be useful not only in its own right, but also by providing a model for more complex systems. So, how far are we from understanding ENS development? At present, it must be admitted that we have only an incomplete understanding, based on a number of independent genetic, descriptive and experimental results (see Figure 9.8). Nevertheless, the power of the techniques already tested on the ENS, together with molecular genetic analyses that use clinically relevant material as their starting point, hold enormous potential for the success of future work.

REFERENCES

Ahrenstedt, O., Knutson, L., Hallgren, R. and Gerdin, B. (1992) Increased luminal release of hyaluronan in uninvolved jejunum in active Crohn's disease but not in inactive disease or in relatives. *Digestion* 52, 6–12.

Alho, A.M. and Underhill, C.B. (1989) The hyaluronic receptor is preferentially expressed on proliferating epithelial cells. *J. Cell Biol.* 108, 1557–1565.

Allan, I.J. and Newgreen, D.F. (1980) The origin and differentiation of enteric neurons of the intestine of the fowl embryo. *Am. J. Anat.* 157, 137–154.

Badner, J.A., Sieber, W.K., Garver, K.L. and Chakravarti, A. (1990) A genetic study of Hirschsprung disease. *Am. J. Hum. Genet.* 46, 568–580.

Barbacid, M. (1993) The *trk* family of neurotrophin receptors: molecular characterization and oncogenic activation in human tumors. In: *Molecular Genetics of Nervous System Tumors* (Eds: A.J. Levine and H.H. Schmidek), pp. 123–135. Wiley: New York.

Baynash, A.G., Hosoda, K., Giaid, A. et al (1994) Interaction of endothelin-3 with endothelin-B receptor is essential for development of epidermal melanocytes and enteric neurons. *Cell* **79**, 1277–1285.

Beaulieu, J.F. and Vachon, P.H. (1994) Reciprocal expression of laminin A-chain isoforms along the crypt–villus axis in the human small intestine. *Gastroenterology* **106**, 829–839.

Beaulieu, J.F., Vachon, P.H. and Chartrand, S. (1991) Immunolocalization of extracellular matrix components during organogenesis in the human small intestine. *Anat. Embryol.* **183**, 363–369.

Birren, S.J., Lo, L. and Anderson, D.J. (1993) Sympathetic neuroblasts undergo a developmental switch in trophic dependence. *Development*, **119**, 597–610.

Bouziges, F., Simon-Assmann, P., Simo, P. and Kedinger, M. (1991) Changes in glycosaminoglycan expression in the rat developing intestine. *Cell Biol. Int. Rep.* **15**, 97–106.

Buj-Bello, A., Buchman, V.L., Horton, A., Rosenthal, A. and Davies, A.M. (1995) GDNF is an age-specific survival factor for sensory and autonomic neurons. *Neuron* **15**, 821–828.

Cass, D. (1986) Hirschsprung's disease: an historical review. *Prog. Pediatr. Surg.* **20**, 199–214.

Cass, D.T., Zhang, A.L. and Morthorpe, J. (1992) Aganglionosis in rodents. *J. Pediatr. Surg.* **27**, 351–356.

Ceccherini, I., Zhang, A.L., Matera, I. et al (1995) Interstitial deletion of the endothelin-B receptor gene in the spotting lethal (sl) rat. *Hum. Mol. Genet.* **4**, 2089–2096.

Chalazonitis, A., Rothman, T.P., Chen, J. et al (1994) Neurotrophin-3 induces neural crest-derived cells from fetal rat gut to develop *in vitro* as neurons or glia. *J. Neurosci.* **14**, 6571–6584.

Chen, Z. and Kataoka, K. (1991) Histogenesis of the mucosa of the descending colon in mouse fetuses. *Arch. Histol. Cytol.* **54**, 221–232.

Ciacci, C., Lind, S.E. and Podolsky, D.K. (1993) Transforming growth factor-β regulation of migration in wounded rat intestinal epithelial monolayers. *Gastroenterology*, **105**, 93–101.

Ciment, G. and Weston, J.A. (1985) Segregation of development abilities in neural-crest-derived cells: identification of partially restricted intermediate cell types in the branchial arches of avian embryos. *Dev. Biol.* **111**, 73–83.

Clavel, C., Gaillard, D., Lallemand, A. and Birembaut, P. (1988) Distribution de la fibronectine et de la laminine au cours du développement des plexus myentériques humains et dans le maladie de Hirschsprung. *Gastroenterol. Clin. Biol.* **12**, 193–197.

Cohn, S.M., Roth, K.A., Birkemeier, E.H. and Gordon, J.I. (1991) Temporal and spatial patterns of transgene expression in aging adult mice provide insights about the origins, organization and differentiation of the intestinal epithelium. *Proc. Natl Acad. Sci. USA* **88**, 1034–1038.

Colony, P.C. and Conforti, J.C. (1993) Morphogenesis in the fetal rat proximal colon: effects of cytochalasin-D. *Anat. Rec.* **235**, 241–252.

Coventry, S., Yost, C., Palmiter, R.D. and Kapur, R.P. (1994) Migration of ganglion cell precursors in the ileoceca of normal and lethal spotted embryos, a murine model for Hirschsprung's disease. *Lab. Invest.* **71**, 82–93.

D'Alessio, A., DeVita, G., Cali, G. et al. (1995) Expression of the RET oncogene induces differentiation of SK-N-BE neuroblastoma cells. *Cell Growth Differ.* **6**, 1387–1394.

Dauça, M., Bouziges, F., Colin, S. et al (1990) Development of the vertebrate small intestine and mechanisms of cell differentiation. *Int. J. Dev. Biol.* **34**, 205–218.

De Arcangelis, A., Neuville, P., Boukamel, et al (1996) Inhibition of laminin α1-chain expression leads to alteration of basement membrane assembly and cell differentiation. *J. Cell Biol.* **133**, 417–430.

Dulac, C. and Le Douarin, N.M. (1993) Phenotypic plasticity of Schwann cells and enteric glial cells in response to the microenvironment. *Proc. Natl Acad. Sci. USA* **88**, 6358–6362.

Duluc, I., Jost, B. and Freund, J.-N. (1993) Multiple levels of control of the stage- and region-specific expression of rat intestinal lactase. *J. Cell Biol.* **123**, 1577–1586.

Duluc, I., Freund, J.-N., Leberquier, C. and Kedinger, M. (1994) Fetal endoderm primarily holds the temporal and positional information required for mammalian intestinal development. *J. Cell Biol* **126**, 211–221.

Durbec, P.L., Larsson-Blomberg, L.B., Schuchardt, A., Costantini, F. and Pachnis, V. (1996) Common origin and developmental dependence on c-ret of subsets of enteric and sympathetic neuroblasts. *Development* **122**, 349–358.

Ebendal, T., Tomac, A., Hoffer, B.J. and Olson, L. (1995) Glial cell line-derived neurotrophic factor stimulates fiber formation and survival in cultured neurons from peripheral autonomic ganglia. *J. Neurosci. Res.* **40**, 276–284.

Eccleston, P.A., Bannerman, P.G.C., Pleasure, D.E. et al (1989) Control of peripheral glial cell proliferation: enteric neurons exert an inhibitory influence on Schwann cell and enteric glial cell DNA synthesis in culture. *Development* **107**, 107–112.

Edery, P., Lyonnet, S., Mulligan, L.M. et al. (1994a) Mutations of the *RET* proto-oncogene in Hirschsprung's disease. *Nature* **367**, 378–380.

Edery, P., Pelet, A., Mulligan, L.M. et al (1994b) Long segment and short segment familial Hirschsprung's disease: variable clinical expression at the *RET* locus. *J. Med. Genet.* **31**, 602–606.

Epperlein, H.H., Krotoski, D., Halfter, W. and Frey, A. (1990) Origin and distribution of enteric neurons in Xenopus. *Anat. Embryol.* **182**, 53–67.

Epstein, M.L., Mikwa, T., Brown, A.M. and McFarlin, D.R. (1994) Mapping the origin of the avian enteric nervous system with a retroviral marker. *Dev. Dyn.* **201**, 236–244.

Fairman, C.L., Clagett-Dame, M., Lennon, V.A. and Epstein, M.L. (1995) Appearance of neurons in the developing chick gut. *Dev. Dyn.* **204**, 192–201.

Fleischman, R.A., Saltman, D.L., Stastny, V. and Znienier, S. (1991) Deletion of the *c-kit* protooncogene in the human developmental defect piebald trait. *Proc. Natl Acad. Sci. USA* **888**, 10885–10889.

Foltzer-Jourdainne, C., Kedinger, M. and Raul, F. (1989) Perinatal expression of brush border hydrolases in rat colon: hormonal and tissue regulations. *Am. J. Physiol.* **257**, G496–G503.

Freund, J.-N., Boukamel, R. and Benazzouz, A. (1992) Gradient expression of *Cdx* along the rat intestine throughout postnatal development. *FEBS Lett* **314**, 163–166.

Furness, J.B. and Bornstein, J.C. (1995) The enteric nervous system and its extrinsic connections. In: *Textbook of Gastroenterology* (Ed.: T. Yamada), pp. 2–18. Lippincott: Philadelphia, PA.

Gallagher, J.T. (1989) The extended family of proteoglycans: social residents of the pericellular zone. *Curr. Opin. Cell Biol.* **1**, 1201–1218.

Gershon, M.D. and Rothman, T.P. (1991) Enteric glia. *Glia* **4**, 195–204.

Gordon, J.I., Schmidt, G.H. and Roth, K.A. (1992) Studies of intestinal stem cells using normal, chimeric, and transgenic mice. *FASEB J.* **6**, 3039–3050.

Graham, A. (1992) Patterning the rostrocaudal axis of the hindbrain. *Sem. Neurosci.* **4**, 307–315.

Hafez, M.M., Hsu, S., Yan, Z., Winawer, S. and Friedman, E. (1992) Two roles for transforming growth factor β1 in colon enterocytic cell differentiation. *Cell Growth and Differ.* **3**, 753–762.

Haffen, K., Lacroix, B., Kedinger, M. and Simon-Assmann, P. (1983) Inductive properties of fibroblastic cell cultures derived from rat intestinal mucosa on epithelial differentiation. *Differentiation* **23**, 226–233.

Haffen, K., Kedinger, M. and Simon-Assmann, P. (1989) Cell contact dependent regulation of enterocytic differentiation. In *Human Gastrointestinal Development* (Ed.: E. Lebenthal), pp. 19–39. Raven Press: New York.

Henning, S.J., Rubin, D.C. and Shulman, R.J. (1994) Ontogeny of the intestinal mucosa. In *Physiology of the Gastrointestinal Tract* (Ed.: L.R. Johnson), 3rd edn, pp. 571–610. Raven Press: New York.

Hofstra, R.M.W., Osinga, J., Tan-Sindhunata, G. et al (1996) A homozygous mutation in the endothelin-3 gene associated with a combined Waardenburg type 2 and Hirschsprung phenotype (Shah–Waardenburg syndrome). *Nature Genetics* **12**, 445–447.

Hohn, A., Leibrock, J., Bailey, R. and Barde, Y.A. (1990) Identification and characterization of a novel member of the nerve growth factor/brain-derived neurotrophic factor family. *Nature* **344**, 339–341.

Hosoda, K., Hammer, R.E., Richardson, J.A. et al. (1994) Targeted and natural (piebald-lethal) mutations of endothelin-B receptor gene produce megacolon with spotted coat color in mice. *Cell* **79**, 1267–1276.

Howlett, A.R. and Bissell, M.J. (1993) The influence of tissue microenvironment (stroma and extracellular matrix) on the development and function of mammary epithelium. *Epith. Cell Biol.* **2**, 79–89.

Huet, C., Sahuquillo-Merino, C., Coudrier, E. and Louvard, D. (1987) Absorptive and mucus secreting subclones isolated from a multipotent intestinal cell line (HT29) provide new models for cell polarity and terminal differentiation. *J. Cell. Biol.* **105**, 345–357.

Hynes, R.O. (1992) Integrins: versatility, modulation, and signalling in cell adhesion. **Cell 69**, 11–25.

Ikadai, H., Fujita, H., Agematsu, Y. and Imamichi, T. (1979) Observation of congenital aganglionosis rat (Hirschsprung's disease rat) and its genetical analysis. *Congen. Anom.* **19**, 31–36.

Ingber, D.E. (1993) Extracellular matrix as a regulator of epithelial polarity, cell growth, and tissue pattern. In *The Pancreas: Biology, Pathobiology, and Disease* (Eds: W. Vay Liang Go et al), 2nd edn, pp. 369–380. Raven Press: New York.

Ito, K. and Sieber-Blum, M. (1993) Pluripotent and developmentally restricted neural crest-derived cells in posterior visceral arches. *Dev. Biol.* **156**, 191–200.

Iwanaga, T., Hoshi, O., Han, H. et al. (1994) Lamina propria macrophages involved in cell death (apoptosis) of enterocytes in the small intestine of rats. *Arch. Histol. Cytol.* **57**, 267–276.

James, R. and Kazenwadel, J. (1991) Homeobox gene expression in the intestinal epithelium of adult mice. *J. Biol. Chem.* **266**, 3246–3251.

Kalcheim, C., Carmeli, C. and Rosenthal, A. (1992) Neurotrophin-3 is a mitogen for cultured neural crest cells. *Proc. Natl. Acad. Sci. USA* **89**, 1661–1665.

Kapur, R., Sweetser, D.A., Doggett, B., Siebert, J.R. and Palmiter, R.D. (1995) Intercellular signals downstream of the endothelin receptor-B mediate colonization of the large intestine by enteric neuroblasts. *Development* **121**, 3787–3795.

Kapur, R., Livingston, R., Doggett, B. et al. (1996) Abnormal microenvironmental signals underlie intestinal aganglionosis in Dominant megacolon mutant mice. *Dev. Biol.* **174**, 360–369.

Kapur, R.P., Yost, C. and Palmiter, R.D. (1992) A transgenic model for studying development of the enteric nervous system in normal and aganglionic mice. *Development* **116**, 167–175.

Kapur, R.P., Yost, C. and Palmiter, R.D. (1993) Aggregation chimeras demonstrate that the primary defect responsible for aganglionic megacolon in lethal spotted mice is not neuroblast autonomous. *Development* **117**, 993–999.

Kedinger, M. (1994) Growth and development of intestinal mucosa. In *Small Bowel Enterocyte Culture and Transplantation* (Ed.: F.C. Campbell), pp. 1–31. Landes: Austin, TX.

Kedinger, M., Simon, P.M., Grenier, J.F. and Haffen, K. (1981) Role of epithelial–mesenchymal interactions in the ontogenesis of intestinal brush-border enzymes. *Dev. Biol.* **86**, 339–347.

Kedinger, M., Simon-Assmann, P.M., Lacroix, B. et al (1986) Fetal gut mesenchyme induces differentiation of cultured intestinal endoderm and crypt cells. *Dev. Biol.* **113**, 474–483.

Kedinger, M., Simon-Assmann, P., Alexandre, E. and Haffen, K. (1987) Importance of a fibroblastic support for in vitro differentiation of intestinal endodermal cells and for their response to glucocorticoids. *Cell. Differ.* **20**, 171–182.

Kedinger, M., Bouziges, F., Simon-Assmann, P. and Haffen, K. (1989) Influence of cell interactions on intestinal brush border enzyme expression. In *Highlights of Modern Biochemistry* (Eds: A. Kotyk, J. Skoda, V. Paces and V. Krostka), pp. 1103–1112. VSP International Science: Zeist.

Kedinger, M., Simon-Assmann, P., Bouziges, F. et al (1990) Smooth muscle actin expression during rat gut development and induction in fetal skin fibroblastic cells associated with intestinal embryonic epithelium. *Differentiation.* **43**, 87–97.

Keshet, E., Lyman, S.D., Williams, D.E. et al (1991) Embryonic RNA expression patterns of the c-kit receptor and its cognate ligands suggest multiple functional roles in mouse development. *EMBO J.* **10**, 2425–2435.

Kirchgessner, A. and Gershon, M.D. (1989) Identification of vagal efferent fibres and putative target neurons in the enteric nervous system of the rat. *J. Comp. Neurol.* **285**, 38–53.

Klein, G., Langegger, M., Timpl, R. and Ekblom, P. (1988) Role of laminin A chain in the development of epithelial cell polarity. *Cell* **55**, 331–341.

Klein, R.M. (1989) Small intestinal cell proliferation during development. In *Human Gastrointestinal Development* (Ed.: E. Lebenthal), pp. 367–392. Raven Press: New York.

Kuritani, S.C. and Kirby, M.L. (1991) Initial migration and distribution of the cardiac neural crest in the avian embryo: an introduction to the concept of the circumpharyngeal crest. *Am. J. Anat.* **191**, 215–227.

Lacroix, B., Kedinger, M., Simon-Assmann, P. et al (1984) Developmental pattern of brush border enzymes in the human fetal colon: correlation with some morphogenetic events. *Early Hum. Dev.* **9**, 95–103.

Lahav, R., Ziller, C., Dupin, E. and Le Douarin, N.M. (1996) Endothelin-3 promotes neural crest cell proliferation and mediates a vast increase in melanocyte number in culture. *Proc. Natl Acad. Sci. USA* **93**, 3892–3897.

Lander, A.D. and Calof, A.L. (1993) Extracellular matrix in the developing nervous system. In *Molecular Genetics of Nervous System Tumours* (Eds: A.J. Levine and H.H. Schmidek), pp. 341–355. Wiley: New York.

Lane, P.W. (1966) Association of megacolon with two recessive spotting genes in the mouse. *J. Hered.* **57**, 29–31.

Lane, P.W. and Liu, H.M. (1984) Association of megacolon with a new dominant spotting gene (*Dom*) in the mouse. *J. Hered.* **75**, 435–439.

Le Douarin, N.M. and Teillet, M.A. (1973) The migration of neural crest cells to the wall of the digestive tract in avian embryo. *J. Embryol. Exp. Morphol.* **30**, 31–48.

Le Douarin, N.M. and Teillet, M.A. (1974) Experimental analysis of the migration and differentiation of neuroblasts of the autonomic nervous system and of neuroectodermal mesenchymal derivatives, using a biological cell marking technique. *Dev. Biol.* **41**, 162–184.

Le Tissier, P.R., Guénet, J.-L., Skidmore, C.J. and Peters, J. (1993) Mapping studies on distal chromosome 2. *Mouse Genome* **91**, 879–881.

Lecoin, L., Gabella, G. and Le Douarin, N. (1996) Origin of the c-kit-positive interstitial cells in the avian bowel. *Development* **122**, 725–733.

Louvard, D., Kedinger, M. and Hauri, H.P. (1992) The differentiating intestinal epithelial cell. Establishment and maintenance of functions through interactions between cellular structures. *Annu. Rev. Cell Biol.* **8**, 157–195.

Lumsden, A., Sprawson, N. and Graham, A. (1991) Segmental origin and migration of neural crest cells in the hindbrain region of the chick embryo. *Development* **113**, 1281–1291.

Lyon, M.F. and Kirby, M.C. (1994) Mouse chromosome atlas. *Mouse Genome* **92**, 19–61.

Lyonnet, S., Bolino, A., Pelet, A. et al (1993) A gene for Hirschsprung disease maps to the proximal long arm of chromosome 10. *Nature Genetics* **4**, 346–350.

MacDonald, T.T., Horton, M.A, Choy, M.Y. and Richman, P.I. (1990) Increased expression of laminin collagen receptor (VLA-1) on epithelium of inflamed human intestine. *J. Clin. Path.* **43**, 313–315.

Maiuri, L., Raia, V., Potter, J. et al (1991) Mosaic pattern of lactase expression by villous enterocytes in human adult-type hypolactasia. *Gastroenterology* **100**, 359–369.

Maiuri, L., Rossi, M., Raia, V. et al (1992) Patchy expression of lactase protein in adult rabbit and rat intestine. *Gastroenterology* **103**, 1739–1746.

Martucciello, G., Favre, A., Takahashi, M. and Jasonni, V. (1995) Immunohistochemical localization of RET protein in Hirschsprung's disease. *J. Pediatr. Surg.* **30**, 433–436.

Mayer, T.C. (1977) Enhancement of melanocyte development from piebald neural crest by a favorable tissue environment. *Dev. Biol.* **56**, 255–262.

McCabe, L., Griffin, L.D., Kinzer, A. et al (1990) Overo lethal white foal syndrome: equine model of aganglionic megacolon (Hirschsprung's disease). *Am. J. Med. Genet.* **36**, 336–340.

Meijers, J.H.C., Tibboel, D., van der Kamp, A.W.M. et al (1987) Cell division in migratory and aggregated neural crest cells in the developing gut: an experimental approach to innervation-related motility disorders of the gut. *J. Pediatr. Surg.* 22, 243–245.

Meijers, J.H.C., Tibboel, D., van der Kamp, A.W.M., Haperen-Heuts, C.C.M. and Molenaar, J.C. (1989) A model for aganglionosis in the chicken embryo. *J. Pediatr. Surg.* 24, 557–561.

Menard, D. and Pothier, P. (1987) Differential distribution of digestive enzymes in isolated epithelial cells from developing human fetal small intestine and colon. *J. Pediat. Gastroenterol. Nutr.* 6, 509–516.

Murch, S.H., MacDonald, T.T., Walker-Smith, J.A. et al (1993) Disruption of sulphated glycosaminoglycans in intestinal inflammation. *Lancet* 341, 711–714.

Nathan, C. and Sporn, M. (1991) Cytokines in context. *J. Cell. Biol.* 113, 981–986.

Newgreen, D.F. (1992) Establishment of the form of the peripheral nervous system. In *Development, Regeneration and Plasticity of the Autonomic Nervous System* (Eds: I.A. Hendry and C.E. Hill), pp. 1–94. Harwood Academic: Basle, Switzerland.

Newgreen, D.F. and Hartley, L. (1995) Extracellular matrix and adhesive molecules in the early development of the gut and its innervation in normal and *Spotting lethal* rat embryos. *Acta Anat.* 154, 243–260.

Newgreen, D.F., Jahnke, I., Allan, I.J. and Gibbins, I.L. (1980) Differentiation of sympathetic and enteric neurons of the fowl embryo in grafts to the chorio-allantoic membrane. *Cell Tiss. Res.* 208, 1–19.

Newgreen, D.F., Powell, M.E. and Moser, B. (1990) Spatiotemporal changes in HNK-1/L2 glycoconjugates on avian embryo somite and neural crest cells. *Dev. Biol.* 139, 100–120.

Nishijima, E., Meijers, J.H.C., Tibboel, D. et al (1990) Formation and malformation of the enteric nervous system in mice: an organ culture study. *J. Pediatr. Surg.* 25, 627–631.

Okamoto, E. and Ueda, T. (1967) Embryogenesis of intramural ganglia of the gut and its relation to Hirschsprung's disease. *J. Pediatr. Surg.* 2, 437–443.

Otto, B. and Wright, N. (1994) Trefoil peptides: coming up clover. *Curr. Biol.* 4, 835–838.

Pachnis, V., Mankoo, B. and Costantini, F. (1993) Expression of the *c-ret* proto-oncogene during mouse embryogenesis. *Development* 199, 1005–1017.

Parikh, D.H., Tam, P.K.H., Velzen, D. and Edgar, D. (1992) Abnormalities in the distribution of laminin and collagen type IV in Hirschsprung's disease. *Gastroenterology* 102, 1236–1241.

Paul, E.C.A., Hochman, J. and Quaroni, A. (1993) Conditionally immortalized intestinal epithelial cells: novel approach for study of differentiated enterocytes. *Am. J. Physiol.* 265, C266–C278.

Paulsson, M. (1992) Basement membrane proteins: structure, assembly, and cellular interactions. *Crit. Rev. Biochem. Molec. Biol.* 27, 93–127.

Payette, R.F., Tennyson, V.M., Pomeranz, H.D. et al (1988) Accumulation of components of basal laminae: association with the failure of neural crest cells to colonize the presumptive aganglionic bowel of *ls/ls* mutant mice. *Dev. Biol.* 125, 341–360.

Pelet, A., Attie, T., Goulet, O. et al (1994) De novo mutations of the *RET* proto-oncogene in Hirschsprung's disease. *Lancet* 344, 1769–1770.

Peters-van der Sanden, M.J.H., Kirby, M.L., Gittenberger-de Groot, A.C. et al (1993a) Ablation of various regions within the avian vagal neural crest has differential effects on ganglion formation in the fore-, mid- and hindgut. *Dev. Dyn.* 196, 183–194.

Peters-van der Sanden, M.J.H., Luider, T.M., van der Kamp, A.W.M., Tibboel, D. and Meijers, C. (1993b) Regional differences between various axial segments of the avian neural crest regarding the formation of enteric ganglia. *Differentiation* 53, 17–24.

Pham, T.D., Gershon, M.D. and Rothman, T.P. (1991) Time of origin of neurons in the murine enteric nervous system: sequence in relation to phenotype. *J. Comp. Neurol.* 314, 789–798.

Phillips, M.T., Kirby, M.L. and Forbes, G. (1987) Analysis of cranial neural crest distribution in the developing heart using quail–chick chimeras. *Circ. Res.* 60, 27–30.

Pichel, J.G., Shen, L., Sheng, H.Z. et al (1996) Defects in enteric innervation and kidney development in mice lacking GDNF. *Nature* 382, 73–76.

Pomeranz, H.D. and Gershon, M.D. (1990) Colonization of the avian hindgut by cells derived from the sacral neural crest. *Dev. Biol.* **137**, 378–394.

Pomeranz, H.D., Rothman, T.P. and Gershon, M.D. (1991a) Colonization of the post-umbilical bowel by cells derived from the sacral neural crest: direct tracing of cell migration using an intercalating probe and a replication-deficient retrovirus. *Development* **111**, 647–655.

Pomeranz, H.D., Sherman, D.L., Smalheiser, N.R., Tennyson, V.M. and Gershon, M.D. (1991b) Expression of a neurally related laminin binding protein by neural crest-derived cells that colonize the gut: relationship to the formation of enteric ganglia. *J. Comp. Neurol.* **313**, 625–642.

Pomeranz, H.D., Rothman, T.P., Chalazonitis, A., Tennyson, V.M. and Gershon, M.D. (1993) Neural crest-derived cells isolated from the gut by immunoselection develop neuronal and glial phenotypes when cultured on laminin. *Dev. Biol.* **156**, 341–361.

Ponder, B.A.J., Schmidt, G.H., Wilkinson, M.M. et al (1985) Derivation of mouse intestinal crypts from single progenitor cells. *Nature* **313**, 689–691.

Postlethwaite, A.E. and Kang, A.H. (1992) Fibroblasts and matrix proteins. In *Inflammation: Basic Principles and Clinical Correlates* (Eds: J.I. Gallin et al), 2nd edn, pp. 747–773. Raven Press: New York.

Probstmeier, R., Martini, R. and Schachner, M. (1990) Expression of J1 tenascin in the crypt villus unit of adult mouse small intestine. Implications for its role in epithelial cell shedding. *Development* **109**, 313–321.

Potten, C.S. and Loeffler, M. (1990) Stem cells – Attributes, cycles, spirals, pitfalls and uncertainties: lessons for and from the crypt. *Development* **110**, 1001–1020.

Puffenberger, E.G., Hosoda, K., Washington, S.S. et al (1994) A missense mutation of the endothelin-B receptor gene in multigenic Hirschsprung's disease. *Cell* **79**, 1257–1266.

Raghow, R. (1994) The role of extracellular matrix in postinflammatory wound healing and fibrosis. *FASEB J.* **8**, 823–831.

Riedl, S.E., Faissner, A., Schlag, P. et al (1992) Altered content and distribution of tenascin in colitis, colon adenoma, and colorectal carcinoma. *Gastroenterology* **103**, 400–406.

Rio, M.C., Chenard, M.P., Wolf, C. et al (1991) Induction of pS2 and hSP genes as markers of mucosal ulceration of the digestive tract. *Gastroenterology* **100**, 375–379.

Romeo, G., Ronchetto, P., Luo, Y. et al (1994) Point mutations affecting the tyrosine kinase domain of the RET proto-oncogene in Hirschsprung's disease. *Nature* **367**, 377–378.

Rothman, T.P. and Gershon, M.D. (1982) Phenotypic expression in the developing murine enteric nervous system. *J. Neurosci.* **2**, 381–393.

Rothman, T.P., Le Douarin, N.M., Fontaine-Perus, J.C. and Gershon, M.D. (1990) Developmental potential of neural crest-derived cells migrating from segments of developing quail bowel back-grafted into younger chick host embryos. *Development* **109**, 411–423.

Rothman, T.P., Goldowitz, D. and Gershon, M.D. (1993) Inhibition of migration of neural crest-derived cells by the abnormal mesenchyme of the presumptive aganglionic bowel of *ls/ls* mice: analysis with aggregation and interspecies chimeras. *Dev. Biol.* **159**, 559–573.

Rothman, T.P., Chen, J. and Gershon, M.D. (1994) Microenvironmental factors in the differentiation of the enteric neurons from neural crest-derived precursors. *Neurosci. Abstr.* **20**, 1492.

Rubin, D.C., Swietlicki, E., Roth, K.A. and Gordon, J.I. (1992) Use of fetal intestinal isografts from normal and transgenic mice to study the programming of positional information along the duodenal-to-colonic axis. *J. Biol. Chem.* **267**, 15122–15133.

Sartor, B.R. (1994) Cytokines in intestinal inflammation: pathophysiological and clinical considerations. *Gastroenterology* **106**, 533–539.

Sastry, S., Horwitz, A.F. (1993) Integrin cytoplasmic domains: mediators of cytoskeletal linkages and extra- and intracellular initiated transmembrane signalling. *Curr. Opin. Cell Biol.* **5**, 819–831.

Schmidt, G.H., Winton, D.J. and Ponder, B.A.J. (1988) Development of the pattern of cell renewal in the crypt–villus unit of chimaeric mouse small intestine. *Development* **103**, 785–790.

Schuchardt, A., D'Agati, V., Larsson-Glombey, L., Costantini, F. and Pachnis, V. (1994) Defects in the kidney and enteric neurons system of mice lacking the tyrosine kinase receptor *ret. Nature* **367**, 380–383.

Schumacher, G. (1993) First attack of inflammatory bowel disease and infectious colitis. *Scand. J. Gastroenterol.* **28**, 1–24.

Serbedzija, G.N., Burgan, S., Fraser, S.E. and Bronner-Fraser, M. (1991) Vital dye labelling demonstrates a sacral neural crest contribution to the enteric nervous system of chick and mouse embryos. *Development* **111**, 857–866.

Sextier-Sainte-Claire Deville, F., Ziller, C. and Le Douarin, N.M. (1994) Developmental potentials of enteric neural crest-derived cells in clonal and mass cultures. *Dev. Biol.* **163**, 141–151.

Sieber-Blum, M. (1991) Role of the neurotrophic factors BDNF and NGF in the commitment of pluripotent neural crest cells. *Neuron* **6**, 949–955.

Simo, P., Simon-Assmann, P., Arnold, C. and Kedinger, M. (1992) Mesenchyme-mediated effect of dexamethasone on laminin in cocultures of embryonic gut epithelial cells and mesenchyme-derived cells. *J. Cell Sci.* **101**, 161–171.

Simon-Assmann, P. and Kedinger, M. (1993) Heterotypic cellular cooperation in gut morphogenesis and differentiation. *Semin. Cell Biol.* **4**, 221–230.

Simon-Assmann, P., Kedinger, M. and Haffen, K. (1986) Immunocytochemical localization of extracellular matrix proteins in relation to rat intestinal morphogenesis. *Differentiation* **32**, 59–66.

Simon-Assmann, P., Bouziges, F., Arnold, C. et al (1988) Epithelial–mesenchymal interactions in the production of basement membrane components in the gut. *Development* **102**, 339–347.

Simon-Assmann, P., Bouziges, F., Vigny, M. and Kedinger, M. (1989) Origin and deposition of basement membrane heparan sulfate proteoglycan in the developing intestine. *J. Cell Biol.* **109**, 1837–1848.

Simon-Assmann, P., Bouziges, F., Freund, J.-N., Perrin-Schmitt, F. and Kedinger, M. (1990a) Type IV collagen mRNA accumulates in the mesenchymal compartment at early stages of murine developing intestine. *J. Cell Biol.* **110**, 849–857.

Simon-Assmann, P., Simo, P., Bouziges, F., Haffen, K. and Kedinger, M. (1990b) Synthesis of basement membrane proteins in the small intestine. *Digestion* **46**, 12–21.

Simon-Assmann, P., Duclos, B., Orian-Rousseau, V. et al (1994) Differential expression of laminin isoforms and $\alpha 6$-$\beta 4$ integrin subunits in the developing human mouse intestine. *Dev. Dyn.* **201**, 71–85.

Simon-Assmann, P., Kedinger, M., DeArcangelis, A., Rousseau, V. and Simo, P. (1995) Extracellular matrix components in intestinal development. *Experientia* **51**, 883–900.

Smith, J., Cochard, P. and Le Douarin, N.M. (1977) Development of choline acetyltransferase and cholinesterase activities in enteric ganglia derived from presumptive adrenergic and cholinergic levels of the neural crest. *Cell Differ.* **6**, 199–216.

Southwell, B. (1982) The origin of enteric neurons in mice. MSc Thesis, University of Melbourne.

Spritz, R.A., Giebal, L.B. and Holmes, S.A. (1991) Dominant negative loss of function mutations in the c-kit (mast cell growth factor receptor) protooncogene in human piebaldism. *Am. J. Hum. Genet.* **50**, 261–269.

Stallmach, A., Schuppan, D., Riese, H.H., Matthes, H. and Riecken, E.O. (1992) Increased collagen type III synthesis by fibroblasts isolated from strictures of patients with Crohn's disease. *Gastroenterology*, **102**, 1920–1929.

Tait, I.S., Evans, G.S., Flint, N. and Campbell, F.C. (1994) Colonic mucosal replacement by syngenetic small intestinal stem cell transplantation. *Am. J. Surg.* **167**, 67–72.

Takiguchi-Hayashi, K. and Yasugi, S. (1990) Transfilter analysis of the inductive influence of proventricular mesenchyme on stomach epithelial differentiation of chick embryos. *Roux' Arch. Dev. Biol.* **198**, 400–466.

Teitelman, G. (1990) Insulin cells of pancreas extend neurites but do not arise from the neurectoderm. *Dev. Biol.* **142**, 368–379.

Tennyson, V.M., Payette, R.F., Rothman, T.P. and Gershon, M.D. (1990) Distribution of hyaluronic acid and chondroitin sulphate proteoglycans in the presumptive aganglionic terminal bowel of *ls/ls* fetal mice: an ultrastructural analysis. *J. Comp. Neurol.* **291**, 345–362.

Tennyson, V.M., Gershon, M.D., Sherman, D.L. et al (1993) Structural abnormalities associated with congenital megacolon in transgenic mice that overexpress the *Hoxa-4* gene. *Dev. Dyn.* **198**, 28–53.

Timpl, R. (1989) Structure and biological activity of basement membrane proteins. *Eur. J. Biochem.* **180**, 487–502.

Traber, P.G. (1994) Differentiation of intestinal epithelial cells: lessons from the study of intestine-specific gene expression. *J. Lab. Clin. Med.* **123**, 467–477.

Treanor, J.J.S., Goodman, L., de Sauvage, F. et al (1996) Characterization of a multicomponent receptor for GDNF. *Nature* **382**, 80–83.

Tucker, G.C., Ciment, G. and Thiery, J.P. (1986) Pathways of avian neural crest cell migration in the developing gut. *Dev. Biol.* **116**, 430–450.

Valentich, J.D. and Powell, D.W. (1994) Intestinal subepithelial myofibroblasts and mucosal immunophysiology. *Curr. Opin. in Gastroenterol.* **10**, 645–651.

Webster, W. (1973) Embryogenesis of the enteric ganglia in normal mice and in mice that develop congenital aganglionic megacolon. *J. Embryol. Exp. Morphol.* **30**, 573–585.

Winton, D.J. and Ponder, B.A.J. (1990) Stem-cell organization in mouse small intestine. *Proc. Roy. Soc. Lond. (Biol.)* **23**, 13–18.

Wolgemuth, D.J., Behringer, R.R., Mostoller, M.P., Brinster, R.L. and Palmiter, R.D. (1989) Transgenic mice overexpressing the mouse homeobox-combining gene *Hox-1.4* exhibit abnormal gut development. *Nature* **337**, 464–469.

Wood, J.D. (1987) Physiology of enteric neurons. In *Physiology of the Gastrointestinal Tract* (Ed.: L.R. Johnson), pp. 1–41. Raven Press: New York.

Wright, N.A., Pike, C. and Elia, G. (1990) Induction of a novel epidermal growth factor-secreting cell lineage by mucosal ulceration in human gastrointestinal stem cells. *Nature* **343**, 82–85.

Xu, H., Christmas, P., Wu, S.R., Wewer, U.M. and Engvall, E. (1994) Lack of M-laminin and defective muscle basement membrane in the dystrophic *dy/dy* mouse. *Proc. Natl Acad. Sci.* **91**, 5572–5576.

Yasugi, S. (1993) Role of epithelial–mesenchymal interactions in differentiation of epithelium of vertebrate digestive organs. *Dev. Growth Differ.* **35**, 1–9.

Yntema, C.L. and Hammond, W.S. (1954) The origin of intrinsic ganglia of trunk viscera from vagal neural crest in the chick embryo. *J. Comp. Neurol.* **101**, 515–541.

Yntema, C.L. and Hammond, W.S. (1955) Experiments on the origin and development of the sacral autonomic nerves in the chick embryo. *J. Exp. Zool.* **129**, 375–414.

Yohn, J.J., Smith, C., Stevens, T. et al (1994) Human melanoma cells express functional endothelin-1 receptors. *Biochem. Biophys. Res. Commun.* **30**, 449–457.

Young, H., Ciampoli, D., Southwell, B.R. and Newgreen, D.F. (1996) Origin of the interstitial cells of Cajal in the mouse intestine. *Dev. Biol.* **180**, 97–107.

Zweibaum, A., Laburthe, M., Grasset, E. and Louvard, D. (1991) The use of cultured cell lines in studies of intestinal cell differentiation and function. In *Handbook of Physiology: The Gastrointestinal, System* (Eds: R. Field and M. Frissell), pp. 223–255. Liss: New York.

Zweibaum, A., Lesuffleur, T., Barbat, A. et al (1993) Colon cancer cell differentiation as related to methotrexate and 5-fluorouracil resistance. In *Cell Biology* (Eds: N. D'Alessandro et al), pp. 1–15. *NATO ASI Series*. Springer Verlag: Berlin.

10 The Head and Face

PETER THOROGOOD

Developmental Biology Unit, Institute of Child Health, London, UK

The vertebrate head and face is a modular structure, with contributions from a range of cell lineages. Its development comprises a sequence of highly co-ordinated patterns of growth and morphogenetic events such as cell migration, fusion of epithelia, tissue invaginations and evaginations, cell polarization, tissue interactions/cell signalling and directed extracellular matrix secretion. All of these events are not only precisely co-ordinated in a spatiotemporal sense but they must also generate a structure in which all the modular contributions are anatomically 'in register' (Noden, 1992) and functionally integrated. Thus, position and timing become critically important at the cell level during craniofacial development. This morphogenetic complexity means that the craniofacial complex is particularly sensitive to perturbation by genetic mutation or environmental teratogens. In fact, one-third of all major birth defects involve the head and face (Gorlin et al, 1990).

The source of the major lineages within the head is fundamentally important. Probably the single most important aspect is the dual source of mesenchyme, from the 'ectomesenchyme' of the **neural crest** and from mesoderm. Indeed, much of the connective tissues and the peripheral nervous system in the head, face and neck is derived from the cephalic neural crest (Le Douarin, 1982; Hall and Horstadius, 1988), with the ectodermal placodes making a significant contribution to the cranial sensory ganglia (Webb and Noden, 1993). This means that the greater part of the skeletal tissue and the cranial ganglia, the odontoblasts of the teeth, the corneal stromal fibroblasts, the fascia of the muscles, the smooth muscle associated with major blood vessels, dermis and melanocytes are all derived from that transient population of cells which emerge from a de-epithelialization event at the margin of the neural tube during neurulation and which proceed to migrate throughout the body of the embryo (Thorogood, 1994; and see Chapter 8). The question of cell lineage and diversity within the crest remains unsettled, with strong evidence from different experimental strategies for both intrinsic multipotency and for cell interactions generating diversity (Selleck et al, 1993; Stemple and Anderson, 1993). In contrast to the crest derivatives, mesodermal mesenchyme (i.e. derived from the internalization of cells during gastrulation) makes a proportionately much smaller contribution, providing a source of angiogenic tissue, a limited amount of connective tissue, the bones of the occipital region of the skull and otic capsule and, importantly, all the striated muscle, including the extrinsic muscles of the eye.

Embryos, Genes and Birth Defects. Edited by P. Thorogood.
© 1997 John Wiley & Sons Ltd.

The emergence of the neural crest as a developmental novelty at some distant time in our evolutionary past (Gans and Northcutt, 1983) not only had a profound effect on the body plan of some now extinct class of primitive chordate but also underpinned the explosive and radiative evolution of the vertebrates as we know them. For the head in particular, it was especially important since cephalization reaches a very advanced level in vertebrates. In a functional sense the head and face is not a single organ system but is a complex of interdependent organs and tissue systems. Here, early craniofacial morphogenesis will be dealt with in a general sense, with emphasis on the human face and referring to other organ systems within the head as and when necessary (for a fuller account of the developmental anatomy, see Larsen, 1993).

DEVELOPMENTAL ANATOMY

DEVELOPMENTAL TOPOGRAPHY OF THE HUMAN FACE

Craniofacial morphogenesis is topographically complex and critical events in craniofacial development take place at stages when the rostral end of the embryonic axis does not resemble a head in any obvious sense. The first outward indication of morphogenesis is a lifting up of the anterior end of the axis from the surrounding extraembryonic tissues, the so-called **head fold**, at the beginning of the fourth week of embryonic life and, by the end of that week, the gradual emergence of a series of bulges and intervening grooves on the ventrolateral aspects of the early head. The most rostral of these (in a virtually terminal location) is a midline process, termed the **frontonasal mass**. Flanking this, and first distinguishable during the fifth week, are the paired **olfactory placodes**, areas of thickened ectoderm that will subsequently invaginate to give rise to much of the olfactory organs, including the chemosensory neurones, and the gonadotrophin-releasing hormone neurones. The medial and lateral edges of these placodes will grow into the paired, bilateral **medial** and **lateral nasal processes** (Figure 10.1), followed by the paired and bilateral **maxillary processes**. These processes or primordia collectively will give rise to the upper and mid-face (Figure 10.1). Moving back along the axis there are a series of paired ventrolateral processes called the **branchial arches**, each separated from its neighbours fore and aft by a groove in the surface ectoderm termed the **branchial groove** and matched by an outpocketing from the foregut internally called the **branchial** or **pharyngeal pouch**. At these points between adjacent arches the surface ectodem and the endoderm lining the foregut are in close approximation.

These arches are remnants of the gill arches of a vertebrate ancestor and, although reduced in number, retain some of their primitive characteristics; likewise, the grooves and pouches together represent the embryonic gill clefts of that ancestor. Thus, each arch and associated pouch originally formed a set of structures (skeletal, vascular, muscular, neural and glandular) comprising a single functional unit in a repeating metameric series. One characteristic of arch

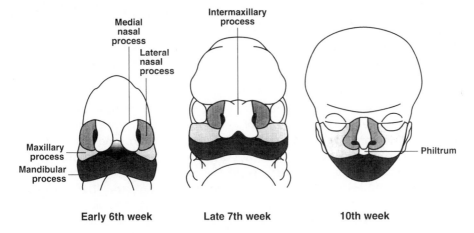

Figure 10.1 Development of the human face from a frontal perspective. Growth of the facial primordia brings them into contact at precise locations and at precise times; fusion, continued growth and epithelial remodelling ensues, generating the basic features of the face by the tenth week of embryonic development. (After Larsen, 1993)

development in modern vertebrates is the specialization of each arch, with its developmental potential being deployed in unique and axial level-specific ways (see later, Table 10.1). The maxillary process, which gives rise to the tissues of the upper jaw, is regarded as an anterior protrusion from the first or **'mandibular'** arch, which itself gives rise to the lower jaw. Thus, the embryonic mouth or **stomodaeum** is surrounded by first arch-derived tissues. Branchial arches are generally numbered 1, 2, 3, 4 and 6, the fifth arch being assumed to have been lost during the course of evolution (see later; Figures 10.4 and 10.6). Another widely held assumption is that the ancestral chordates possessed an arch anterior or rostral to what we currently regard as the first arch. This 'pre-mandibular' arch is thought to have swung forward during the course of evolution to give rise to the anterior part of the skull base, the **trabeculae cranii**, functioning to support the new anterior additions to the ancestral brain, structures that we now regard as the fore- and midbrain or prosencephalon and mesencephalon respectively. Continuing with this evolutionary perspective, the progressive shift forward of the ancestral second arch, which we now regard as arch 1 or the mandibular arch, permitted the development of a biting and masticatory function. At a later stage, proximal elements from this arch and from the second or **'hyoid'** arch became secondarily modified as the conductive elements of the middle ear. It can thus be seen that the changing morphology and pattern of these arch elements, arising as development novelties generated by mutational changes to the mechanisms controlling their development, provided the foundation for the explosive evolution of the vertebrates from a primitive chordate ancestor and, ultimately, for the development of the human face.

During the sixth week, as the olfactory placodes thicken and invaginate to form the **nasal pits**, the frontonasal mass, comprising largely neural crest derived from the anterior mesencephalon (and possibly prosencephalon – see later), grows forward and downward. The lateral and medial margins of the invaginating placodes grow and, as the lateral and medial nasal processes, contact the maxillary primordia on each side at a timepoint during the seventh week (Figure 10.1). The three-branched contact seam so formed is the site at which adhesion and fusion occur. Remodelling of the ectoderm at the points of contact eliminates the seams and generates epithelial continuity across the forming upper face. The combination of these three processes on each side of the forming face will provide the cheeks and the wings or alae of the nostrils (Figure 10.1). Failure of fusion at these points, for any reason, will result in **unilateral** or **bilateral facial clefting** (see later), from the mouth up towards the forming eye(s). Coincident with the formation of the maxillary region, the frontonasal mass grows to provide a body of tissue between the medial nasal processes, the so-called **intermaxillary process**, which will provide the mid-facial tissue including much of the nose and the **philtrum**. Again, a failure to attain a critical mass for any of the processes/primordia involved will result in facial clefting, in this case **midline clefting** (see later) with the two sides of the face continuing to develop in a semi-autonomous fashion but with the lack of midline union causing an often wide midline cleft.

The mandibular process, which will give rise to the lower jaw, is rarely affected by clefting since fusion is not a feature of its development. Nevertheless a pattern of growth co-ordinated with that of the upper and mid-face is essential to provide a balanced physiognomy and functional integration. For example, both **hypo-** and **hyperplastic mandibles** will be dysfunctional with regard to dental occlusion. In rare instances, lateral clefting back from the angle of the mouth to the external meatus of the ear is seen but the aetiology is not always clear since fusion is not a feature of the development of this region and such clefts may reflect some vascular crisis earlier in development (see later).

The first branchial cleft, that is, between the first and second branchial arches, deepens and sinks inwards to develop into the **external auditory canal** or **meatus**; internally the corresponding first branchial pouch grows into the **tubotympanic recess** which will subsequently become the tympanic cavity of the middle ear and the Eustachian tube with its maintained continuity to the oropharynx. Intimately linked with this is the derivation of the **auditory ossicles** of the middle ear from the proximal mesenchyme of the first arch, which provides the **incus** and **malleus**, and from the second arch, providing the **stapes**. Concomitant with this, during the fourth to seventh weeks of development, the **otic placode** invaginates, sinks inwards and starts to form the vestibular system of the inner ear. The ossicles themselves form within loose mesenchyme which becomes engulfed by the expanding tympanic cavity and, whilst the stapes comes to lie adjacent to the oval window of the inner ear, the endodermal lining of the tympanic cavity and the ectoderm of the meatus, with a small fibrous layer sandwiched between, develop into the **tympanic membrane** or eardrum. The external **auricle** of the ear is formed from a number of condensations of tissue from both first and second arches, which surround the proximal part of the cleft. As the cleft itself sinks inwards to form the meatus, these **auricular**

hillocks grow, fuse and undergo a poorly understood morphogenesis to produce an appendage that functions to funnel airborne vibrations into the meatus and along the canal to the tympanic membrane. From their initially low position on the embryonic neck the auricles migrate progressively dorsalward co-ordinate with the morphogenesis of the meatus. Given the developmental complexity of forming the inner, middle and external parts of the ear, this organ is predictably susceptible to disruption. Thus, first arch syndromes (see later) can affect ossicle development as well as components of the jaw, and result in conductive deafness. Even relatively mild disturbances to this sensitive event may result in misshapen, small auricles (**microtia**) or absent auricles (**anotia**). Growth of the auricular hillocks and their morphogenesis into an auricle takes place largely during the fetal stages, even though the hillocks are themselves first distinguishable at the sixth week of embryogenesis.

Caudal to the first branchial arch, the arch series becomes progressively obscured by the caudalward extension of the second arch. During the sixth week, it grows backwards, in a sheet-like manner, over the third, fourth and sixth arches to fuse with the body wall at a point adjacent to the position of the descending heart primordium. The individual fates of these arches are summarized in Table 10.1. The transient space enclosed by this second arch-derived process, which is normally lost in tissue remodelling, may persist as a **lateral cervical cyst**, sometimes with fistulae draining externally, internally (into the oropharynx) or both.

By early fetal stages the landmarks of the human face have been established; during the second and third trimesters, allometric growth will transform it into the more familiar face of the neonate. However, the dramatic events producing the external topography are paralleled by an equally complex internal morphogenesis involving the oropharynx and the branchial pouches.

MORPHOGENESIS OF THE STOMODAEUM AND OROPHARYNX

In the initial stages of first arch development, the primitive mouth/buccal cavity or **stomodaeum** is separated from the foregut by a layer of apposed ectoderm externally and endoderm internally. This **buccopharyngeal membrane** breaks down late during the fourth week of development thereby creating continuity with the primitive foregut; the through cavity so formed is termed the **oropharynx**. The tongue forms on the floor of the oropharynx with contributions from arches 1, 2 and 4 and from the occipital somites (see later). During the fifth week, a small endodermal invagination from the dorsal surface of the tongue primordium grows and migrates downwards into the developing neck where the cells will form the thyroid gland at a site anterior to the future larynx. Physical continuity with the dorsum of the tongue is briefly maintained as the **thyroglossal duct** but this connection is lost as development proceeds; small foci of ectopic thyroid tissue occasionally result from fragmentation of the primordium as it descends into the neck.

During the late third week of embryonic life, a placodal structure on the roof of the stomodaeum invaginates dorsally towards the underside of the overlying

Table 10.1 Embryological development of branchial arches. (After Larsen, 1993)

Branchial arch	Arch artery	Skeletal elements	Muscles	Cranial nerve
1	Terminal branch of maxillary artery	Derived from arch cartilages (originating from neural crest) From maxillary cartilage: alisphenoid, incus From mandibular (Meckel's cartilage: malleus Derived by direct ossification from arch dermal mesenchyme: maxilla, zygomatic, squamous portion of temporal bone, mandible	Muscles of mastication (temporalis, masseter and pterygoids), mylohyoid, anterior belly of the digastric, tensor tympani, tensor veli palatini (originate from cranial somitomere 4)	Maxillary and mandibular divisions of trigeminal (V)
2	Stapedial artery (embryonic), corticotympanic artery (adult)	Stapes, styloid process, stylohyoid ligament, lesser horns and upper rim of hyoid (derived from the second-arch, Reichert's cartilage; originate from neural crest)	Muscles of facial expression (orbicularis oculi, orbicularis oris, risorius, platysma, auricularis, fronto-occipitalis, and buccinator), posterior belly of the digastric, stylohyoid, stapedius (originate from cranial somitomere 6)	Facial (VIII)
3	Common carotid artery, root of internal carotid	Lower rim and greater horns of hyoid (derived from the third-arch cartilage; originate from neural crest)	Stylopharyngeus (originates from cranial somitomere 7)	Glossopharyngeal (IX)
4	Arch of aorta, right subclavian artery, original sprouts of pulmonary arteries	Laryngeal cartilages (derived from the fourth-arch cartilage; originate from lateral plate mesoderm)	Constrictors of pharynx, cricothyroid levator veli palatini (originates from occipital somites 2 to 4)	Superior laryngeal branch of vagus (X)
6	Ductus arteriosus, roots of definitive pulmonary arteries	Laryngeal cartilages (derived from the sixth-arch cartilage; originate from lateral plate mesoderm)	Intrinsic muscles of larynx (originate from occipital somites 1 and 2)	Recurrent laryngeal branch of vagus (X)

forebrain. This structure, known at this stage as **Rathke's pouch**, becomes associated with a ventral downgrowth from the forebrain, known as the **infundibulum**, and together they will form the **pituitary gland**. Initially, the site of invagination of Rathke's pouch can be seen on the roof of the stomodaeum but this continuity is soon lost as pituitary development proceeds. Rathke's pouch itself gives rise to the **adenohypophysis** and **pars intermedia** while the **neurohypophysis** forms from the infundibulum.

Initially the nasal cavity and oropharynx are continuous, with only a posterior extension of intermaxillary process-derived tissue, the **primary palate**, separating them rostrally. Full anatomical separation of the two is achieved by the formation of the secondary palate from the bilateral **palatal shelves** which grow ventromedially into the oropharynx from the medial surface of the maxillary processes (Figure 10.2). Initially the shelves project almost ventrally and lie lateral to the tongue primordium. However, starting at the eighth week they rotate through 90° to point medially, and grow to fuse in the midline. The nasal cavity thereby becomes separated from the oropharynx except at the posterior extreme, and is divided into two passages by the concomitant downward growth of the nasal septum. Like so many other phenomena during craniofacial development, morphogenesis of the palate is highly sensitive to perturbation for a variety of reasons. Reduced growth of the mesenchyme within the shelves, or an oversized tongue primordium impeding their rotation, will both cause **palatal clefting**. Given the interrelationship with maxillary development, and with development of the primary palate from the intermaxillary process, it is not surprising that cleft palate may often accompany facial clefting (see later).

Rather more complex is the fate of the tissue lining the pouches. The morphogenesis and growth of the first pouch to form the tubotympanic recess (and subsequently the tympanic cavity and the Eustachian tube) has already

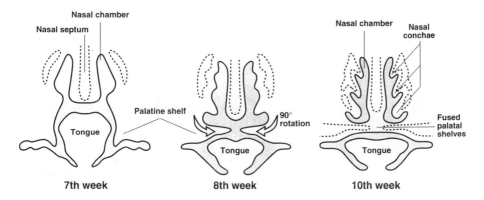

Figure 10.2 Morphogenesis of the palatal shelves during development of the oropharynx. Note how the paired palatal shelves, initially growing ventrally on either side of the tongue primordium, rotate through 90° at about the eighth week into a horizontal plane, to fuse in the midline, thereby creating the secondary palate. (After Larsen, 1993)

been dealt with but even from that brief account it is evident that allometric growth and tissue relocations are an integral feature. With the development of the remaining pouches these phenomena are even more dramatic, with some cell populations being relocated to sites in the lower neck and even the chest (Figure 10.3). The endoderm and associated mesenchyme of the second pouch give rise to the **palatine tonsils**, differentiating from the end of the third trimester onwards. During weeks 5–7, endodermal cells from the third and fourth pouches descend through the forming neck to give rise to the **inferior** and **superior parathyroid gland** respectively (the third pouch-derived cells descending further than their more caudal counterparts to an inferior location). Starting at 6 weeks, a similar route of descent is exhibited by the cells of what is variously interpreted as a pocket of the fourth pouch or, more controversially, as a vestigial fifth pouch, to give rise to **parafollicular** or **calcitonin-producing cells** of the thyroid. The precise derivation of these cells, from pouch endoderm, associated mesenchyme or groove ectoderm, is still to be determined. The most dramatic of all of these descents is that displayed by the cells that will form the stroma of the **thymus**. These originate from tissue proliferations at the distal tip of each third pouch during weeks 4–5 and subsequently relocate in the anterior chest wall where full morphogenesis of the thymus gland ensues.

During the fourth week, the **respiratory diverticulum** grows out as an evagination from the underside of the foregut. During the following week it branches for the first time; the left and right branches will go on to form the right and left **bronchial buds**, which branch progressively to form the respiratory tree, and the stem develops into the trachea and larynx. The epithelial lining of the respiratory tract is thus endodermal in origin although the surrounding stroma is mesodermal. Rostral to the opening of the respiratory diverticulum, at the

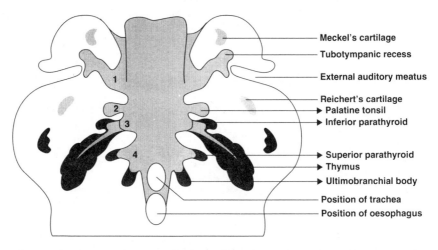

Figure 10.3 Coronal plane of section through the oropharynx illustrating the fate of the branchial pouches, numbered 1–4 with the principal derivatives indicated by arrows. The angular midline object at the top of the figure is the tongue seen in a dorsal perspective. (After Larsen, 1993)

approximate level of the fourth arch, the **epiglottis** develops from about 6 weeks onwards; the tissue derivation of this structure and its supportive cartilages is not entirely clear.

MORPHOGENESIS OF THE MUSCULOSKELETAL SYSTEM

Given the focused nature of this chapter, accounts of most organ systems cannot be included and the reader is directed to several insightful reviews on patterning of the various tissue systems in the head (Noden, 1991; Le Douarin, 1993). However, given the relative importance of the musculoskeletal system in head morphogenesis, and its involvement in birth defects, it seems appropriate to cover a few aspects that are essential to an appreciation of the later parts of the chapter.

The major part of the skull is produced by ectomesenchymal cells of neural crest origin. In fact, the mesodermal contribution, which was thought to include the bones of the cranial vault, has recently been reassessed. The first five somites, the **occipital somites**, together with the non-segmented cephalic mesoderm, become incorporated into the skull to form the occipital bones and a major part of the otic capsule. All of the remaining parts of the skull, including the rostral part of the cranial base, the facial skeleton and jaws, a minor part of the otic capsule, the bones of the cranial vault and the cells of the sutures are derived from the neural crest (Couly et al, 1993). A combination of epigenetic tissue interactions (in the neurocranium) and genetic specification (in the viscerocranium; see later) seems to be involved in determining the intricate patterns of skeletogenic differentiation that subsequently take place (Hanken and Thorogood, 1993; Thorogood, 1993).

Paraxial mesoderm, including the occipital somites, is the sole source of myogenic cells in the head (Noden, 1983a; Couly et al, 1992). Like myogenic cells elsewhere in the body, these cells have no intrinsic pattern specification of their own and when heterotopically grafted develop according to the site of grafting (Trainor et al, 1994). Facial musculature appears to be patterned entirely by the crest-derived connective tissue cells (Noden, 1983a) in a manner resembling the patterning of (somite-derived) limb musculature by (flank-derived) connective tissue cells (see Chapter 7). The mechanism by which this patterning is specified is completely unknown.

MAIN CLASSES OF CRANIOFACIAL DEFECT

Given the high proportion of major birth defects that affect the head or face, there is a predictable diversity of phenotype and of aetiology. Even today the causes of the majority (60%) of birth defects are largely unknown, with single gene mutations accounting for 7.5%, chromosomal anomalies 6% and multifactorial traits 20%, with maternal factors such as diabetes accounting for the remainder (Moore, 1995). Traditionally, birth defects have been classified according to phenotype. However, as modern genetic analyses progress, it becomes clear that, though essential clinically, such classifications are inevitably simplistic when it comes to understanding aetiology. In the case of single gene defects, belief in a one gene/one syndrome relationship is not necessarily justified (see Chapter 1), as exemplified by the craniosynostoses (Mulvihill, 1995). Furthermore, the 'unknown' and 'multifactorial' categories remain by far the largest and, given that they may contain a combination of environmental and predisposing genetic factors, unravelling the aetiology can be exceedingly complex (see Chapter 5). Thus, explanation based on phenotype, or genetics or environmental factors alone will be distorted, simply because of the complexity of the biological situation and the incompleteness of our current understanding. Here, a classification of the major craniofacial defects is presented, based on the particular embryonic event or developmental mechanisms likely to have been perturbed, whether by genetic or environmental factors or a combination of both. Selective examples are provided, but for comprehensive accounts, see Gorlin et al (1990), Ferguson (1991) and Winter and Baraitser (1993).

FOREBRAIN/FRONTONASAL MASS DEFECTS

Impaired forebrain development, coupled with an insufficient frontonasal mass and intermaxillary process, results in midline defects. The various phenotypes are collectively referred to as the **holoprosencephalies**. In a mild form this type of defect may be seen in **fetal alcohol syndrome**, characterized by a short, upturned nose, a shallow or absent philtrum, highly arched palate, a short retracted lower jaw and a degree of mental retardation (indeed, alcohol consumption is estimated to be the most common cause of congenital mental retardation in the West; Larsen, 1993). Where there are different degrees of failure of the prosencephalon to cavitate and develop correctly (hence 'holoprosencephaly'), a progressive series of defects can be recognized; these involve progressive reduction of the ventromedial forebrain structures and of crest-derived mesenchyme in the frontonasal region. Thus, mid-face structures derived from the intermaxillary process, such as the philtrum, may be absent, resulting in **mid-facial clefting**. Further deficiency, coupled with the narrower midbrain and a suspected failure of midline definition of the bilateral olfactory placodes, goes beyond clefting to produce a facies with reduced nasal structures, sometimes manifest as a small nose with a single nostril (**cebocephaly**). Further reduction results in a complete absence of nose and olfactory structures (including olfactory bulbs, tracts and cortex), with eyes developing much closer to the midline (**hypotelorism**). Finally, in the most extreme cases, the aberrant development of the floor of the forebrain produces only a single midline optic cup and **cyclopia** results (see note added in proof).

EPITHELIAL FUSION DEFECTS

This class of defect includes all those cases where there has been a failure of facial processes or primordia to grow, contact a neighbouring process, fuse and remodel to produce tissue continuity across the previous contact seam. Primarily it includes failure in the events involved in building the upper face, resulting in **unilateral** or **bilateral facial clefting**, and in building the secondary palate, producing a **cleft palate**; these events can be isolated or syndromic. The aetiology of clefting is exceedingly complex (Johnston and Bronsky, 1995) and, ironically, far more effort has been expended in elucidating the cause of palatal clefting than facial clefting although it may well be that some of the lessons learned from the former may apply to the latter. Three main types of cause can be recognized at a broad embryological level. First, inadequately sized primordia, where growth may have failed or been impaired for any one of a number of genetic or environmental reasons, will fail to make contact with neighbouring processes at the appropriate developmental time; fusion and subsequent events will fail as a consequence. Secondly, epithelial differentiation itself may be impaired such that appropriate adhesive molecules are not expressed and the epithelial surfaces, although in physical contact, cannot progress beyond this and fuse. Thirdly, there may be non-specific physical reasons why fusion fails. For example, the size and position of the tongue within the oropharynx can impede the rotation of the palatal shelves; an overly wide head may mean that, even if rotation is successfully accomplished, medial growth does not quite bring the medial edges of the shelves into contact for fusion to proceed.

VASCULAR CRISIS DEFECTS

Although sometimes difficult to corroborate, it does now appear that disruptions in the orderly development of the blood vascular system in the head and neck can, through the localized ischaemia and the tissue necrosis that results, produce some of the more common craniofacial defects. Thus, the lateral clefting from the gape of the mouth back towards the auditory meatus mentioned earlier is thought to be the consequence of a haematoma within the stapedial artery that supplies blood to the maxillary and mandibular processes, the resultant ischaemic necrosis giving rise to undersized primordia. The **hemifacial microsomias**, such as **Goldenhar syndrome**, are thought to arise by a comparable vascular disturbance but, whereas the lateral clefting may be absent or minimal, the mandible, the temporomandibular joint, associated musculature and (outer and inner) ear may all be undersized, dysmorphic or missing. Similar events may underlie other apparently spontaneous craniofacial defects but the ability of embryonic tissue to repair lesions caused by ischaemia may partially or wholly conceal the original cause.

SKELETAL DYSPLASIA DEFECTS

In some instances, genetic or environmental perturbations that are tissue type-specific will inevitably affect craniofacial development if that tissue is present in the head. Thus, **achondroplasia**, an autosomal dominant mutation affecting the function of the epiphyseal growth plates in the long bones of the appendicular skeleton, also affects the function of the synchondroses in the cranial base, resulting in a reduced growth of the mid-face. A 'bossing' or prominence of the frontal bones results as the cranium grows normally but disproportionately to the reduced facial skeleton. In other instances, although the target tissue may be skeletal, the defects may be largely confined to skeletal tissues within the head as seen in the majority of the (autosomally dominant) **craniosynostoses**, where the growth function of the cranial sutures is terminated when they prematurely differentiate into bone; the continued growth of the cranium, co-ordinated with that of the growing brain, is prevented. The resultant increase in intracranial pressure can distort the shape of the cranium and cause neuropathological damage. Generally, such localization of defects to the head is seen in **Crouzon**, **Pfeiffer** and **Saethre–Chotzen syndromes** but not in **Apert syndrome**, where oligosyndactyly of the hands and feet is a characteristic feature additional to the craniosynostosis.

BRANCHIAL ARCH DEFECTS

In this large and diverse category are all those defects thought to result from an impairment of neural crest migration, of branchial arch growth and/or correct specification of arch morphogenetic fate. Superficially some may resemble phenotypes arising from vascular crises (see earlier) but here the aetiology is distinctly different and the phenotype generally bilateral. A dysmorphic lower face with an underdeveloped lower jaw (**micrognathia**), palatal clefting and abnormal external ears, sometimes with conductive deafness due to absent or dysmorphic ossicles, are features of the single biggest group of syndromes within this class, known collectively as **mandibulofacial dysostosis**. Examples of those known to have a genetic basis are **Treacher–Collins** and **Hallerman–Streif syndromes**, known to be autosomal dominant and autosomal recessive respectively. Mandibulofacial dysostosis is also a response to a variety of environmental insults during the first 6 weeks of development, including the potent craniofacial teratogen, retinoic acid (Lammer et al, 1985; and see later). Other syndromes affecting arch derivatives are known, perhaps the most common being **DiGeorge syndrome**, where not only are there craniofacial problems similar to those described for mandibulofacial dysostosis but both the thymus and parathyroids are either absent or reduced and there are cardiovascular anomalies including persistent truncus arteriosus and dysmorphic aortic vessels. Parathyroid and thymic anomalies are likely consequences of disruption to third and fourth branchial pouches associated with some defect in neural crest development and arch morphogenesis; the cardiovascular problems are thought to result from disruption to the 'cardiac neural crest' which emerges from the posterior hindbrain (see Chapter 11).

DEFORMATION AND DISRUPTION DEFECTS

A number of non-specific physical factors, such as fetal compression from **oligohydramnios** (reduced amniotic cavity) and **amniotic bands** (folds of the amnion that entangle the fetus, constricting, and sometimes cutting through, fetal tissue) can generate craniofacial defects. However, since they are sporadic in their occurrence and random in their effects on craniofacial morphogenesis, they will not be considered further here.

CELLULAR AND MOLECULAR MECHANISMS CONTROLLING CRANIOFACIAL DEVELOPMENT

Over the last 20 years our understanding of the developmental mechanisms involved in the building of the head and face has changed enormously. The development of new technologies and their application, in novel analytical strategies, to the traditional animal models (chiefly avian and murine) have generated fresh paradigms; consequently, determining the mechanisms controlling craniofacial development is no longer the rather intractable problem that it was once thought to be.

THE BRANCHIAL REGION (AND LOWER FACE)

This comprises those axial levels approximating to the hindbrain or rhombencephalon and the branchial arches. It is dealt with first because recent molecular advances relating to this part of the head underpin much of what has ensued regarding the more rostral regions (see later). Tissue recombination experiments, in which the ectodermal and mesenchymal components of facial primordia were interchanged, demonstrated that the specification of growth and morphogenetic fate in the arches resides in the mesenchymal component (Richman and Tickle, 1989). The focus of attention therefore becomes the rhombencephalic crest which gives rise to most of the branchial arch mesenchyme (with the exception of the myogenic lineage, see earlier). Given that much of the mid- and lower face, and the jaw skeleton, is arch-derived, hindbrain crest is clearly profoundly important in the formation of the face. Furthermore, as will become apparent, it is the mode of rhombencephalic crest migration, imposed by the organization of the hindbrain, that ensures anatomical registration between axial structures and the metameric array of branchial arches.

The hindbrain itself is now recognized as a truly segmental structure (Lumsden and Keynes, 1989) with eight neuromeres known as **rhombomeres** (identified as R1–8) which constitute units of lineage restriction, i.e. early commitment to particular developmental fates (Fraser et al, 1990). A very significant step forward was made with the discovery that certain regulatory genes display expression domains that coincide with rhombomere boundaries (e.g. Wilkinson et al, 1989). In particular, the more 3' genes of the **Hox gene family**, homologous to the *antennapedia* gene family in *Drosophila* and containing a homeobox sequence (see Chapter 1), display expression domains within the hindbrain that have anterior cut-offs arranged in a staggered array at successive rhombomere boundaries. Given that these segmental units represent units of (neuroepithelial) lineage restriction, this highly ordered pattern of gene expression might therefore constitute part of a mechanism whereby morphogenetic specification is established (McGinnis and Krumlauf, 1992; Wilkinson, 1993). Four clusters of Hox genes are found within the vertebrate genome, existing on different chromosomes and all derived from a common ancestral cluster by cluster duplication events back in the evolutionary past (Graham et al, 1989). There are two important points to note. First, the order of the cut-offs along the rostrocaudal axis of the hindbrain maps with the sequential position of a particular Hox gene within its cluster along the 3' to 5' polarity of a chromosome. This topographical correlation is usually termed **structural co-linearity** and, since the 3'-most genes within each cluster are also the first to be expressed, a **temporal co-linearity** also exists (Duboule and Dollé, 1989). Second, as a result of common origin from a gene in the ancestral Hox cluster, there is an equivalence between individual genes in different clusters due to their sequence homology and relative 3' to 5' position within their respective clusters (see later, Figure 10.5). These are collectively termed **paralogous groups,** and it is significant that paralogous genes also share identical expression domains (Figure 10.4). Thus, *Hox-A3* is paralogous to *Hox-B3* and *Hox-D3* in that they display a very conserved sequence homology, occupy equivalent positions within their respective Hox clusters on mouse genes 6, 11 and 2 respectively, and all three display anterior cut-offs at the boundary between R4 and R7.

However, in parallel to these discoveries, other important and complementary relationships have emerged. First, rhombencephalic crest cells from particular axial levels migrate into particular branchial arches. Thus, R1 and R2 crest cells migrate into the first arch, R4 crest cells into the second arch and crest cells from R6 into the third arch (Lumsden et al, 1991). It should be noted that R3 and R5 apparently produce little if any neural crest and this coincides with the occurrence of programmed cell death in the mid-dorsal region of these rhombomeres (Graham et al, 1993). (There is an alternative interpretation that R3 and R5 crest cells, although relatively small populations, migrate to join the streams of crest cells emerging from the adjacent even-numbered rhombomeres; Sechrist et al, 1993.) Not only is there a precision of migration route but the crest cells initially carry with them a pattern of Hox gene expression identical to that expressed in the rhombomere from which they originated (Figure 10.4). Consequently, the crest-derived mesenchyme of each arch expresses a different and arch-specific combination of Hox genes. This constitutes what has some-times been referred to as a **branchial Hox code**, with the implication that this combinatorial code is somehow involved in transmitting morphogenetic specification from the hindbrain to the branchial arches (Hunt et al, 1991). Similar codes have been described for the vertebral column (Kessel and Gruss, 1991; see Chapter 13) and the limb (Duboule, 1992; see Chapter 7). In the case of the arches, the axial level-specific code is thought to be secondarily imposed upon the initially naive ectoderm and any mesoderm within an arch, thereby establishing a unique identity for each arch. In this way, genetic 'information' that is specific to a particular rostrocaudal level and assumed to have a role in the specification of positional identity is conveyed from the axial structures, in this case the neural tube, to the periphery – the branchial arches. Such a scenario, if correct, provides a mechanism ensuring a degree of anatomical registration and

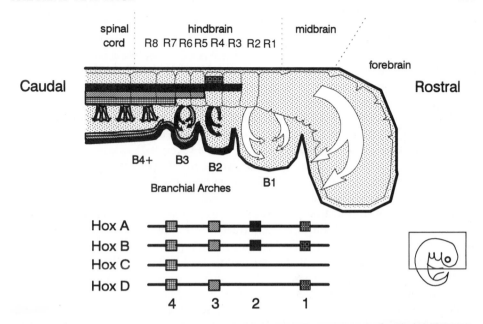

Figure 10.4 The Branchial Hox code as elucidated in the mouse embryo, illustrating the relationship between expression domains of the 3'-most Hox genes in the rhombomeres (R1–8) in the developing hindbrain and branchial arches (B1–B4+), and their position within their respective clusters (labelled A–D) on individual chromosomes. Paralogous groups are defined vertically across the clusters and these 3'-most paralogous groups are numbered 1–4; note the correspondence in hatching between an individual gene in its cluster, its paralogues in other clusters, and their spatial expression domain in the rhombomere, in streams of migrating crest cells (arrows) and in the ectodermal covering of each arch (migration of crest cells from particular axial levels is indicated by arrows). Spatial co-linearity is seen in the rostral-to-caudal sequence of anterior cut-offs (from right to left) and the location of the individual genes 3' to 5' along each chromosome (also from right to left). Note that no Hox genes are expressed in those crest cells migrating from the first two rhombomeres into the first arch or in those migrating rostrally from the mesencephalon and prosencephalon. The location of the diagram *vis-à-vis* the rest of the embryo is shown in the inset. (Diagram supplied by Paul Hunt)

a molecular basis for the earlier finding that morphogenetic specification resides in the mesenchyme of the arches (Richman and Tickle, 1989).

If Hox genes, or at least their combinatorial expression, have such a role, then transgenic technology provides a means of functionally testing such hypotheses. Both loss-of-function and gain-of-function transgenic mouse lines have been created for this purpose and a few selected examples, illustrating both the advantages and the limitations of the transgenic approach, will be reviewed. For a variety of reasons, it is believed that it is the anterior region of the expression domains which is the most critical. A very clear demonstration of the usefulness of gain-of-function mutants is provided by extending rostrally the expression of a Hox gene, *Hox-D4*, into the occipital region of the forming head. The anterior cut-off for *Hox-D4* is normally at the level of the first cervical vertebra. By placing the gene under the control of a promoter that extends this cut-off rostrally, the occipital bones of the skull are transformed into extra cervical vertebrae (Lufkin et al, 1992). Significantly, the original cervical vertebrae display a normal phenotype, supporting the belief that it is the anterior cut-off (in this case, a new one) that is critical in morphogenetic specification of the cells at that position. The outcome of this transgenic manipulation reveals something fundamental, not only about the role of such genes in skull development but also about the evolution of the craniovertebral junction (see Chapter 13). It was noted earlier that during embryogenesis, the first five (occipital) somites are normally lost due to incorporation into the occipital skull, presumably reflecting a caudalward extension of the skull during evolution; this genetic manipulation produces an atavistic reversal of that phenomenon.

Direct evidence supporting the proposed role of a branchial Hox code comes from transgenic inactivation of a gene normally expressed within the branchial arches. Transgenic knockout of *Hoxa-2*, normally expressed with a cut-off between R2 and R3 and expressed in the second arch, results in a deletion of second arch structures. In their place are seen duplicated first arch structures, with a second Meckel's cartilage forming adjacent to the otic capsule and duplication of the malleus, a first arch-derived auditory ossicle (Gendron-Maguire et al, 1993). It will have been apparent from Figure 10.4 that no Hox genes are expressed in the first arch, where first arch morphology may reflect some kind of 'default' property (Noden, 1983b). Here, elimination of *Hoxa-2* expression from the second arch, and with no other paralogous groups expressed at this axial level, a default value seems to have been imposed on second arch tissue, in spite of the persisting expression of the only paralogue, *Hoxb-2*.

However, transgenic phenotypes can sometimes be quite perplexing. A loss-of-function mutant of *Hoxa-3* (formerly called *Hox-1.5*) displays a phenotype that has been interpreted as a model for DiGeorge syndrome. Embryos homozygous for the inactivated gene are athymic and aparathyroid, have reduced thyroid tissue and display cardiac and arterial anomalies (Chisaka and Capecchi, 1991; Manley and Capecchi, 1995). These abnormalities are in accord with the known expression domain for this gene, which displays an anterior cut-off at the interface between the second and third arches and with the known derivatives from within this domain. However, there are a number of craniofacial defects in tissues derived from first and second arches, that is, anterior to the normal expression domain. In this case, relating the altered genotype to the altered phenotype is not straightforward and suggests that an element of 'cross-talk' between *Hox-A3* and other regulatory genes may be taking place. Furthermore, there are reports of single Hox gene knockouts where there is no detectable effect on craniofacial phenotype. These have been explained by redundancy between members of a paralogous group, such that if one is knocked out, the remaining paralogues continue to maintain the function of that group. Currently, double knockouts where two paralogues are simultaneously inactivated are being developed to pursue this question (Condie and Capecchi, 1994). Clearly, the relationship between Hox gene expression and morphogenetic specification of the arches is not on a straightforward one-to-one basis.

Some progress in understanding this relationship comes from a rather different approach, that of experimental embryology and the use of tissue grafting and ablation techniques. Ablation of the hindbrain neural crest has revealed a surprising degree of regenerative potential within the neuro-epithelium of the neural tube, with crest being regenerated and proceeding to migrate normally (Scherson et al, 1993). Furthermore, such cells display a branchial Hox code appropriate for their axial level and go on to form normal viscerocranial skeletal structures (Hunt et al, 1995). It would appear that the neuroepithelial cells have changed their fate and, if so, then morphogenetic specification across the dorsoventral axis of the neural tube is clearly still plastic at this stage of development. In contrast, the fact that the regenerated cells express Hox genes appropriate to their axial level of origin within the recon-structed neural tube indicates that rostrocaudal specification is fixed at an earlier stage and persists through regeneration. Since the skeletogenic derivatives of the hindbrain crest still form correctly from these regenerated crest cells, the relationship between axial level of origin of crest, Hox gene expression and morphogenetic fate survives this particular perturbation. Rotation of hindbrain crest through 180° to confront the cells with a novel and inappropriate axial environment is also revealing. Whilst rhombomeric Hox gene expression is maintained and apparently fixed, within the migrating neural crest cells it can modulate, suggesting that crest cells can alter Hox gene expression in response to environmental signals (Saldivar et al, 1996). Such changes correlate with a re-specification of morphogenetic fate of the cells concerned (Hunt et al, 1996). Collectively, such results demonstrate that the morphogenetic specification of the arches, or at least of the hindbrain neural crest cells that colonize them, is not a simple matter of a fixed pre-pattern determined by axial level in the hindbrain and maintained autonomously within the migrating crest cells. They also indicate that positional input from the axial environment may have an additional role in determining the code as it is expressed within the arches.

All of this data from analysis of animal models would be of little use in understanding human craniofacial development if the branchial Hox code was different in humans or not deployed in the same way. Recently, the **human branchial Hox code** has been defined using material from a human embryo bank and probes specific to human Hox genes for in-situ hybridization analysis of the expression domains of the 3'-most genes. Human Hox genes are organized into four clusters just as in any other vertebrate and the relationship of the various paralogous groups to the ancestral complex, represented by the *Drosophila* HOM-C complex, can be traced (Figure 10.5) (Acampora et al, 1989). Eight members of paralogous groups 1, 2, 3 and 4 known to be expressed in the mouse hindbrain and branchial arches were studied and found to be expressed in comparable spatiotemporal patterns in the human embryo at 4 weeks (Figure 10.6). The combinatorial patterns of expression representing the first three groups parallel the patterns described for their homologues in the mouse and bird, demonstrating a high degree of conservation of the branchial Hox code (Figure 10.7). (Expression of group 4 genes had not previously been described for any other vertebrate, so issues of conservation can only be assumed for this

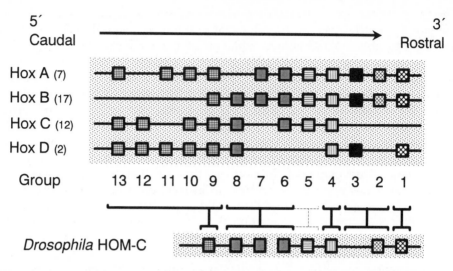

Figure 10.5 Genomic organization of the human *HOX* genes with clusters A, B, C and D on chromosomes 7, 17, 12 and 2 respectively. Conventions used are identical to those in Figure 10.4. Note the equivalence in organization between paralogous groups 1–4 here, for the human, and in Figure 10.4, for the mouse. The lower part of the figure illustrates the assumed relatedness to genes in the HOM-C complex, the single gene cluster in *Drosophila* thought to resemble the single ancestral cluster. (Diagram supplied by Paul Hunt)

paralogous group.) Furthermore, it was demonstrated that, as development proceeds, individual paralogues of a single group, which initially share a common expression domain, are differentially down-regulated in a tissue-, organ- or site-specific fashion (Vieille-Grosjean et al, 1997).

Although the data tell us nothing about conservation of function (see Chapter 1), the tight correlations with the published data from animal models suggest that the repertoire of Hox gene expression serves an equivalent function in the embryonic assembly of the head and face in the human and the mouse. Furthermore, the results allow assessment of the extent to which the mouse can justifiably be used as a model system to understand human craniofacial development and its dysmorphogenesis. On the basis of the similarities found it would seem reasonable to assume that models of normal craniofacial development based on Hox gene function, generated by work on the mouse, can be safely extrapolated to the human (Vieille-Grosjean et al, 1997). However, to what extent transgenic manipulation of Hox gene expression can be used to model dysmorphic syndromes is a more contentious issue (see later).

Definition of a Hox code does not in itself provide an explanation for morphogenetic specification during craniofacial development. The code constitutes just one level of control within a genetic hierarchy but does provide us with a 'window' through which we can identify the upstream control elements (i.e. what sets up the code?) and the downstream targets (i.e. what are the target genes for the various homeoproteins?). In other words, knowledge of the code

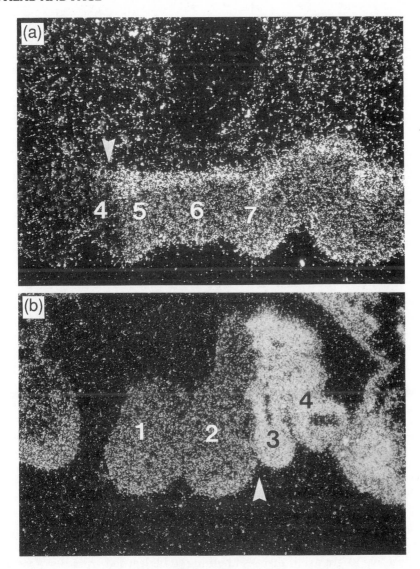

Figure 10.6 In-situ hybridization preparations showing *HOXA3* expression in (a) hindbrain and (b) branchial arches. Both sections are in coronal plane, rostral is to the left and caudal to the right, with the midline approximately following the top edge of each plate; rhombomeres 4–7 and branchial arches 1–4 are labelled. Anterior cut-offs for the expression domain, indicated by the white arrowheads, are clearly seen at the R4/R5 interface and at the arch 2/arch 3 interface in the hindbrain and branchial region respectively. Dark field. (From Vieille-Grosjean et al, 1996)

provides an opportunity to identify the other genetic components within the hierarchy. However, despite considerable research activity, we are still largely ignorant about both aspects although perhaps slightly more progress has been made in identifying upstream control elements. Given the similarities in

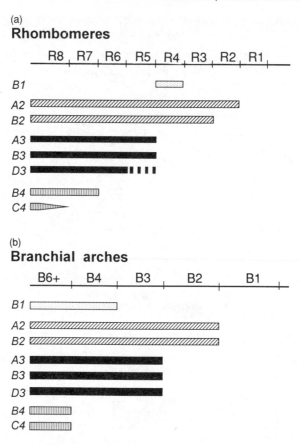

Figure 10.7 Summary of the human branchial Hox code illustrating the spatial expression domains for eight of the 3′-most *HOX* genes in (a) rhombomeres and (b) branchial arches. As with the mouse, paralogues generally show equivalent expression domains. (From Vieille-Grosjean et al, 1997)

chromosomal organization in clusters, co-linearity of expression, and genetic function generally between the Hox genes in the mouse and the HOM-C genes in *Drosophila*, we might ask if there is anything to be learned from our (extensive) knowledge of upstream regulation in *Drosophila*. However, fundamental differences in very early development exclude this possibility; expression of genes of the HOM-C homeotic complex is established before cellularization and in response to gradients of morphogens set up in the ooplasm during maturation of the oocyte. In vertebrates, Hox genes become expressed in cell populations where extensive division, migration and morphogenetic movements are taking place and it is likely that vertebrates have evolved different strategies for regulation of the Hox complex genes (Krumlauf, 1994). Not only this but the experimental strategies that can be used to screen for the relevant genes in an organism like *Drosophila* are not generally feasible in vertebrates and so there has been a reliance on cell lines and transgenics. Although such transgenic manipulation has been used very creatively (see earlier), there remains some concern that normal regulation of an individual Hox gene might be lost when it is manipulated in isolation; in some unknown way, cluster organization may be important and regulation of a Hox gene in a non-clustered context may produce patterns of expression that are incomplete or abnormal (Krumlauf, 1994).

Nevertheless, some progress has been made in identifying upstream regulators. The discovery that some murine Hox genes expressed in the hindbrain contain multiple regulatory regions that individually drive expression of the gene in a segment-specific fashion, has permitted identification of at least one upstream controlling gene. The murine *Hoxb-2* gene contains distinct regulatory elements that separately drive expression in R4 and in R3/R5 (Sham et al, 1993). It is now known that the zinc-finger regulatory gene **Krox-20** controls the R3/R5 expression of *Hoxb-2*, and the Krox-20 protein has been shown, by in-vitro assay, to bind to three regions of the *Hoxb-2* gene (Sham et al, 1993). Thus ectopic expression of *Krox-20* can activate *Hoxb-2* in locations where it would not normally be expressed and loss-of-function transgenics for *Krox-20*, although initially displaying R3 and R5 expression of *Hoxb-2*, fail to maintain it (Swiatek and Gridley, 1993). Reassessment of the phenotype in the *kreisler* mouse, originally identified through an inner ear anomaly, has revealed that hindbrain segmentation is abnormal, with R5 and R6 absent. *Krox-20* is not expressed at all in its R5 domain and there are predictable downstream changes in hindbrain Hox gene expression (McKay et al, 1994), supporting the idea that *Krox-20* is indeed upstream of Hox genes. At this stage the full range of *Krox-20* targets is not known and it is quite conceivable that other (Hox) genes may also be targeted and that *Krox-20* will prove to have an even greater role in hindbrain patterning. The consequences for the branchial Hox code and branchial arch morphogenesis are obvious.

The *sonic hedgehog* (*shh*) gene encodes a signal protein that has been shown to be involved in the patterning of several systems (Johnson and Tabin, 1995) including the neural tube (see Chapter 8), the somites and the limb (see Chapter 7). In the limb, *shh* can mimic the effect of the zone of polarizing activity and appears to be part of the upstream regulation of Hox gene expression. Given that shh peptides are also present in the branchial arches (Marti et al, 1995), then *shh* is a further candidate for upstream regulation (see note added in proof).

However, considerable interest is focused on the role of **retinoids** (isoforms of vitamin A) in the upstream control of Hox genes. It has long been known that retinoids are not only necessary for normal development but that at elevated levels they are potent craniofacial teratogens in both animal model systems and humans (Lammer et al, 1985). Indeed, the treatment of amphibian and mouse embryos causes either truncations of more rostral tissues in the embryonic head or their transformation to a more caudal specification (Durston et al, 1989; Marshall et al, 1992). Moreover, retinoids have been shown to alter patterns of Hox gene expression in cultured cell lines in an ordered, concentration-dependent fashion, such that the more 3' Hox genes, normally expressed rostrally, display greater sensitivity to retinoic acid, with the more 5' genes being progressively less sensitive (Simeone et al, 1992); in other words there is a co-linearity of sensitivity to retinoic acid that parallels the temporal and spatial co-linearity of gene expression discussed earlier.

The effects of retinoids are mediated by two families of nuclear receptors, the **retinoic acid receptors** (RARs) and the **retinoid X receptors** (RXRs). Retinoic acid-bound RARs are transcription factors that operate by binding to the **retinoic acid response elements** (RAREs) in the promoter region of the target gene; significantly, a number of Hox genes have now been demonstrated to contain such RAREs. Intracellular availability of retinoid for binding to the nuclear receptors is determined by cytoplasmically located retinoid binding proteins and these, like the nuclear receptors, display a regional distribution during craniofacial morphogenesis (e.g. Gustafson et al, 1993). The roles of the binding proteins include the processing and catabolism of retinoids, thereby determining quantitative availability. It is thought that it is the balance, and types, of binding protein and nuclear receptor present within cells which determines tissue-specific sensitivity to retinoids (Morriss-Kay, 1993). The RARs constitute a large family of genes and clearly there is a degree of functional redundancy amongst family members since it has taken the creation of double knockouts to produce phenotypes that parallel the features seen in vitamin A-deficient fetuses (Lohnes et al, 1994). Most of the dysmorphic craniofacial features generated by retinoid deficiency or excess involve crest-derived structures and, predictably, exogenous retinoic acid disrupts the orderly migration and axial identity of hindbrain crest (Lee et al, 1995). Although some aspects of the abnormal crest migration might be ascribed to physicochemical influences on cell motility and the surrounding extracellular matrix (Moro Balbás et al, 1993), the majority of defects are thought likely to be the consequence of mis-specification of morphogenetic fate, mediated by inappropriate upstream regulation of Hox genes.

Far less progress has been made with regard to downstream targets. There is evidence from several sources for 'cross-talk' between Hox genes (e.g. Zappavigna et al, 1991), so we can anticipate that a number of regulatory genes will be downstream targets for Hox gene products. However, we might reasonably expect some target genes to be those encoding structural proteins such as extracellular matrix proteins and their receptors, peptide growth factors and receptors, cell adhesion molecules and cytoskeletal proteins: in other words those types of molecule which are directly involved in building the morphology apparently specified by the Hox genes. The fragmentary picture that has emerged to date only partly fits this prediction. For instance, the full significance of the identification of a mouse homologue (*mgl-1*) of a *Drosophila* tumour suppressor gene as a downstream target for *Hox-C8* (Tomotsune et al, 1993) is unclear, although the authors speculate that *Hox-C8* may be one of several Hox genes involved in the regulation of *mgl-1* in the embryonic spinal cord. In contrast, the possibility that genes encoding cell adhesion molecules might constitute downstream targets is confirmed by the report that **N-CAM** (neural cell adhesion molecule) expression can be regulated by certain Hox genes (Jones et al, 1992). To date no target genes have been unequivocally identified for the more 3' Hox genes expressed in the branchial arches, although clearly this is an issue of great interest and it can be anticipated that candidates will be identified in the very near future.

THE ROSTRAL HEAD (AND UPPER FACE)

Far less is known about the genetic specification of more rostral head structures (i.e. the mid- and upper face) forming at the levels of the fore- and midbrain. It has been proposed that this part of the head represents an additional module, evolved on the front end of a primitive *Amphioxus*-like ancestral chordate (Gans and Northcutt, 1983), and rostral to the anterior end of the original notochord. Indeed some of the most evolutionarily advanced and complex parts of the brain arise from the prosencephalon. The proposal has revived the traditional debate as to whether this rostral region of the head is in any way segmented, an issue that molecular biology may finally resolve. Recently, we have even seen the orientation of the rostral axis itself being reassessed. Recognition that the axis itself becomes distorted as a result of flexure during neural tube morphogenesis, such that the original anterior extremity becomes folded into a more ventral location (Puelles and Rubenstein, 1993), is critically important since any segmental or neuromeric organization at these axial levels would otherwise be overlooked. Hox genes appear to have no role to play in the morphogenetic specification of either the CNS or peripheral, crest-derived structures at these more anterior levels, given that the most anterior cut-off is the expression of paralogous group 2 genes in R3 and the second arch (see earlier). However, that does not mean that homeobox-containing genes in general do not have a role. In fact, recently, a number of such genes from several gene families have been implicated in the development of the anterior head. Once again, these are related to homeotic genes first identified in *Drosophila*, where they have been demonstrated to play a key role in the development of the anterior head segments. Exploration of vertebrate genomes with *Drosophila*-derived probes has revealed vertebrate homologues through conservation of sequence, with comparable anterior expression domains and apparently some functional conservation too.

In *Drosophila*, maternally derived message from the regulatory *bicoid* gene is laid down in a gradient fashion during oogenesis, with the high point being anterior. Downstream targets for the bicoid protein include **orthodenticle** (*otd*), **empty spiracle** (*ems*) and **buttonhead** (*btd*), all so named because of the effect that mutation in these homeobox genes has on the fly phenotype (reviewed by Finkelstein and Boncinelli, 1994). For example, a loss-of-function mutation in *otd* results in loss of antennal segment-derived sensory organs.

In the vertebrate CNS, anterior neuromeres, if they exist, are difficult to distinguish on the basis of morphology alone. The recent reassessment of the orientation of the axis within the forebrain has enabled a more rational analysis of possible segmentation, which has been aided by gene expression data and possible correlations between domain boundaries and neuromere interfaces within the forebrain (Figdor and Stern, 1993; Puelles and Rubenstein, 1993). Thus, the expression of the vertebrate homologues of *otd* and *ems* (*Otx1*, *Otx2*; *Emx1*, *Emx2*) reveals domains that are precisely defined in the fore- and midbrain, and in a way that might be interpreted as segmental. These domains are also nested in a fashion not dissimilar to the Hox genes (Simeone et al, 1992), but in this case have both anterior and posterior cut-offs (Figure 10.8). Furthermore,

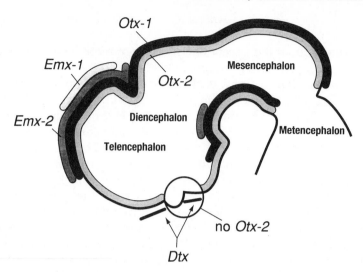

Figure 10.8 Section in midline vertical plane, illustrating the nested expression domains of the *Otx*, *Emx* and *Dtx* genes within the forebrain and midbrain of the mouse. In contrast to Hox genes, note the posterior cut-offs, the most caudal of which are at the midbrain/hindbrain boundary. (After Finkelstein and Boncinelli, 1994)

there is a temporal component to expression as well as a spatial ordering, in that *Otx2* is expressed first (throughout the epiblast initially, then confined to the node and finally to the anterior neuroectoderm) and the others follow in the sequence *Otx1*, *Emx2* and finally *Emx1*.

Given the conservation of sequence, the comparable expression domains at the anterior end of the axis in both vertebrates and *Drosophila* and the demonstration of functional conservation of other regulatory genes in other systems (see Chapter 1), it is appropriate to ask if function in this system has also been conserved in any way, despite the dramatic differences in phenotype. Different experimental strategies have been very revealing. Over-expression in *Xenopus* embryos, achieved by injecting mRNA for the *Xenopus Otx2* homologue into early embryos, results in expansion of the head at the expense of trunk/tail structures and the formation of ectopic and additional rostral organs such as the 'cement gland' (Blitz and Cho, 1995; Pannese et al, 1995). Knocking out the function of the *Otx2* gene by transgenic mutagenesis in the mouse has profound effects on development of the rostral head, leaving the branchial level and trunk relatively unscathed. Homozygous knockouts actually lack the rostral head completely (Acampora et al, 1995) with truncation of the axis at the level of R3 (Matsuo et al, 1995). Analysis of the heterozygotes reveals that the craniofacial phenotype, comprising a loss or reduction of the lower jaw, loss of eyes and dysmorphic olfactory apparatus, resembles otocephaly (Matsuo et al, 1995). From this, it has been concluded that the phenotypes can be attributed to haploid insufficiency and it is argued that, since some of the defects can be attributed to a failure of neural crest development at diencephalic and mesencephalic levels,

Otx2 and related genes are fundamentally important in the development and evolution of the masticatory jaw apparatus and the anterior neurocranium. The recent demonstration that, in mammals, the forebrain as well as the anterior midbrain generates crest that contributes significantly to the frontonasal mass (Osumi-Yamashita et al, 1994) together with the acknowledged posterior midbrain contribution to the first arch (Tan and Morriss-Kay, 1985; Imai et al, 1996) supports such an interpretation. Thus, although the comparative data are still far from complete, a degree of conservation appears to have been maintained. There also remains the interesting possibility that variations in control of *Otx* and *Emx* expression might underpin the evolutionary plasticity of fore- and midbrain development amongst different vertebrate groups (Holland et al, 1992).

Even though it is only *Otx2* that has been experimentally studied in detail to date, it seems reasonable to assume that members of both the *Otx* and *Emx* gene families are likely to be pivotal in the development of this part of the body plan. If that is the case, then what establishes (and regulates) these expression domains? Mechanisms and genetic signalling hierarchies within the rostral head are largely unknown to date. However, it is known that anterior (i.e. prechordal) mesoderm induces *Otx2* expression, and posterior mesoderm inhibits it, in explants of mouse embryonic tissues (Ang et al, 1994). Significantly, given its craniofacial teratogenicity, the inhibitory effect can be mimicked by exogenous retinoic acid (Ang et al, 1994), which also abolishes *Otx2* expression to create anterior defects in *Xenopus* embryos (Pannese et al, 1995). *Lim1*, a homeobox gene expressed initially in Hensen's node and subsequently in the anterior head mesoderm, is a candidate gene for upstream control since *Lim1* knockouts fail to develop anterior head structures (Shawlot and Behringer, 1995) and *Otx2* expression is dependent upon anterior mesoderm. A second candidate is *noggin*, which encodes a secreted polypeptide capable of inducing *Otx2* in explants of amphibian ectoderm and switching on various anterior neural markers, as well as inducing cement glands (Lamb et al, 1993). Currently we can say little more than that there is likely to be an interesting cross-talk between *Lim1* and *Otx2* and that *noggin* may well be involved in the upstream control of *Otx2*. Downstream targets remain unknown at this stage.

Although the thrust of the analytical work has been on elucidating *Otx2* function (given its early and appropriate expression), another member of this group of genes has been directly implicated in a dysmorphic syndrome. The gene EMX2 has been shown to be mutated in patients with **schizencephaly**, a rare mediolateral clefting defect of the cerebral cortex (Brunelli et al, 1996). Certainly animal studies have shown *Emx2* to be expressed in the correct location for such a cortical defect and it is speculated that the gene may have a role in neuroblast proliferation and/or migration. Such a role fits precisely with what might be predicted for the functions of this gene in forebrain development (Finkelstein and Boncinelli, 1994). It is likely that identification of further syndromes involving these genes, and the creation of transgenic models of *Otx1*, *Emx1* and *Emx2*, will shortly begin to reveal much more about the molecular control of rostral head morphogenesis.

HOW DO WE LEARN ABOUT MECHANISMS UNDERLYING ABNORMAL DEVELOPMENT?

Much of the tremendous increase in our understanding of the molecular and cellular mechanisms underlying craniofacial morphogenesis has been achieved within the last 5 to 6 years. However, in spite of intense effort, there are still major questions that are unresolved, reflecting the complexity of the system. In this sense, the application of new paradigms emerging from developmental biology to the elucidation of clinical craniofacial dysmorphogenesis remains in its infancy. The true value of some undoubtedly significant molecular advances in basic science to the clinical dysmorphologist remains unclear. Thus, initial excitement over the possibility of Hox gene mutations being responsible for a number of dysmorphic syndromes (e.g. Redline et al, 1992) has not been vindicated. In fact, it is striking that Hox genes have not been implicated directly in any human craniofacial syndrome although secondary, downstream involvement cannot be excluded. Instead, the Pax gene family has proved to be much more fertile ground in identifying mutations responsible for dysmorphic syndromes (see Chapters 1, 8, 13 and 14), and a diverse range of unpredicted genes involved in transcriptional regulation or encoding growth factors, their receptors or structural proteins have recently been implicated in craniofacial dysmorphogenesis (Winter, 1995).

Progress has been largely achieved through two approaches. The more productive approach has been gene mapping and mutational analysis of possible candidate genes in the region of interest (Moore, 1995; Winter, 1995, 1996). In some cases this can reveal previously unsuspected developmental mechanisms. The identification of the fibroblast growth factor receptor (FGFR) genes in the major craniosynostosis syndromes is a case in point. Prior to the unequivocal identification of *FGFR1* and *FGFR2* as the loci for Crouzon, Apert, Pfeiffer and Jackson–Weiss syndromes (Reardon and Winter, 1995), developmental biologists working on craniofacial development had little if any reason to consider the roles of these receptors and their ligands in skull development in general or in sutural morphogenesis in particular. Now that this group of growth factors have been implicated in skull development, there are considerable efforts being made to define their functional role in normal development and, through this knowledge, to relate the mutated genotype to the dysmorphic phenotype. One expectation is that elucidation of the basic biology of normal suture growth and differentiation will open up new avenues of therapeutic/corrective strategy.

Occasionally genes have been identified by traditional, labour-intensive positional cloning approaches, aided by the existence of balanced translocations. The recent identification of *Treacle*, encoding a novel protein of unknown function, as the gene for Treacher–Collins syndrome exemplifies this strategy (Treacher Collins Syndrome Collaborative Group, 1996). More typically though, it is clues from the expression patterns of known genes deemed to be 'developmentally significant', and which happen to map within the region of interest, that assist the dysmorphologist.

Ironically, the use of transgenic technology has been less revealing about clinical dysmorphology than might have been expected. Although a significant proportion of transgenics display a craniofacial phenotype, the majority of these transgenic manipulations have not been made with the primary intention of modelling a human dysmorphic condition. Any parallel with human syndromes is typically made retrospectively and is a secondary consequence of experiments that were designed primarily to understand the basic biological role of the gene of interest in normal (mouse) development. A typical case in point is the *Hoxa-3* knockout which, on the basis of the phenotype, has been proposed as a model for DiGeorge syndrome (Chisaka and Capecchi, 1991; Manley and Capecchi, 1995). In fact, given the location of the Hox A cluster on human chromosome 7, it now seems likely that, at best, *HOXA3* serves to regulate the unidentified DiGeorge genes at 22q11 and 10p13. Thus, in one sense, the use of transgenics to study dysmorphogenesis has been historically different from their use to understand inherited metabolic disorders where transgenic modelling of a particular disease may be the primary goal.

At the cellular level, the precision of cell lineage definition and tissue derivation has facilitated a more informed interpretation of the dysmorphic phenotype and how it has been created (e.g. Johnston and Bronsky, 1995). A scheme has been proposed relating faulty segmentation at the hindbrain level to abnormalities in specific arches and their derivatives, for a range of branchial arch syndromes (Couly et al, 1994). The earlier suggestion by numerous workers (e.g. Lammer et al, 1985) that perturbation of cephalic neural crest development might constitute a relatively common dysmorphogenic mechanism has been thoroughly vindicated, for both genetic and teratogenic disruption of developmental mechanisms. Neural crest development is sensitive to perturbation at a multiplicity of levels:

- faulty induction at the open neural plate stage
- abnormal axial/morphogenetic specification upon leaving the neural primordium
- disturbed migration of the cells (defects in cell motility, adhesion molecules, extracellular matrix)
- inadequate proliferation or excessive (apoptotic) cell death
- failure of normal differentiation (e.g. through failure of a cell signalling event)
- defects in those tissues upon which crest-derived cells are dependent (e.g. a vascular crisis with ensuing ischaemia)

It is evident that many craniofacial defects are attributable to such disturbances in crest development and earlier still in the development of the brain, not only at the rhombencephalic/branchial levels but, as is increasingly evident, at the levels of prosencephalon and mesencephalon too. In this sense, the claim that 'the face reflects the brain' (Winter, 1996) is amply justified.

AN AGENDA FOR THE FUTURE

Given that progress in research is rarely gradual and likely to be revolutionized by paradigm shifts in understanding and perceptions, proposing an agenda is a risky undertaking. The following list comprises a mixture of items, some of which emerge from contemporary work and others that are long overdue and only now do we have the technologies and understanding to tackle them.

- Elucidation of the role of the endoderm in determining the position and metamerism of the branchial arches; little has been done since the early work using amphibian model systems (Balinsky, 1981).
- Analysis of the differentiation of epithelial diversity in the mouth and buccal cavity; there are at least six epithelial domains, including the vermilion of the lips, yet with the exception of the secondary palate (e.g. Dixon et al, 1993) we have no knowledge of how this diversity is generated and maintained.
- Analysis of the cell biology of facial morphogenesis; data are now emerging for the expression of adhesion molecules on the epithelia (Lüning et al, 1994), and for growth factor and mitogen expression in the mesenchyme (Francis-West et al, 1994), of the facial primordia. A full assessment of the adhesive properties and growth specification of the facial primordia seems almost overdue.
- Creative use of the *Cre/loxP* system (see Chapter 4) to create conditional transgenic knockouts whereby a gene can be controlled in a stage- or tissue-specific manner, making it easier to distinguish the primary effects of changed expression from the secondary and tertiary ones. It is likely that this will be paralleled by the increasing use of antisense oligonucleotide strategies to specifically inactivate message in controlled ways since this approach has already been used productively in the study of tooth and mandibular development (Slavkin, 1995).
- Elucidation of how temporal and structural co-linearity of Hox gene expression is achieved during craniofacial development; this remains a fundamental problem for all of the fields in which expression co-linear with the 3' to 5' orientation of the gene cluster is seen (Krumlauf, 1994).
- Elucidation of the putative upstream role of retinoids in the in-vivo regulation of Hox genes during early head development.
- Clarification of the respective roles of the other regulatory genes that are currently being identified as critical in various aspects of craniofacial development (Richman and Mitchell, 1996). These include *AP2* (Schorle et al, 1996), *twist* (Chen and Behringer, 1995), *Msx-1* (Satoka and Maas, 1994) and *goosecoid* (Yamada et al, 1995).
- Clarification of the apparent default value in the first branchial arch (see earlier). The homeobox gene *Dlx-2* appears to have a function in development of the first arch (Qiu et al, 1995), where no Hox genes are expressed. It may therefore have a role in morphogenetic specification of the arch series along with the Hox genes. If so, then predictions about *Dlx-2* expression can be tested in those transgenics where the second arch is transformed to a first arch identity.

Progress will be dependent upon the integration of these and other items into a unified model of craniofacial development. Any such model should be able to explain not only normal development of the head and face but also the range of craniofacial phenotypes seen phylogenetically and the dysmorphologies encountered by the clinician.

ACKNOWLEDGEMENT

I am most grateful to Paul Hunt, who kindly supplied the diagrams used in Figures 10.4 and 10.5.

REFERENCES

Acampora, D., D'Esposito, M., Faiella, A. et al (1989) The human HOX gene family. *Nucleic Acids Res.* **17**, 10385–10402.

Acampora, D., Mazan, S., Lallemand, Y. et al (1995) Forebrain and midbrain regions are deleted in *Otx2-/-* mutants due to a defective anterior neuroectoderm specification during gastrulation. *Development* **121**, 3279–3290.

Ang, S.-L., Conlon, R.A., Jin, O. and Rossant, J. (1994) Positive and negative signals from mesoderm regulate the expression of mouse *Otx2* in ectoderm explants. *Development* **120**, 2979–2989.

Balinsky, B. (1981) *An Introduction to Embryology*, 5th edn, pp. 465–466. Saunders College: New York.

Blitz, I.L. and Cho, K.W.Y. (1995) Anterior neurectoderm is progressively induced during gastrulation: the role of the *Xenopus* homeobox gene *orthodenticle*. *Development* **121**, 993–1004.

Brunelli, S., Faiella, A., Capra, V. et al (1996) Germline mutations in the homeobox gene *EMX2* in patients with severe schizencephaly. *Nature Genetics* **12**, 94–96.

Chen, Z.-F. and Behringer, R.R. (1995) *Twist* is required in head mesenchyme for cranial neural tube morphogenesis. *Genes Dev.* **9**, 686–699.

Chisaka, O. and Capecchi, M.R. (1991) Regionally restricted developmental defects resulting from targeted disruption of the mouse homeobox gene *hox-1.5*. *Nature* **350**, 473–479.

Condie, B.G. and Capecchi, M.R. (1994) Mice with targeted disruptions in the paralogous genes hoxa-3 and hoxd-3 reveal synergistic interactions. *Nature* **370**, 304–307.

Couly, G.F., Coltey, P.M. and Le Douarin, N.M. (1992) The developmental fate of the cephalic mesoderm in quail-chick chimeras. *Development* **114**, 1–15.

Couly, G.F., Coltey, P.M. and Le Douarin, N.M. (1993) The triple origin of skull in higher vertebrates: a study in quail-chick chimeras. *Development* **117**, 402–429.

Couly, G., Coltey, P., Chéron, G. et al (1994) Rhombomères, code Hox, crête neurale et malformations de la face. *La Recherche* **10**, 151–162.

Dixon, M.J., Carette, M.J.M., Moser, B.B. and Ferguson, M.J.W. (1993) Differentiation of isolated murine embryonic palatal epithelium in culture. *In vitro cell. Dev Biol.* **29A**, 51–61.

Duboule, D. (1992) The vertebrate limb: a model system to study the *hox*/HOM gene network during development and evolution. *BioEssays* **14**, 375–384.

Duboule, D. and Dollé, P. (1989) The structural and functional organisation of the murine HOX gene family resembles that of *Drosophila* homeotic genes. *EMBO J.* **8**, 1497–1505.

Durston, A., Timmermans, J., Hage, W. et al (1989) Retinoic acid causes an anteroposterior transformation in the developing central nervous system. *Nature* **340**, 140–144.

Ferguson, M.W.J. (1991) The orofacial region. In *Textbook of Fetal and Perinatal Pathology* (Eds: J.S. Wigglesworth and D.B. Singer), vol. 1, pp. 843–879.

Figdor, M.C. and Stern, C.D. (1993) Segmental organisation of embryonic diencephalon. *Nature* **363**, 630–633.

Finkelstein, R. and Boncinelli, E. (1994) From fly head to mammalian forebrain: the story of *otd* and *Otx*. *Trends Genet.* **10**, 310–315.

Francis-West, P.H., Tatla, T. and Brickell, P.M. (1994) Expression patterns of the bone morphogenetic protein genes *Bmp-4* and *Bmp-2* in the developing chick face suggest a role in outgrowth of the primordia. *Dev. Dynam.* **201**, 168–178.

Fraser, S., Keynes, R. and Lumsden, A. (1990) Segmentation in the chick hindbrain is defined by cell lineage restrictions. *Nature* **344**, 431–435.

Gans, C. and Northcutt, R.G. (1983) Neural crest and the origin of vertebrates. *Science* **220**, 268–274.

Gendron-Maguire, M., Mallo, M., Zhang, M. and Gridley, T. (1993) *Hoxa-2* mutant mice exhibit homeotic transformation of skeletal elements derived from cranial neural crest. *Cell* **75**, 1317–1331.

Gorlin, R.J., Cohen, M.M. and Levine, L.S. (1990) *Syndromes of the Head and Neck*, 3rd edn. Oxford University Press: New York and Oxford.

Graham, A., Papalopulu, N. and Krumlauf, R. (1989) The murine and Drosophila homeobox gene complexes have common features of organisation and expression. *Cell* **57**, 367–378.

Graham, A., Heyman, I. and Lumsden, A. (1993) Even-numbered rhombomeres control the apoptotic elimination of neural crest cells from odd-numbered rhombomeres in the chick hindbrain. *Development* **119**, 233–245.

Gustafson, A.-L., Dencker, L. and Eriksson, U. (1993) Non-overlapping expression of CRBP 1 and CRABP 1 during pattern formation of limbs and craniofacial structures in the early mouse embryo. *Development* **117**, 451–460.

Hall, B.K. and Horstadius, S. (1988) *The Neural Crest*. Oxford University Press: Oxford.

Hanken, J. and Thorogood, P. (1993) Evolution of the skull: a problem in pattern formation. *Trends Ecol. Evol.* **8**, 9–15.

Holland, P., Ingham, P. and Krauss, S. (1992) Mice and flies head to head. *Nature* **358**, 627–628.

Hunt, P., Gulisano, M., Cook, M. et al (1991) A distinct Hox code for the branchial region of the vertebrate head. *Nature* **353**, 861–864.

Hunt, P., Ferretti, P., Krumlauf, R. and Thorogood, P. (1995) Restoration of normal hox code and branchial arch morphogenesis after extensive deletion of hindbrain neural crest. *Dev. Biol.* **168**, 584–597.

Hunt, P., Buxton, P., Ferretti, P. and Thorogood, P. (1997) Plasticity of the neural crest and the branchial arch hox code after crest migration. In press.

Imai, H., Osumi-Yamashita, N., Ninomiya, Y. and Eto, K. (1996) Contribution of early-emigrating midbrain crest cells to the dental mesenchyme of mandibular molar teeth in rat embryos. *Dev. Biol.* **176**, 151–165.

Johnston, M.C. and Bronsky, P.T. (1995) Prenatal craniofacial development: new insights on normal and abnormal mechanisms. *Crit. Rev. Oral Biol. Med.* **6**, 25–79.

Johnston, R.L. and Tabin, C. (1995) The long and the short of *hedgehog* signalling. *Cell* **81**, 313–316.

Jones, F.S., Predinger, E.A., Bittner, D.A. et al (1992) Cell adhesion molecules as targets for *Hox* genes: neural cell adhesion molecule promoter activity is modulated by co-transfection with *Hox-2.5* and *-2.4*. *Proc. Natl Acad. Sci. USA* **89**, 2086–2090.

Kessel, M. and Gruss, P. (1991) Homeotic transformations of murine vertebrae and concomitant alterations of Hox codes induced by retinoic acid. *Cell* **67**, 89–104.

Krumlauf, R. (1994) *Hox* genes in vertebrate development. *Cell* **78**, 191–201.

Lamb, T.M., Knecht, A.K., Smith, W.C. et al (1993) Neural induction by the secreted polypeptide Noggin. *Science* **262**, 713–718.

Lammer, E.J., Chen, D.T., Hoar, R.M. et al (1985) Retinoic acid embryopathy. *New Engl. J. Med.* **313**, 832–841.

Larsen, W.J. (1993) *Human Embryology*. Churchill Livingstone: New York.

Le Douarin, N.M. (1982) *The Neural Crest*. Cambridge University Press: Cambridge.

Le Douarin, N.M. (1993) Patterning of neural crest derivatives in the avian embryo: *in vivo* and *in vitro* studies. *Dev. Biol.* **159**, 24–49.

Lee, Y.M., Osumi-Yamashita, N., Ninomiya, Y. et al (1995) Retinoic acid stagedependently alters the migration pattern and identity of hindbrain neural crest cells. *Development* **121**, 825–837.

Lohnes, D., Mark, M., Mendlesohn, C. et al (1994) Function of the retinoic acid receptors (RARs) during development: (I) Craniofacial and skeletal abnormalities in RAR double mutants. *Development* **120**, 2723–2748.

Lufkin, T., Mark, M., Hart, C.P. et al (1992) Homeotic transformation of the occipital bones of the skull by ectopic expression of a homeobox gene. *Nature* **359**, 835–841.

Lumsden, A. and Keynes, R. (1989) Segmental patterns of neuronal development in the chick hindbrain. *Nature* **337**, 424–428.

Lumsden, A., Sprawson, N. and Graham, A. (1991) Segmental origin and migration of neural crest cells in the hindbrain region of the chick embryo. *Development* **113**, 1281–1291.

Lüning, C., Rass, A., Rozell, B., Wroblewski, J. and Obrink, B. (1994) Expression of E-cadherin during craniofacial development. *J. Craniofac. Genet. Dev. Biol.* **14**, 207–216.

Manley, N.R. and Capecchi, M.R. (1995) The role of Hoxa-3 in mouse thymus and thyroid development. *Development* **121**, 1989–2003.

Marshall, H., Nonchev, S., Sham, M.-H. et al (1992) Retinoic acid alters hindbrain *Hox* code and induces transformation of rhombomeres 2/3 into a 4/5 identity. *Nature* **360**, 737–741.

Marti, E., Takada, R., Bumcrot, D.A., Sasaki, H. and McMahon, A. (1995) Distribution of Sonic Hedgehog peptides in the developing chick and mouse embryo. *Development* **121**, 2537–2547.

Matsuo, I., Kuratani, S., Kimura, C., Takeda, N. and Aizawa, S. (1995) Mouse *Otx2* functions in the formation and patterning of rostral head. *Genes Dev.* **9**, 2646–2658.

McGinnis, W. and Krumlauf, R. (1992) Homeobox genes and axial patterning. *Cell* **68**, 283–302.

McKay, I., Muchamore, I., Krumlauf, R. et al (1994) The *kreisler* mouse: a hindbrain segmentation mutant that lacks two rhombomeres. *Development* **120**, 2199–2211.

Moore, G.E. (1995) Molecular genetic approaches to the study of human craniofacial dysmorphologies. *Int. Rev. Cytol.* **158**, 215–277.

Moro Balbás, J.A., Gato, A., Alonso Revuelta, J.F., Represa, J.J. and Barbosa, E. (1993) Retinoic acid induces changes in rhombencephalic neural crest cell migration and extracellular matrix composition in chick embryos. *Teratology* **48**, 197–206.

Morriss-Kay, G.M. (1993) Retinoic acid and craniofacial development: molecules and morphogenesis. *BioEssays* **15**, 9–15.

Mulvihill, J.J. (1995) Craniofacial syndromes: no such thing as a single gene disease. *Nature Genetics* **9**, 101–103.

Noden, D.M. (1983a) The embryonic origins of avian cephalic and cervical muscles and associated connective tissues. *Am. J. Anat.* **168**, 257–276.

Noden, D.M. (1983b) The role of neural crest in patterning of avian cranial skeletal, connective and muscle tissue. *Dev. Biol.* **96**, 296–312.

Noden, D.M. (1991) Cell movements and control of patterned tissue assembly during craniofacial development. *J. Craniofac. Genet. Dev. Biol.* **11**, 192–213.

Noden, D.M. (1992) Spatial integration among cells forming the cranial peripheral nervous system. *J. Neurobiol.* **24**, 248–261.

Osumi-Yamashita, N., Ninomiya, Y., Doi, H. and Eto, K. (1994) The contribution of both forebrain and midbrain crest cells to the mesenchyme in the frontonasal mass of mouse embryos. *Dev. Biol.* **164**, 409–419.

Pannese, M., Polo, C., Andreazzoli, M. et al (1995) The *Xenopus* homologue of *Otx2* is a maternal homeobox gene that demarcates and specifies anterior body regions. *Development* **121**, 707–720.

Puelles, L. and Rubenstein, J.L.R. (1993) Expression patterns of homeobox and other putative regulatory genes in the embryonic mouse forebrain suggest a neuromeric organisation. *Trends Neurosci.* **16**, 472–479.

Qiu, M., Bulfone, A., Martinez, S. et al (1995) Null mutation of *Dlx-2* results in abnormal morphogenesis of proximal first and second branchial arch derivatives and abnormal differentiation in the forebrain. *Genes Dev.* **9**, 2523–2538.

Reardon, W. and Winter, R. (1995) The molecular pathology of syndromic craniosynostosis. *Molec. Med. Today* **1**, 432–437.

Redline, R.W., Neish, A., Holmes, L. and Collins, T. (1992) Biology of disease: homeobox genes and congenital malformations. *Lab. Invest.* **66**, 659–670.

Richman, J.M. and Mitchell, P.J. (1996) Craniofacial development: knockout mice take one on the chin. *Curr. Biol.* **6**, 364–367.

Richman, J.M. and Tickle, C. (1989) Epithelia are interchangeable between facial primordia of chick embryos and morphogenesis is controlled by the mesenchyme. *Dev. Biol.* **136**, 201–210.

Saldivar, J.R., Krull, C.E., Krumlauf, R., Ariza-McNaughton, L. and Bronner-Fraser, M. (1996) Rhombomere of origin determines autonomous versus environmentally regulated expression of *Hoxa3* in the avian embryo. *Development* **122**, 895–904.

Satokata I. and Maas, R. (1994) *Msx1* deficient mice exhibit cleft palate and abnormalities of craniofacial and tooth development. *Nature Genetics* **6**, 348–355.

Scherson, T., Serbedzija, G., Fraser, S. and Bronner-Fraser, M. (1993) Regulative capacity of the cranial neural tube to form neural crest. *Development* **118**, 1049–1061.

Schorle, H., Meier, P., Buchert, M., Jaenisch, R. and Mitchell, P.J. (1996) Transcription factor AP-2 essential for cranial closure and craniofacial development. *Nature* **381**, 235–238.

Sechrist, J., Serbedzija, G.N., Scherson, T., Fraser, S. and Bronner-Fraser, M. (1993) Segmental migration of the hindbrain neural crest does not arise from segmental generation. *Development* **118**, 691–703.

Selleck, M.A.J., Scherson, T.Y. and Bronner-Fraser, M. (1993) Origins of neural crest cell diversity. *Dev. Biol.* **159**, 1–11.

Sham, M.-H., Vesque, C., Nonchev, S. et al (1993) The zinc finger gene *Krox-20* regulates *Hox-B2* during hindbrain segmentation. *Cell* **72**, 183–196.

Shawlot, W. and Behringer, R.R. (1995) Requirements for *Lim1* in head-organiser function. *Nature* **374**, 425–430.

Simeone, A., Acampora, D., Gulisano, M., Stornaluolo, A. and Boncinelli, E. (1992) Nested expression domains of four homeobox genes in developing rostral brain. *Nature* **358**, 687–690.

Slavkin, H.C. (1995) Antisense oligonucleotides: an experimental strategy to advance a causal analysis of development. *Int. J. Dev. Biol.* **39**, 123–126.

Stemple, D.L. and Anderson, D.J. (1993) Lineage diversification of the neural crest; *in vitro* investigations. *Dev.. Biol.* **159**, 12–23.

Swiatek, P.J. and Gridley, T. (1993) Perinatal lethality and defects in hindbrain development in mice homozygous for a targeted mutation of the zinc finger gene *Krox 20*. *Genes Dev.* **7**, 2071–2084.

Tan, S.-S. and Morriss-Kay, G.M. (1985) The development and distribution of the cranial neural crest in the rat embryo. *Cell Tissue Res.* **240**, 403–416.

Thorogood, P. (1993) The differentiation and morphogenesis of cranial skeletal tissues. In *The Vertebrate Skull* (Eds: J. Hanken and B.K. Hall), vol. 1, pp. 112–152.

Thorogood, P. (1994) Craniofacial development and the neural crest. In *Early Fetal Growth and Development* (Eds: R.H.T. Ward, S.K. Smith and D. Donnai), pp. 111–120. Royal College of Obstetricians and Gynaecologists: London.

Tomotsune, D., Shoji, H., Wakamatsu, Y., Kondoh, H. and Takahashi, N. (1993) A mouse homologue of the *Drosophila* tumour suppressor gene *l(2)gl* controlled by Hox-C8 *in vivo*. *Nature* **365**, 69–72.

Trainor, P., Tan, S.-S. and Tam, P.P.L. (1994) Cranial paraxial mesoderm: regionalisation of cell fate and impact on craniofacial development in mouse embryos. *Development* **120**, 2397–2408.

Treacher Collins Syndrome Collaborative Group (1996) Positional cloning of a gene involved in the pathogenesis of Treacher Collins syndrome. *Nature Genetics* **12**, 130–136.

Vieille-Grosjean, I., Hunt, P., Massimo, G., Boncinelli, E. and Thorogood, P. (1997)

Branchial *HOX* gene expression and human craniofacial development. *Developmental Biology* (in press).

Webb, J.F. and Noden, D.M. (1993) Ectodermal placodes: contributions to the development of the vertebrate head. *Am. Zool.* **33**, 434–447.

Wilkinson, D.G. (1993) Molecular mechanisms of segmental patterning in the vertebrate hindbrain and neural crest. *BioEssays* **15**, 499–505.

Wilkinson, D.G., Bhatt, S., Cook, M., Boncinelli, E. and Krumlauf, R. (1989) Segmental expression of Hox-2 homeobox-containing genes in the developing mouse hindbrain. *Nature* **341**, 405–409.

Winter, R.M. (1995) Recent molecular advances in dysmorphology. *Hum. Molec. Genet.* **4**, 1669–1704.

Winter, R.M. (1996) What's in a face? *Nature Genetics* **12**, 124–129.

Winter, R.M. and Baraitser, M. (1993) *The London Dysmorphology Database*, 3rd edn. Oxford University Press: Oxford.

Yamada, G., Mansouri, A., Torres, M. et al (1995) Targetted mutation of the murine goosecoid gene results in craniofacial defects and neonatal death. *Development* **121**, 2917–2922.

Zappavigna, V., Renucci, A., Ispizua-Belmonte, J. et al (1991) *Hox-4* genes encode transcription factors with potential auto- and cross-regulatory capacities. *EMBO J.* **10** 4177–4188.

NOTE IN PROOF

The human *Sonic hedgehog* (*SHH*) gene has recently been identified as a gene responsible for holoprosencephaly (Belloni et al, 1996, *Nature Genetics* **14**, 353–360) and the transgenic knock-out produces a phenotype with a number of midline defects including cyclopia and the floor of the brain (Chiang et al, 1996, *Nature* **383**, 407–413). Clearly, Shh signalling has a major role in craniofacial development, at least part of which stems from its function in patterning the CNS.

11 The Heart

MARGARET L. KIRBY

Developmental Biology Program and Heart Development Group, IMMAG, Medical College of Georgia, Augusta, USA

DEVELOPMENTAL ANATOMY

The heart forms from the **cardiogenic plate** at the cranial end of the germ disc (Figure 11.1). Angioblasts appear in clusters that later form vesicles which join to create a network of channels; these channels enlarge to become two endothelial tubes which fuse craniocaudally. The **primary heart tube** is formed when this endothelial tube is invested by **myocardium** – the cell layer destined to form the heart muscle. The myocardium secretes an expansive extracellular matrix referred to as **cardiac jelly** (Markwald et al, 1985), which forms a third layer between the endothelial and myocardial cell layers. Thus, the primitive heart tube consists of a homogeneous myocardial layer, several cells thick, and an endocardial layer separated from the myocardium by cardiac jelly (Figure 11.2a; Manasek, 1968). The primary heart tube quickly develops expansions and sulci that divide it into primitive, functional chambers. Since the heart begins to beat very early during its morphogenesis, it is important to establish a working arrangement to support the metabolic needs and vascular growth of the embryo while the transformation from a primitive tube into an adult heart with four chambers is taking place. The tube elongates and **loops** to the right, at the same time pivoting to the right on the anteroposterior axis (Manasek et al, 1972).

The convexity of the loop, called the **bulboventricular** or **primary fold**, demarcates the inflow from the outflow portion of the looped tube. The **inflow portion** consists of the sinus venosus, primitive atrium, atrioventricular canal and proximal portion of the primitive ventricle. The **outflow portion** of the looped tube consists of the distal portion of the primitive ventricle and the outflow tract which includes a slender non-trabeculated tube comprising the conus cordis, proximally, and the truncus arteriosus, distally (Figure 11.2b). The truncus arteriosus is the most distal part of the tube invested with myocardium, and its junction with the aortic sac is the region where the aortic and pulmonary semilunar valves will form. The most distal part of the outflow tract is the aortic sac although it develops in association with the pharynx rather than as a part of the original looped tube.

A series of aortic arch arteries connect the aortic sac bilaterally with the left and right dorsal aortae (Figure 11.2b). The aortic arch arteries traverse and

Embryos, Genes and Birth Defects. Edited by P. Thorogood.
© 1997 John Wiley & Sons Ltd.

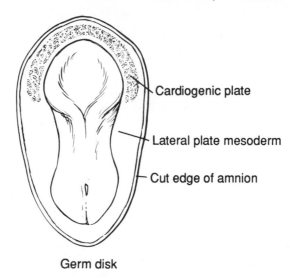

Germ disk

Figure 11.1 Dorsal view of a developing mammalian embryo showing the cardiogenic plate in the cranial region of the lateral plate mesoderm. The myocardium and perhaps endocardium of the initial heart tube differentiate from this area of mesoderm

develop from tissue located in the pharyngeal arches (Figure 11.3). In both the atrioventricular and conotruncal regions, bulges called cardiac cushions form in the lumen of the heart tube. After looping, the heart continues rearrangment of the inflow and outflow tracts such that they are **aligned** correctly with respect to the developing left and right ventricles (Figure 11.4). As the alignment is adjusted, various **septation** events divide the chambers and outflow vessels.

While the sinus venosus and venous system are originally bilaterally symmetrical, regression of specific veins causes a shift of the central venous return to the right side of the primitive atrium. The sinus venosus is incorporated into the nascent right atrium and interatrial septum, which divides the cavity of the primitive atrium into definitive right and left atria. The atrioventricular canal is converted into right and left channels by growth and fusion of **endocardial cushions** arising from the dorsal and ventral walls of the tube. The primitive ventricle is divided into right and left ventricular chambers by inward growth of a muscular ventricular septum (Figure 11.2c). During the process of septation, the outflow tract (conus arteriosus, truncus arteriosus and aortic sac) will be converted into the parts of the right and left ventricles just below the semilunar valves, the region of the valves, and the proximal parts of the aorta and pulmonary trunk (Figure 11.2d,e). Outflow septation begins in the aortic sac by growth of a partition between the fourth and sixth aortic arch arteries. This partition is continued into the truncal and conal cushions, progressively separating a **pulmonary** from **systemic circulation**. A final fusion of the conal part of the

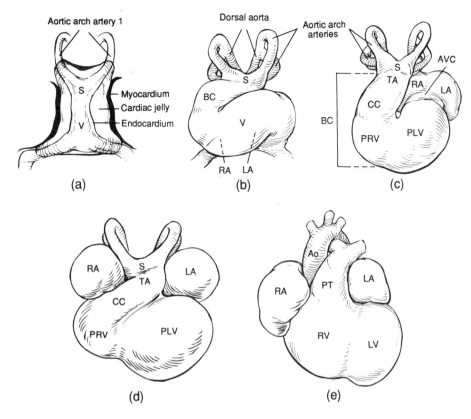

Figure 11.2 Progressive stages in heart development from the initial tubular heart (a) to a fully septated adult-type heart (e). In (a) the forming heart tube (V) connects distally with the aortic sac (S) from which arise a pair of aortic arch arteries that connect with the dorsal aorta. The heart tube has only three layers at early stages of development, which are designated endocardium, myocardium and cardiac jelly. Expansion and looping of the heart tube shown in (b) result in identifiable regions of the tubular heart. The regions that become right and left atria (RA and LA) are shown. The ventricle (V) becomes the presumptive left ventricle while the bulbus cordis (BC) gives rise to the outflow portion of the looped tube. In (c) the bulbus cordis has become the presumptive right ventricle (PRV), conus cordis (CC) and truncus arteriosus (TA). The regions that form the right and left atria have shifted and absorption of the sinus venosus into the presumptive right atrium contributes to shifting that chamber toward the right, probably by expansion. AVC, atrioventricular canal. (d) shows the chambers in their correct locations, but septation is not complete as can be seen in (e). The most prominent sign of septation externally is division of the aortic sac into the aorta (Ao) and pulmonary trunk (PT) above the valves, the truncus arteriosus into aortic and pulmonary semilunar valves, and the conus cordis into the infundibulum and vestibule which are portions of the ventricles just proximal to the semilunar valves

septum with the ventricular septum and atrioventricular cushion tissue completes ventricular septation. The ventricular conduction system develops concomitant with ventricular septation to ensure simultaneous contraction of both ventricles (Moorman and Lamers, 1995).

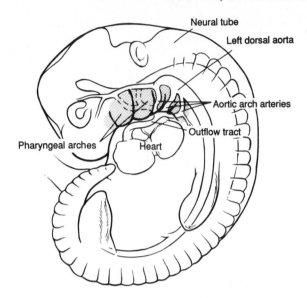

Figure 11.3 Left side of a human embryo showing the relationship of the heart with its outflow tract connecting to the dorsal aorta via a series of aortic arch arteries. Aortic arch arteries 1 and 2 located in pharyngeal arches 1 and 2 regress relatively early in development while the caudal three arch arteries persist as major arterial vessels in the thorax

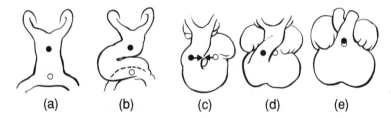

Figure 11.4 Development of the heart proceeds by looping of the primitive heart tube followed by alignment of the inflow and outflow portions. The open circle is at the venous pole (inflow region) while the closed circle is in the outflow region

CELLS NEEDED FOR NORMAL HEART DEVELOPMENT

Four groups of cells are necessary for normal structural development of the heart: myocardium, endocardium, epicardium and neural crest-derived ecto-mesenchymal cells. The **myocardium** is derived from lateral plate mesoderm. During gastrulation the cells are spatially ordered so that the cells which will form the myocardium of the outflow tract migrate through the primitive streak first, followed by presumptive ventricular, atrial and finally sinus venosus cells (Rosenquist, 1970). In the axolotl, the heart field forms as the anterior lateral plate mesoderm migrates over the underlying pharyngeal endoderm and the mid-ventral and lateral walls of the pharyngeal cavity have been shown to have inductive capacity (Easton et al, 1994).

While the origin of the myocardium has been clearly shown, the derivation of the **endocardium** is unclear. Initial studies have not identified cardiogenic plate cells except in myocardium so it is possible that atrial and ventricular endocardium are not derived from the cardiogenic plate (Mikawa et al, 1992). The endocardium of the outflow region has been mapped to the cephalic paraxial and lateral plate mesoderm underlying and slightly rostral and lateral to the otic placode (Noden, 1991), and these cells become interspersed with atrial and ventricular endocardium during the initial stages of cardiogenesis.

The **epicardium** grows from mesothelial protrusions from the dorsal mesocardium on the right ventral wall of the sinus venosus (Ho and Shimada, 1978; Hiruma and Hirakow, 1989). The protrusions touch the dorsal wall of the atrioventricular groove, adhere and begin to form a sheet-like epicardium that ultimately invests the entire myocardium with the outflow tract last. Cells that accompany the epicardium from the liver form the cardiac vascular plexus, which is transformed into the adult coronary vessels (Poelmann et al, 1993). The cardiac plexus extends towards the outflow tract and vessels grow into the aortic wall to form the main coronary arteries (Bogers et al, 1989; Waldo et al, 1990).

The last major contribution to heart development is made by cells derived from the **neural crest** (Kirby, 1993). While the neural crest extends from the mid-diencephalon to the tail of the embryo and participates in craniofacial and peripheral nervous system development (see Chapters 8 and 10), only cells originating from the caudal rhombencephalon participate in structural development of the heart (Figure 11.5). The cells originate from rhombomeres 6, 7 and 8 located between the mid-otic placode and somite 3. The neural crest cells migrate from the neural folds and pause in the circumpharyngeal region while pharyngeal arches 3, 4 and 6 form, and then as each arch forms it is populated by

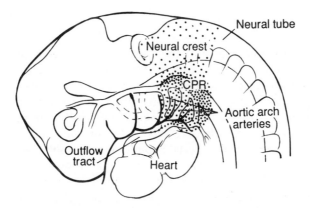

Figure 11.5 Pharyngeal region of a human embryo showing the migration of neural crest cells into the circumpharyngeal region (CPR) and then into the developing caudal pharyngeal arches to surround the aortic arch arteries. Cells then migrate into the outflow tract of the heart where they will participate in outflow septation

cells migrating from the circumpharyngeal region (Kuratani and Kirby, 1991). These ectomesenchymal cells support development of the aortic arch arteries in the pharyngeal arches and form the tunica media of the persisting arch vessels (Le Lièvre and Le Douarin, 1975). A population of cells continue migrating from pharyngeal arches 3, 4 and 6 into the outflow tract, where they will participate in septation (Figure 11.5).

MAIN CLASSES OF CARDIOVASCULAR DEFECTS

The major structural defects of heart development can be classified into the following groups:

(1)   Defects of alignment
(2)   Defects of septation
(3)   Interruption, stenosis and atresia

DEFECTS OF ALIGNMENT

These defects include malalignment of either inflow or outflow portions of the heart. Inflow malalignments include **straddling tricuspid valve** and **double-inlet left ventricle. Tricuspid atresia** may also be classified with inflow malalignments. The outflow tract can also be malaligned in defects that include **double-outlet right ventricle, tetralogy of Fallot** and **Ebstein's anomaly.** Another form of malalignment occurs in transposition of the great vessels, in which the aorta and pulmonary trunks arise from incorrect ventricles (Figure 11.6). This defect is almost immediately fatal at birth, unless there also exist septation defects that allow blood from the pulmonary circulation to mix with blood from the systemic circulation.

DEFECTS OF SEPTATION

Failure of development of any of the septa in the four-chambered heart can occur. Thus there can be failure of the primary septa of the initial atrial cavity to make left and right atria (**common atrium** or **atrial septal defect**), of the atrioventricular canal to divide the region of the atrioventricular valves into right and left channels (**atrioventricular canal**), and of the muscular ventricular septum that divides the primitive ventricle into left and right ventricles (**muscular ventricular septal defect**). Septation of the outflow tract is complex and involves division of the conal and truncal parts of the heart into left and right channels, and division of the aortic sac into the proximal parts of the major vessels emanating from the left and right ventricles, the aorta and pulmonary trunk (Figure 11.6). Defects in outflow septation result in **ventricular septal defect** where there is a small to moderate-sized defect below the semilunar valves or persistent truncus arteriosus where the entire outflow below the semilunar valves and above is a single large vessel.

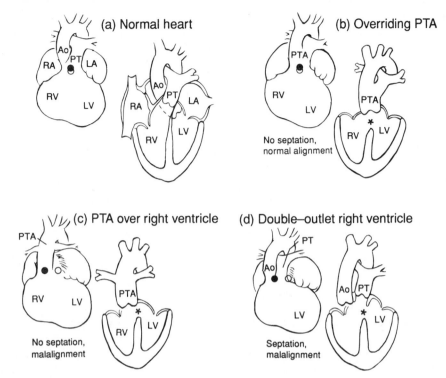

Figure 11.6 Alignment and septation defects of the outflow tract. The open and closed circles show the position of the outflow and inflow regions as seen in Figure 11.4. (a) Normal alignment and septation. (b) Persisting truncus arteriosus (PTA) overriding the ventricular septum. In this case septation has not occurred but the alignment of the outflow tract is normal. Compare this configuration with (c), showing a PTA originating completely from the right ventricle, a malalignment. In (d), septation has occurred but the two outflow vessels, the aorta and pulmonary trunk originate from the right ventricle, a malalignment. RA and LA, right and left atria; RV and LV, right and left ventricles; Ao, aorta; PT, pulmonary trunk

INTERRUPTION, STENOSIS AND ATRESIA

Valves and the outflow portion of the ventricles can be narrowed or stenotic, and veins coming into the heart or arteries leaving the heart can undergo atresia. **Interrupted aorta** is a form of atresia in which a portion of the aorta has probably formed but then regressed abnormally (Figure 11.7). The specific term **aortic atresia** is applied to a condition in which the aortic semilunar valve and base of the aorta have disappeared.

SYNDROMES INVOLVING CARDIOVASCULAR DEFECTS

Many heart anomalies are present as part of a complex or syndrome. For example, in **DiGeorge syndrome, persistent truncus arteriosus** (a septation

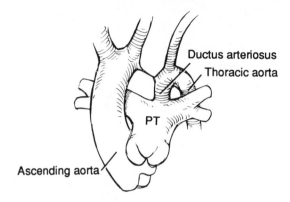

Figure 11.7 One form of interruption or atresia. In this case the aorta is interrupted between two of its branches (the left carotid and left subclavian arteries, not marked). The remarkable ability of the cardiovascular system to make do with what is available is shown by the pulmonary trunk (PT) providing the major blood supply to the dorsal (or thoracic) aorta in place of the missing piece of the aorta

defect) and interrupted aortic arch accompany aplasia or hypoplasia of the thymus, parathyroids and/or thyroid glands with facial dysmorphology. Many chromosomal deletions or trisomies are also accompanied by heart defects. For example, **Down syndrome** (trisomy 21) is characterized by craniofacial dysmorphology, mental retardation, hypotonia, short metacarpals and phalanges, and about 25% incidence of atrioventricular canal (a septation defect).

CONTEMPORARY STUDIES OF HEART DEVELOPMENT

Because it is one of the earliest systems to function in development, our understanding of the major events in normal heart development comes largely from descriptive or perturbation studies of the cardiovascular system in amphibian and chick embryos. With the advent of molecular techniques, mouse embryo culture systems, transgenic mice and more fully characterized mutant mice, it is now feasible to study normal and perturbed cardiovascular development in mammalian embryos to determine whether the same processes are fundamental to placental and non-placental animals.

EARLY DIFFERENTIATION AND REGIONALIZATION OF THE HEART

At the present time, relatively little is known about the molecular cues involved in induction of cells in the cardiogenic plate to form a heart. The **heart morphogenetic field** is induced by the pharyngeal endoderm as the anterior lateral plate mesoderm migrates over it. While no factor is yet a candidate for this induction, it is probably a diffusible substance. A much broader field of mesoderm is exposed to the inductive signal from the pharynx than actually forms the presumptive heart mesoderm (Smith and Armstrong, 1993; Easton et al, 1994). Easton et al (1994) have proposed that both an activator and an inhibitor are produced by the precardiac mesoderm in response to the inductive signal from the pharyngeal endoderm. The activator triggers initial expression of the myocardial (and perhaps endocardial) phenotype while the inhibitor suppresses heart formation in the remainder of the field.

One of the most exciting benefits of the 'molecular age' has been, and continues to be, the discovery of certain genes and classes of genes that are conserved through invertebrates and vertebrates. *Csx* (cardiac-specific homeobox) is a homeobox-containing gene that is expressed specifically in the developing mouse heart (Komuro and Izumo, 1993). The *Csx* homeodomain sequence diverges from that of the Hox genes but is similar to that of *Drosophila msh-2* (*tinman*), which plays a role in *Drosophila* heart formation. *Csx* expression can be detected in the presomitic embryo when mesoderm differentiates into promyocardium. Its expression precedes that of cardiac-specific genes in embryonic stem cells that develop into beating myocytes. The temporal and spatial pattern of expression of *Csx*, coupled with the fact that it is most likely a transcription factor, suggests the possibility that it may play a role in differentiation of cardiac cells (Komuro and Izumo, 1993).

Each region of the heart has its own intrinsic rate of contraction from the onset of myocardial contractility. The differences in contractile properties are probably generated on the basis of regional differences in the developmental genetic programme. A great deal of attention has been focused on identifying differences in the cardiac genetic programme that generate these region-specific properties within the differentiating heart tube. The differential expression of regulatory genes suggests that the looped tube is composed of four basic segments: atria, atrioventricular canal, ventricle and outflow tract. Significantly, two genes with homeodomains, *Msx-1* (formerly *Hox-7*) and *Msx-2* (formerly *Hox-8*), are differentially expressed in the heart. *Msx-1* is associated with cells undergoing epithelial-to-mesenchymal transition in the atrioventricular region and outflow tract to form the endocardial cushions. *Msx-2* is expressed in myocardial cells that will become the cardiac conduction system which co-ordinates myocardial contractions (Chan-Thomas et al, 1993).

MYOCARDIAL CONTRACTILE PROTEINS

In the adult heart, **cardiac myocytes** form a functional syncytium via tight, low-resistance junctions between binucleated myocytes. Although myogenesis in the heart has some resemblance to that in skeletal muscle, there are some significant differences. The first phase is proliferation of the non-differentiated precursor cells called **myoblasts**. In the next stage the myoblasts elongate and initiate synthesis of muscle-specific proteins culminating in the appearance of striations (**myofibrils**) and muscle contractions. Cytodifferentiation in the heart is not synchronized and myoblasts coexist with myocytes initially. As more cells synthesize contractile proteins, all acquire myofibrils and the myocytes are transformed to fully functioning myocytes. Mitosis still occurs in cardiac myocytes even at advanced stages of cytodifferentiation (Bugaisky and Zak, 1986).

In skeletal muscle, members of the **MyoD family** have been found to initiate and control myogenesis. A similar family of controller genes has not been identified in cardiac myogenesis and so far no expression of the MyoD family has been observed in developing heart (Buckingham et al, 1992). Members of the MyoD family heterodimerize via helix-loop-helix domains with tissue-specific factors to regulate gene expression positively or negatively via target DNA consensus sites called E-boxes (Murre et al, 1989). Cardiac progenitor cells appear to be committed to the cardiac myocyte lineage at gastrulation when ventricular myosin heavy chain 1 (*VMHC1*) is expressed. This myocyte marker appears long before differentiation of the tubular beating heart (Bisaha and Bader, 1991; Montgomery et al, 1994). Another early appearing transcript, *CMF-1*, has a basic helix-loop-helix motif that can bind the enhancer of the muscle creatine kinase gene in an E box-dependent manner, interacts with E2A heart proteins and competes with E box-binding activity. It may be one of the factors controlling differentiation of the cardiogenic mesoderm (Yutsey and Bader, 1995). Another helix-loop-helix factor, *Id* (inhibitor of differentiation), is highly expressed in proliferating myoblasts. Id is expressed in neonatal cardiac cells and appears to down-regulate expression of E box-specific complexes (Evans and O'Brien, 1993). *Id* is expressed at high levels in proliferating mesenchymal and epithelial tissues and is down-regulated as differentiation proceeds. *Id* shows striking overlaps with expression of *twist*, a mesodermal marker in *Drosophila*, and *Msx-1* (Robert et al, 1989; Wolf et al, 1991) in that high levels of all three are associated with development of the cardiac cushions (Evans and O'Brien, 1993). Clearly, there are complex and dynamic interactions with other proteins, in association with promoter elements, that remain to be elucidated.

Looping is associated with onset of expression of many contractile proteins and onset of circulation. Before looping, the primary myocardium expresses both α and β **myosin heavy chains**. After looping, atrial and ventricular segments of fast-conducting working myocardium develop, which express either α or β myosin heavy chain. **Smooth muscle α-actin** is up-regulated prior to looping and turned off in the primitive ventricle during looping and before the appearance of sarcomeric (skeletal and cardiac) α-actin proteins. The **sarcomeric actins** are expressed coincident with the onset of circulation (Ruzicka and Schwartz, 1988; McQuinn and Schwartz, 1995). The myocardial cuff surrounding the distal outflow tract retains smooth muscle α-actin expression distinguishing it from the rest of the tube. As with smooth muscle α-actin, many contractile proteins are expressed in all the cardiac chambers in early development with regional specificity acquired later. Some atrial and ventricular specific genes (i.e. **myosin light chain-1a, myosin light chain-1v** and **atrial natriuretic factor**) acquire regional specificity relatively late (post-septation or after parturition). Recent data show that some contractile proteins are regionally restricted from their first appearance. For example, **myosin light chain-2v** is expressed exclusively in the ventricle. By contrast, **myosin light chain-2a** is expressed throughout the early myocardium and is then restricted to the atrium by down-regulation in the ventricle preceding septation (Kubalak et al, 1994).

In addition to the contractile proteins, some of the early expressed genes are co-expressed with neuroectodermal or neuroendocrine tissues (e.g. *HNK-1*, *ANP*, *EAP-300*, *N-CAM*, *GIN* and several neurofilament peptides). Most of these are also expressed throughout the tubular heart and become increasingly restricted during septation (Moorman and Lamers, 1995). The significance of the expression patterns of these genes is currently under investigation.

Terminal differentiation of the myocardial cell phenotype requires expression of the tumour suppressor, retinoblastoma (Rb) protein. The level of phosphory-lation of Rb protein controls differentiation probably by lengthening the cell cycle but perhaps also by interacting with the promoters of genes expressed in mature myocytes. p107 can substitute for Rb as a co-factor for differentiation but cannot maintain the terminally differentiated state in myocytes lacking Rb protein (Schneider et al, 1994).

CELL–SUBSTRATE INTERACTIONS AND CARDIAC CUSHION FORMATION

Many events in cardiac morphogenesis depend on co-ordinated expression of cell surface receptors mediating cell–cell associations or cell–substrate interactions. **Cell–cell interaction** is essential to establish the endothelial tubes as well as the myocardial cell layer investing the initial endothelial tubes. Subsequently, migration of many cells will be required at critical stages during cardiac morphogenesis, such as the epicardial migration on the surface of the heart, neural crest cell migration to form the outflow septation complex and the migration accompanying the epithelial–mesenchymal transformation to make the cardiac cushions. The **cardiac jelly** provides the milieu for many of these activities. There are three major families of adhesion receptors: the integrins, the cadherins and members of the immunoglobulin superfamily. Cardiac jelly is rich in molecules found in basement membranes including collagens, fibronectin, laminins, hyaluronic acid, chondroitin sulphate and other glycoproteins (Kitten et al, 1987; Little et al, 1989). **Integrins** are heterodimeric proteins mediating cell–extracellular matrix and cell–cell adhesion (Albelda and Buck, 1990; Hynes and Lander, 1992), and are essential in interactions of cells with the molecules found in cardiac jelly. Agents that interfere with interactions of integrins with the extracellular matrix disrupt morphogenetic movement of cells (Linask and Lash, 1988; Bronner-Fraser, 1993). In the integrin family alone, a total of 14 α subunits and 8 β subunits have been described that make approxi-mately 30 different heterodimeric receptors (Baldwin and Buck, 1994). The expression pattern varies during development, indicating a requirement for dynamic patterns to orchestrate events. As an example, a change in integrin expression is required for cells to make the transition from a stationary to migrating cell phenotype (Baldwin and Buck, 1994). With the availability of targeted gene inactivation, it is now possible to determine the function and/or functional redundancy of integrin subunits. If either fibronectin or its receptor (an integrin subunit) is inactivated, a tubular heart develops but the embryos die because of circulatory failure (George et al, 1993; Yang et al, 1993). Embryos null for vascular endothelial cell adhesion molecule (V-CAM), which is one of the ligands for the $\alpha 4\beta 1$ and $\alpha 4\beta 7$ integrins, die at 10.5–12 days with thin atrial and ventricular myocardium, no endocardial cushions and absent or hypoplastic ventricular septation (Baldwin and Buck, 1994).

The cardiac jelly is important for the development of cardiac function; it not only serves to maintain anterograde blood flow as well as shape in the avalvular heart, but also provides a medium for transfer of signals from myocardium to endocardium and vice versa (Baldwin and Solursh, 1989). In two segments, the atrioventricular canal and outflow tract, the myocardium secretes **EDTA-soluble proteins** (ES proteins) that induce endothelial cells to transform into mesenchymal cells that produce the swellings called the cardiac cushions. The ES proteins are delivered to the endothelium via particulate complexes that are associated with fibronectin. Arrival of the complexes at the endothelium is associated with epithelial–mesenchymal transformation of the endothelium. The epithelial–mesenchymal transformation and delamination of endocardial cells is a multi-step process that includes: cellular hypertrophy, expression of *Msx-1*, influx of Ca^{2+}, loss of cell–cell adhesion by decreased expression of neural cell adhesion molecule (N-CAM), increased expression of substrate adhesion molecules, transforming growth factor-β (TGFβ) and urokinase-type plasminogen activator. The activated endothelial cells invade the cardiac jelly to form cushion tissue (Rezaee et al, 1993). In fact, c-*fos* may be a regulator of the epithelial–mesenchymal transformation. Immunohistochemical studies have shown a complex of ES1 antigens localized as extracellular particulates involved in the transformations. One of the components of these particulates is ES/130, a novel protein that plays a role in the epithelial–mesenchymal transformations. Blocking the expression of ES/130 prevents the transformation (Rezaee et al, 1993).

EXTRACARDIAC FACTORS IN HEART DEVELOPMENT

Kirby et al (Kirby, 1989; Kirby et al, 1997) have proposed that there are three critical periods in neural crest-supported heart development. The first is when the neural crest cells are located in the neural folds, are specified as to axial level of origin and are preparing to migrate. Other regions of the neural crest are not capable of substituting for the cardiac neural crest in supporting the normal processes involved in outflow septation and alignment (Kirby, 1989). The cardiac neural crest cells are specified by three different **Hox codes** that are expressed in rhombomeres 6, 7 and 8 in the hindbrain (Hunt et al, 1991). These codes are carried by the neural crest cells into pharyngeal arches 3, 4 and 6. If the Hox codes are disrupted using antisense oligonucleotides, the pattern of development and/or persistence of the pharyngeal arch (or aortic arch) arteries is abnormal (Kirby et al, 1997). During the second critical period the neural crest cells are in the pharyngeal region and support development of the aortic arch arteries and other pharyngeal derivatives, i.e. thymus, parathyroid and thyroid glands. The development of the persisting arch arteries is important for cardiovascular development in general and may be critical in maintaining the configuration of the looped tube. In the third critical period neural crest cells from pharyngeal arches 3, 4 and 6 migrate into the outflow tract where they are necessary for normal development of the outflow septation complex.

Normal alignment of the inflow and outflow portions of the four-chambered heart begins at the looped tube stage of development. It is critical that the inflow and outflow portions of the looped tube move medially and in close proximity to allow each access to both ventricles. Removal of the premigratory cardiac neural crest cells results in persisting truncus arteriosus in mid-incubation chicks. In persisting truncus arteriosus no division of the outflow tract occurs and a single common outflow vessel takes the place of the normal aorta and pulmonary trunk. Removal of a smaller amount of cardiac neural crest can result in malalignment defects (with or without defective septation) such as double-outlet right ventricle and tetralogy of Fallot (Kirby, 1993). It is thought that the malalignment defects are due to dilation of the ventricular portion of the looped tube to maintain normal cardiac output (Leatherbury et al, 1991; Tomita et al, 1991). The dilation prevents normal completion of looping which results in malalignments of the inflow and/or outflow tracts. Although the dilation is possibly due to events in the pharyngeal region, other factors have been shown to be significant in malalignment defects. If the cervical flexure is prevented by inserting a tiny rod in the neural tube prior to closure, embryos frequently develop with double-outlet right ventricle (Manner et al, 1993).

Recent genetic studies have shown that deletion of the q11 region of chromosome 22 results in DiGeorge and velo-cardio-facial syndromes in humans (Driscoll et al, 1992a,b, 1993; Emanuel et al, 1993; Halford et al, 1993). Both syndromes are characterized by outflow tract defects coupled with defective development of the glandular and aortic derivatives of the pharyngeal arches and abnormal facial characteristics. One of the genes from this region may be a transcriptional control protein and is similar to the beta-transducin/enhancer of split (TLE) family that has been most extensively studied in *Drosophila* (Halford et al, 1993). However, there are several more genes to be characterized from this region.

MUTANT AND TRANSGENIC MODELS OF CONGENITAL HEART DEVELOPMENT

Several null mutations have been mentioned previously. **Splotch** (*Sp*) mutant alleles have long been known to disrupt neural crest development in the mouse, resulting in defects of neural crest derivatives including melanocytes and dorsal root ganglia (Auerbach, 1986). Recently, it was demonstrated that Sp^{2H} homozygotes also develop persistent truncus arteriosus (Franz and Kothary, 1993) with accompanying ventricular septal defect (Conway et al, 1995). About 50% of *Splotch* embryos die at around 13.5 days of gestation (Conway et al, 1996). *Splotch* mutations disrupt the *Pax-3* gene (Epstein et al, 1991) which encodes a DNA-binding transcription factor. The Sp^{2H} mutation involves a 32-bp deletion in the homeodomain, one of the two main DNA-binding regions of the Pax-3 protein. DNA-binding studies in vitro have shown that an expressed protein with structure similar to the predicted truncated Pax-3 protein in Sp^{2H} has reduced DNA binding activity with an altered specificity for target sequences (Chalepakis et al, 1994). Thus, the Sp^{2H} mouse model provides an opportunity to investigate both the molecular and cellular basis of neural crest participation in the pathogenesis of persistent truncus arteriosus, and to investigate the cause of the increased lethality associated with the heart defect.

Neurofibromatosis type 1 is an autosomal dominant disease with phenotypic manifestations resulting from abnormalities of neural crest-derived tissues (Riccardi, 1991). The neurofibromatosis type-1 gene (*NF1*) is a tumour suppressor gene with extensive homology with two negative regulators of *Ras*, *IRA1* and *IRA2* (Ballester et al, 1990; Buchberg et al, 1990; Xu et al, 1990). *NF1* shares homology with the domain of mammalian GAP that encodes the GTPase-activation function. The GAP domain negatively regulates Ras by catalysing the conversion of active GTP-bound form of Ras (active) to the inactive GDP-bound form (Hall, 1990). Targeted disruption of *NF1* causes in-utero death between 13.5 and 14.5 days of gestation. The death may partially be due to the presence of heart defects resembling double-outlet right ventricle (Brannan et al, 1994).

The **Talpid 3** (ta^3) mutation in chick embryos results in abnormal cell death (Hinchliffe and Thorogood, 1974). Limb development in *talpid* homozygous embryos has been studied extensively because of the interesting malformations resulting from the absence of cell death during formation of the digits (Hinchliffe and Ede, 1967) and the disruption to the normal limb hox codes (Izpisua-Belmonte et al, 1992). Although these embryos survive only for 5–6 days of development, even at this stage it is clear that they are in the process of forming persistent truncus arteriosus (P.V. Thorogood and M.L. Kirby, unpublished observation). This will be a fascinating model to study because the mutant gene, although currently unidentified, is one that is common to limb, craniofacial and heart development. These three fields frequently develop abnormally in human congenital malformation syndromes.

These are just three examples of the new models of congenital heart defects that have appeared recently. Others have been mentioned elsewhere in the text. We can expect a great many more as an increasing number of the genes involved in normal heart development are silenced in transgenic animals.

CONTRIBUTION OF CURRENT RESEARCH TO UNDERSTANDING ABNORMAL CARDIOVASCULAR DEVELOPMENT

The recent contributions to our understanding of looping and septation events are obviously critically important in understanding normal and abnormal heart development. Since the heart must function throughout the major events in morphogenesis, the myocardial developmental genetic programme unfolds in a continuously changing environment. The interactions of that environment with the myocardial programme are not understood at all. However, it has been shown that myocardial development is altered during defective heart development after ablation or malfunction of the cardiac neural crest such that myocardial function is diminished (Aiba and Creazzo, 1992; Creazzo et al, 1994; Conway et al, 1996). While the reason for this alteration is unknown, it occurs prior to the time when the neural crest would reach the outflow tract, or some time during the first two critical periods in neural crest-related heart development. The changes so induced alter efficiency of myocardial function at the cellular level which directly relates to the broader context of cardiovascular function. Changes in cardiovascular function probably feed back on the myocardium which again may adjust its developmental programme. That this happens in clinical cardiovascular defects is clear since children with heart defects have subtle changes in myocardial function and plasticity. Thus, it is important to understand the developmental programme of the 'pump' as well as the development of the 'plumbing'.

THE FUTURE

There are a number of basic questions that remain unanswered in heart development. The factors that are involved in looping are still almost a complete mystery. Factors intrinsic to the heart appear to initiate looping, although which factor(s) might be most important or what the interaction of factors might be has never been determined. Baldwin and Solursh (1989) showed that hyaluronic acid, the major component of the cardiac jelly, is not essential for looping. Most recently Easton et al (1992) have proposed that a morphogen promotes looping and is produced at the anterior end of the precardiac region, while the cessation of looping is controlled by a morphogen secreted by the posterior end of the precardiac mesoderm. In addition to establishing the factors that initiate and stop the looping process, it is important to discover the factors involved in maintaining normal looping such that the alignment process is normal. While progress in understanding the molecular nature of atrioventricular septation has been made recently, the molecular contributions to outflow tract septation remain obscure. One of the more common outflow defects in children, **transposition of the great arteries**, is not produced in chick embryos but can be produced in mice by exposure to retinoic acid. Retinoic acid, a teratogen (and a morphogen; see Chapters 7, 10 and 13), has the potential to disrupt formation of the heart tube, myocardium, or neural crest migration. Treatment of chick embryos with retinoic acid causes double-outlet right ventricle while treatment of mouse embryos with retinoic acid results in transposition of the great arteries (Nakajima et al, 1995; A.C. Gittenberger de Groot, personal communication). Awareness of the relative strengths and weaknesses of the different model systems used for experimental analysis therefore becomes critical.

Clearly, understanding the intrinsic programme of the developing pump, in the context of its functional requirements, and the extrinsic factors that influence the programme, is essential to an understanding, and the treatment, of children with congenital heart defects.

ACKNOWLEDGEMENTS

My thanks to Karen Waldo for designing and executing the drawings for this chapter, and to Karen and Dr Tony Creazzo for comments and discussion on the manuscript.

REFERENCES

Aiba, S. and Creazzo, T.L. (1992) Calcium currents in hearts with persistent truncus arteriosus. *Am. J. Physiol.* **262**, H1182–H1190.

Albelda, S.M. and Buck, C.A. (1990) Integrins and other cell adhesion molecules. *FASEB J.* **4**, 2868–2880.

Auerbach, R. (1986) Analysis of the developmental effects of a lethal mutation in the house mouse. *J. Exp. Zool.* **127**, 305–329.

Baldwin, H.S. and Buck, C.A. (1994) Integrins and other cell adhesion molecules in cardiac development. *Dev. Biol.* **121**, 220–236.

Baldwin, H.S. and Solursh, M. (1989) Degradation of hyaluronic acid does not prevent looping of the mammalian heart *in situ. Dev. Biol.* **136**, 555–559.

Ballester, R., Marchuk, D., Boguski, M. et al (1990) The *NF1* locus encodes a protein functionally related to mammalian GAP and yeast *IRA* proteins. *Cell* **63**, 851–859.

Bisaha, J.G. and Bader, D. (1991) Identification and characterization of a ventricular-specific avian myosin heavy chain, VMHC1: expression in differentiating cardiac and skeletal muscle. *Dev. Biol.* **148**, 355–364.

Bogers, A.J.J.C., Gittenberger-de Groot, A.C., Poelmann, R.E. and Huysmans, H.A. (1989) Development of the origin of the coronary arteries, a matter of ingrowth or outgrowth? *Anat. Embryol.* **180**, 437–441.

Brannan, C.I., Perkins, A.S., Vogel, K.S. et al (1994) Targeted disruption of the neurofibromatosis type-1 gene leads to developmental abnormalities in heart and various neural crest-derived tissues. *Genes Dev.* **8**, 1019–1029.

Bronner-Fraser, M. (1993) Mechanisms of neural crest cell migration. *BioEssays* **15**, 221–230.

Buchberg, A.M., Cleveland, L.S., Jenkins, N.A. and Copeland, N.G. (1990) Sequence homology shared by neurofibromatosis type-1 gene and *IRA-1* and *IRA-2* negative regulators of the RAS cyclic AMP pathway. *Nature* **347**, 291–294.

Buckingham, M.E., Lyons, G.E., Ott, M.-O. and Sassoon, D.A. (1992) Myogenesis in the mouse. In *Post-implantation Development in the Mouse*, pp. 111–124. Wiley: Chichester.

Bugaisky, L. and Zak, R. (1986) Biological mechanisms of hypertrophy. In *The Heart and Cardiovascular System* (Eds: H.A. Fozzare et al), pp. 1491–1506. Raven Press: New York.

Chalepakis, G., Goulding, M., Read, A., Strachan, T. and Gruss, P. (1994) Molecular basis of splotch and Waardenburg *Pax-3* mutations. *Proc. Natl. Acad. Sci. USA* **91**, 3685–3689.

Chan-Thomas, P.S., Thompson, R.P., Robert, B., Yacoub, M.H. and Barton, P.J.R. (1993) Expression of homeobox genes *Msx-1* (*Hox-7*) and *Msx-2* (*Hox-8*) during cardiac development in the chick. *Dev. Dyn.* **197**, 203–216.

Conway, S.J., Henderson, D.J. and Copp, A.J. (1995) Pax 3 expression in the mouse heart. *Genet. Res.* **65**, 234.

Conway, S.J., Godt, R.E., Greene, C. et al (1996) Neural crest is involved in development of abnormal myocardial function. Submitted.

Creazzo, T.L., Burch, J., Redmond, S. and Kumiski, D. (1994) Myocardial enlargement in defective heart development. *Anat. Rec.* **239**, 170–176.

Driscoll, D.A., Budarf, M.L. and Emanuel, B.S. (1992a) A genetic etiology for DiGeorge syndrome: consistent deletions and microdeletions of 22q11. *Am. J. Hum. Genet.* **50**, 924–933.

Driscoll, D.A., Spinner, N.B., Budarf, M.L. et al (1992b) Deletions and microdeletions of 22q11.2 in velo-cardio-facial syndrome. *Am. J. Med. Genetics* **44**, 261–268.

Driscoll, D.A., Salvin, J., Sellinger, B. et al (1993) Prevalence of 22q11 microdeletions in DiGeorge and velocardiofacial syndromes: implications for genetic counselling and prenatal diagnosis. *J. Med. Genet.* **30**, 813–817.

Easton, H., Veini, M. and Bellairs, R. (1992) Cardiac looping in the chick embryo: the role of the posterior precardiac mesoderm. *Anat. Embryol.* **185**, 249–258.

Easton, H.S., Armstrong, J.B. and Smith, S.C. (1994) Heart specification in the Mexican axolotl (*Ambystoma mexicanum*). *Dev. Dyn.* **200**, 313–320.

Emanuel, B.S., Driscoll, D., Goldmuntz, E. et al (1993) Molecular and phenotypic analysis of the chromosome 22 microdeletion syndromes. *Curr. Top. Microbiol. Immunol.* **184**, 207–224.

Epstein, D.J., Vekemans, M. and Gros, P. (1991) Splotch (Sp^{2H}), a mutation affecting development of the mouse neural tube, shows a deletion within the paired homeodomain of *Pax-3*. *Cell* **67**, 767–774.

Evans, S.M. and O'Brien, T.X. (1993) Expression of the helix-loop-helix factor Id during mouse embryonic development. *Dev. Biol.* **159**, 485–499.

Franz, T. and Kothary, R. (1993) Characterization of the neural crest defect in Splotch (Sp^{1H}) mutant mice using a lacZ transgene. *Dev. Brain Res.* **72**, 99–105.

George, E.L., Georges-Labouesset, E.N., Patel-King, R., Rayburn, H. and Hynes, R.O. (1993) Defects in mesoderm, neural tube and vascular development in mouse embryos lacking fibronectin. *Development* **119**, 1079–1091.

Halford, S., Wadey, R., Roberts, C. et al (1993) Isolation of a putative transcriptional regulator from the region of 22q11 deleted in DiGeorge syndrome, Shprintzen syndrome and familial congenital heart disease. *Hum. Molec. Genet.* **2**, 2099–2107.

Hall, A. (1990) *ras* and *GAP* – who's controlling whom? *Cell* **61**, 921–923.

Hinchliffe, J.R. and Ede, D.A. (1967) Limb development in the polydactylous talpid^3 mutant of the fowl. *J. Embryol. Exp. Morphol.* **17**, 385–404.

Hinchliffe, J.R. and Thorogood, P. (1974) Genetic inhibition of mesenchymal cell death and the development of form and skeletal pattern in the limbs of *talpid*^{3} (*ta*^{3}) mutant chick embryos. *J. Embryol. Exp. Morphol.* **31**, 747–760.

Hiruma, T. and Hirakow, R. (1989) Epicardium formation of chick embryonic heart: computer-aided reconstruction, scanning, and transmission electron microscopic studies. *Am. J. Anat.* **184**, 129–138.

Ho, E. and Shimada, Y. (1978) Formation of the epicardium studied with the scanning electron microscope. *Dev. Biol.* **66**, 579–585.

Hunt, P., Whiting, J., Muchamore, I., Marshall, H. and Krumlauf, R. (1991) Homeobox genes and models for patterning the hindbrain and branchial arches. *Development* **112** Suppl. 1, 187–196.

Hynes, R.O. and Lander, A.D. (1992) Contact and adhesive specificities in the associations, migrations, and targeting of cells and axons. *Cell* **68**, 303–322.

Izpisua-Belmonte, J.C., Ede, D.A., Tickle, C. and Duboule, D. (1992) The mis-expression of posterior *Hox-4* genes in talpid (*ta*^{3}) mutant wings correlates with the absence of anteroposterior polarity. *Development* **114**, 959–963.

Kirby, M. (1989) Plasticity and predetermination of the mesencephalic and trunk neural crest transplanted into the region of cardiac neural crest. *Dev. Biol.* **134**, 402–412.

Kirby, M.L. (1993) Cellular and molecular contributions of the cardiac neural crest to cardiovascular development. *Trends Cardiovasc. Med.* **3**, 18–23.

Kirby, M.L. and Waldo, K.L. (1990) Role of the neural crest in congenital heart disease. *Circulation* **82**, 332–340.

Kirby, M.L., Hunt, P., Wallis, K. and Thorogood, P. (1997) Abnormal patterning of the aortic arch arteries does not evoke cardiac malformations. *Developmental Dynamics* **208**, 34–47.

Kitten, G.T., Markwald, R.R. and Bolender, D.L. (1987) Distribution of basement membrane antigens in cryopreserved early embryonic hearts. *Anat. Rec.* **217**, 379–390.

Komuro, I. and Izumo, S. (1993) Csx: a murine homeobox-containing gene specifically expressed in the developing heart. *Proc. Natl. Acad. Sci. USA* **90**, 8145–8149.

Kubalak, S.W., Miller-Hance, W.C., O'Brien, T.X., Dyson, E. and Chien, K.R. (1994) Chamber specification of atrial myosin light chain-expression precedes septation during murine cardiogenesis. *J. Biol. Chem.* **269**, 16961–16970.

Kuratani, S.C. and Kirby, M.L. (1991) Initial migration and distribution of the cardiac neural crest in the avian embryo: an introduction to the concept of the circumpharyngeal crest. *Am. J. Anat.* **191**, 215–227.

Le Lièvre, C.S. and Le Douarin, N.M. (1975) Mesenchymal derivatives of the neural crest: analysis of chimaeric quail and chick embryos. *J. Embryol. Exp. Morphol.* **34**, 125–154.

Leatherbury, L., Connuck, D.M., Gauldin, H.E. and Kirby, M.L. (1991) Hemodynamic changes and compensatory mechanisms during early cardiogenesis after neural crest ablation in chick embryos. *Pediatr. Res.* **30**, 509–512.

Linask, K.K. and Lash, J.W. (1988) A role for fibronectin in the migration of avian precardiac cells. I. Dose-dependent effects of fibronectin antibody. *Dev. Biol.* **129**, 315–323.

Little, C.D., Piquet, D.M., Davis, L.A., Walters, L. and Drake, C.J. (1989) Distribution of laminin, collagen type IV, collagen type I and fibronectin in chicken cardiac jelly/basement membrane. *Anat. Rec.* **224**, 417–425.

Manasek, F.J. (1968) Embryonic development of the heart. I. A light and electron microscope study of myocardial development in the early chick embryo. *J. Morphol* **125**, 329–366.

Manasek, F.J., Burnside, M.B. and Waterman, R.E. (1972) Myocardial cell shape change as a mechanism of embryonic heart looping. *Dev. Biol.* **29**, 349–371.

Manner, J., Seidl, W. and Steding, G. (1993) Correlation between the embryonic head flexures and cardiac development: an experimental study in chick embryos. *Anat. Embryol.* **188**, 269–285.

Markwald, R.R., Krug, E.L., Runyan, R.B. and Kitten, G.T. (1985) Proteins in cardiac jelly which induce mesenchyme formation. In *Cardiac Morphogenesis* (Eds: F.J. Ferrans, G. Rosenquist and C. Weinstein), pp. 60–69. Elsevier: New York.

McQuinn, T.C. and Schwartz, R.J. (1995) Positive and negative promoter elements regulating α-smooth muscle actin gene expression in cardiac myocytes. In *Developmental Mechanisms of Heart Disease* (Eds: E.B. Clark, R.R. Markwald and A. Takao), pp. 47–56. Futura: Armonk, NY.

Mikawa, T., Borisov, A., Brown, A.M.C. and Fischman, D.A. (1992) Clonal analysis of cardiac morphogenesis in the chick embryo using a replication-defective retrovirus. I. Formation of the ventricular myocardium. *Dev. Dyn.* **193**, 11–23.

Montgomery, M.O., Litvin, J., Gonzalez-Sanchez, A. and Bader, D. (1994) Staging of commitment and differentiation of avian cardiac myocytes. *Dev. Biol.* **164**, 63–71.

Moorman, A.F.M. and Lamers, W.H. (1995) Topography of cardiac gene expression in the embryo: from pattern to function. In *Developmental Mechanisms of Heart Disease* (Eds: E.B. Clark, R.R. Markwald and A. Takao), pp. 261–268. Futura: Armonk, NY.

Murre, C., McCaw, P.S., Vassin, H. et al (1989) Interactions between heterologous helix-loop-helix proteins generate complexes that bind specifically to a common DNA sequence. *Cell* **58**, 537–544.

Nakajima, Y., Morishima, M., Yasui, H., Nakazawa, M. and Momma, K. (1995) Molecular mechanisms of complete transposition of the great arteries produced by all-trans-retinoic acid in mouse embryos. In *Developmental Mechanisms of Heart Disease* (Eds: E.B. Clark, R.R. Markwald and A. Takao), pp. 315–318. Futura: Armonk, NY.

Noden, D.M. (1991) Origins and patterning of avian outflow tract endocardium. *Development* **111**, 867–876.

Poelmann, R.E., Gittenberger-de Groot, A.C., Mentink, M.M.T., Bôkenkamp, R. and Hogers, B. (1993) Development of the cardiac coronary vascular endothelium, studied with anti-endothelial antibodies, in chicken–quail chimeras. *Circ. Res.* **73**, 559–568.

Rezaee, M., Isokawa, K., Halligan, N., Markwald, R.R. and Krug, E.L. (1993) Identification of an extracellular 130-kDa protein involved in early cardiac morphogenesis. *J. Biol. Chem.* **268**, 14404–14411.

Riccardi, V.M. (1991) Neurofibromatosis: past, present and future. *New Engl. J. Med.* **324**, 1283–1285.

Robert, B., Sassoon, D., Jacq, B., Gehring, W. and Buckingham, M. (1989) *Hox-7*, a mouse homeobox gene with a novel pattern of expression during embryogenesis. *EMBO J.* **8**, 91–100.

Rosenquist, G.C. (1970) Location and movements of cardiogenic cells in the chick embryo: the heart-forming portion of the primitive streak. *Dev. Biol.* **22**, 461–475.

Ruzicka, D.L. and Schwartz, R.J. (1988) Sequential activation of alpha-actin genes during avian cardiogenesis: vascular smooth muscle alpha-actin gene transcripts mark the onset of cardiomyocyte differentiation. *J. Cell Biol.* **107**, 2575–2586.

Schneider, J.W., Gu, W., Zhu, L., Mahdavi, V. and Nadal-Ginard, B. (1994) Reversal of terminal differentiation mediated by p107 in *Rb-/-* muscle cells. *Science* **264**, 1467–1471.

Smith, S.C. and Armstrong, J.B. (1993) Reaction–diffusion control of heart development: evidence for activation and inhibition in precardiac mesoderm. *Dev. Biol.* **160**, 535–542.

Tomita, H., Connuck, D.M., Leatherbury, L. and Kirby, M.L. (1991) Relation of early hemodynamic changes to final cardiac phenotype and survival after neural crest ablation in chick embryos. *Circulation* **84**, 1289–1295.

Waldo, K.L., Willner, W. and Kirby, M.L. (1990) Origin of the proximal coronary artery stem and a review of ventricular vascularization in the chick embryo. *Am. J. Anat.* **188**, 109–120.

Wolf, C., Thisse, C., Stoetzel, C. et al (1991) The *M-twist* gene of *Mus* is expressed in subsets of mesodermal cells and is closely related to the Xenopus *X-twi* and the Drosophila *twist* genes. *Dev. Biol.* **143**, 363–373.

Xu, G., Lin, B., Tanaka, K. et al (1990) The catalytic domain of the neurofibromatosis type 1 gene product stimulates *ras*GTPase and complements *ira* mutants of S. cerevisiae. *Cell* **63**, 835–841.

Yang, J.T., Rayburn, H. and Hynes, R.O. (1993) Embryonic mesodermal defects in a_5 integrin-deficient mice. *Development* **119**, 1093–1105.

Yutsey, K.E. and Bader, D. (1995) Regulation of cardiomyogenic differentiation and diversification. In *Developmental Mechanisms of Heart Disease* (Eds: E.B. Clark, R.R. Markwald and A. Takao), pp. 41–46. Futura: Armonk, NY.

12 The Skin

ANNE REEVES HAAKE and LOWELL A. GOLDSMITH

Department of Dermatology, University of Rochester School of Medicine and Dentistry, Rochester, USA

The skin is a complex tissue that elaborates several different specialized structures and is composed of many cell types of varied embryonic origin. As a continually renewing epithelium the epidermis of the skin must recapitulate some developmental events throughout life. It is easy to appreciate, therefore, that the birth defects involving the skin are both numerous and heterogeneous. Abnormalities can result from defects at many levels in the hierarchical development of the skin, from initial establishment of the primary germ layers and migrations of different cell types into the embryonic epidermis, to the morphogenesis and terminal differentiation of the epidermis and its appendages. To understand the developmental mechanisms underlying these malformations it is necessary and informative to consider them within a framework of normal skin development. In this chapter, we will first set out the major developmental events in the morphogenesis and differentiation of normal human skin and then attempt to identify specific developmental processes that may be sensitive to genetically caused malformations or environmental disruptions. In each case, specific skin defects or malformation syndromes involving the skin will be given as examples to illustrate possible aetiology and to suggest new avenues of investigation. It must be stressed that, although descriptive reports of human birth defects involving the skin are abundant, much of the nosology is based on clinical manifestations, and the underlying cellular or molecular mechanisms have only been defined in a few cases.

DEVELOPMENTAL ANATOMY

EMBRYONIC ORIGIN OF THE INTEGUMENT

The structure of the developing human skin (Holbrook, 1991) and the developmental anatomy of the human integument within the context of the entire programme of human embryogenesis (Larsen, 1993) have been reviewed in detail. Only the major features and events of skin development will be highlighted here. The integument, consisting of the skin and its associated appendages, the **pilosebaceous structures**, eccrine sweat glands, apocrine

Embryos, Genes and Birth Defects. Edited by P. Thorogood.
© 1997 John Wiley & Sons Ltd.

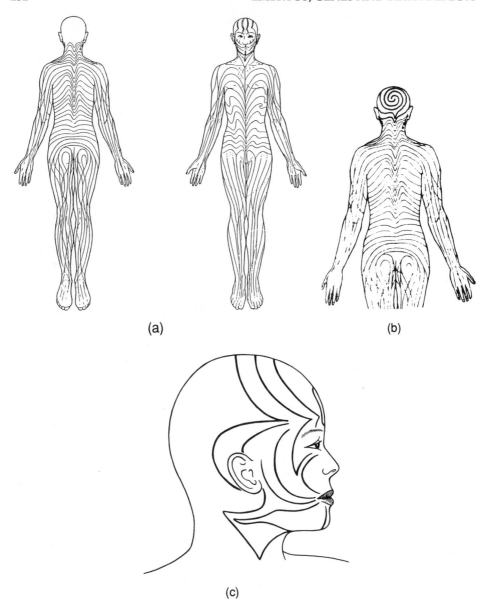

(a)   (b)

(c)

Figure 12.1 Blaschko's lines. (a) As originally described. (b), (c) As modified by Happle (1985) and Bolognia et al (1994), respectively. (Reprinted with permission from Bolognia et al, 1994)

glands and nails, is formed from cells of varied embryonic origin. Skin is composed of two tissues: the **epidermis**, derived from surface ectoderm, and the dermis. The **dermis** is predominantly a derivative of lateral plate mesoderm and the dermatomes of the somites. An exception to this is the dermis of the head and anterior neck, which forms from cephalic neural crest (Larsen, 1993; Gilbert,

1994). In addition to the major ectodermally derived cell type of the epidermis, the **keratinocyte**, the epidermis is colonized by immigrant cells of different embryonic origin including melanocytes, Langerhans cells and Merkel cells.

Melanocytes, responsible for pigmentation of the epidermis, are of neural crest origin. Neural crest cells detach from the neural tube in the sixth week and melanocytic precursors migrate through the developing dermis into the epidermis where they have been detected as early as 6–7 weeks (Holbrook, 1991). **Langerhans cells** are bone marrow-derived cells that function as antigen-presenting dendritic cells of the skin. Like melanocytes, Langerhans cells are first present in the epidermis at about 7 weeks and continually repopulate the epidermis throughout life. Immunocompetence of the fetal epidermis appears to be related to an early function of Langerhans cells in contact hypersensitivity and immune surveillance (Larsen, 1993). The embryonic origin of **Merkel cells**, first present in the human fetal epidermis at 8–12 weeks of gestation (Moll et al, 1986), remains under debate (discussed by Holbrook, 1991). A neural crest origin has been suggested for these cells, which function as mechanoreceptors and associate with underlying dermal nerve fibres. A second hypothesis is that Merkel cells are derived from epidermal cells (Munger, 1965), and they do share characteristics with keratinocytes such as expression of keratin intermediate filaments and formation of desmosomes (Hashimoto, 1972; Holbrook, 1991). Transplantation studies of fetal skin to the nude mouse prior to the appearance of Merkel cells and subsequent development of these cells in the transplanted epidermis support the theory of an epidermal origin (Moll et al, 1990).

MAJOR DEVELOPMENTAL EVENTS OF HUMAN SKIN MORPHOGENESIS AND DIFFERENTIATION

Early embryogenesis: the significance of gastrulation, X-chromosome inactivation and neurulation

Early embryonic processes such as gastrulation establish the body plan and therefore greatly influence later events such as skin organogenesis. Gastrulation not only serves to organize the three primary germ layers, but also establishes the midline/bilateral symmetry and brings diverse populations of cells into contact with each other so that subsequent inductive interactions can function. Another important normal developmental event occurring at this time (late blastula to early gastrula) that can affect skin development is X-chromosome inactivation, also known as **Lyonization** (Lyon, 1961). The morphogenetic movements occurring near, or at the time of, gastrulation, and random X-inactivation in skin precursor cells, together contribute to the formation on the surface of the human body of a system of lines known as **Blaschko's lines** (Figure 12.1). These lines are believed to be anatomical markers of normal skin development that can only be seen in the heterozygous state of various X-linked gene defects or other types of genetic mosaics. According to one theory (Happle, 1985), Blaschko's lines, clearly distinct from the system of dermatomes, 'originate from precursor cells localized along the primitive streak, and they reflect the coherent dorsoventral outgrowth of two functionally different clones during early embryogenesis'. It has also been suggested that these lines are related to metamerism (segmentation) and may follow visceral afferents or may simply represent patterns of skin stretching (discussed by Bolognia et al, 1994).

Establishment of the midline precedes formation of the skin. The development of the dorsal midline and neurulation result in separation of the neuroectoderm from the surface ectoderm and fusion of surface ectoderm (primitive epidermis) over the midline. The ventral midline is formed during the complex process of embryonic folding in the fourth week. The ectodermal, mesodermal and endodermal layers on each side of the germ disc fuse with the corresponding layers on the other side. This results in an ectodermal covering, which will eventually give rise to the epidermis, over the entire embryo (Larsen, 1993).

Differentiation of the ectoderm into primitive epidermis and stratification

The primitive epidermis initially is one cell thick but becomes stratified during the fourth week of gestation by the addition of the **periderm**. This cell layer probably arises through proliferation of basal cells of the primitive epidermis (Holbrook, 1991) but migration of extraembryonic amniotic ectodermal cells over the primitive epidermis has also been hypothesized as the origin of the periderm, on the basis of antigenic similarity between amnion and periderm cells (Lane et al, 1987).

Beginning in the 9th–11th week of gestation, depending on the region, the basal layer proliferates to give rise to the first intermediate layer, so named because of its position between basal cells and the periderm. Additional intermediate cell layers are added throughout the second trimester. The second trimester is a period of development that involves extensive growth of the skin, as both stratification and horizontal expansion to cover the rapidly developing fetus are required (Holbrook, 1991).

Appendage morphogenesis

Simultaneously with the onset of stratification, morphogenesis of specialized structures begins in a regionally specific manner. The development of the hair follicles, sweat glands, sebaceous glands and nails is directed by reciprocal epithelial–mesenchymal interactions. The nature and timing of the tissue interactions that direct appendage morphogenesis in chick and mouse embryos have been characterized through many elegant tissue recombination experiments (Rawles, 1963; Sengel, 1976; Sawyer, 1983; Hardy, 1992). The developing **hair follicle** (Figure 12.2) has been most intensively studied and serves as an example that can be generalized, in many aspects, to other appendages, although the precise mechanisms of tissue interaction are probably specific to each appendage type (Rawles, 1963). The dermis induces the formation of the **hair germ**, which first appears as a discrete group of columnar basal epidermal cells (**epidermal placode**) that have undergone slight invagination. Regionally specific instructive interactions from the dermis establish the type of epidermal appendage and the

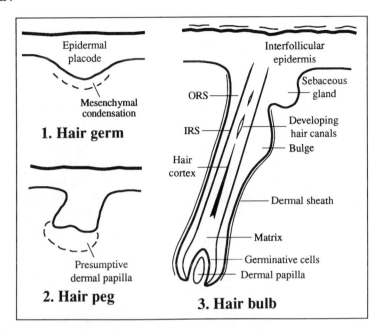

Figure 12.2 Major stages and functionally distinct cell populations in the developing hair follicle. ORS, outer root sheath; IRS, inner root sheath

pattern of appendages within the skin (Rawles, 1963; Sengel, 1976; Sawyer, 1983; Hardy, 1992). The hair germ proliferates and continues invagination into the dermis to form the **hair peg**.

Morphogenesis of the follicle reaches the hair bulb stage as the tip of the hair peg encloses a specialized dermal structure, the **dermal papilla**. Functional regions of the hair follicle have been defined through tissue recombination studies and by analysis of mechanisms controlling the hair cycle (Hardy, 1992; Jahoda and Reynolds, 1993). Proliferative keratinocytes located within the hair matrix are considered to be transient amplifying cells that rapidly divide and differentiate to form the hair during each successive hair cycle. These cells are believed to be derived from slow cycling stem cells located in the hair follicle bulge (Cotsarelis et al, 1990) and are induced by the dermal papilla to proliferate and populate the hair matrix. The dynamics of the hair cycle and its control have been integrated with the stem cell concept in a model coined the **bulge-activation hypothesis** (Sun et al, 1991).

Epidermal terminal differentiation and cornification

Biochemical differentiation precedes morphological differentiation in human fetal skin (Dale et al, 1985; Holbrook, 1991). The stratified fetal epidermis early in the second trimester, consisting of basal cells, several intermediate cell layers and periderm (Figure 12.3a), does not yet resemble the mature epidermis of the adult. However, the biochemical profiles of many of the terminal differentiation

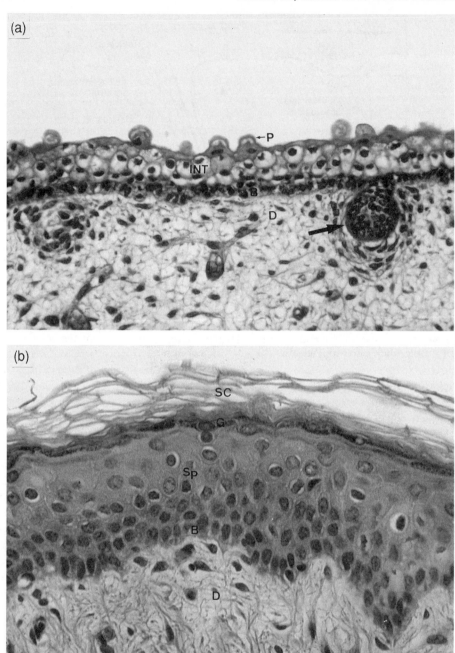

Figure 12.3 (a) Human fetal skin (16 weeks estimated gestational age) showing the major cell types present at this stage. P, periderm; INT, intermediate cell layers; B, basal cell layer; D, dermis; arrow, developing hair follicle. (b) Human neonatal skin showing the characteristic strata of the differentiated epidermis. SC, stratum corneum; G, granular cell layer; Sp, spinous cell layers; B, basal cell layer; D, dermis. Haematoxylin and eosin

markers, typical of the adult epidermis, are seen as early as 8 weeks of gestation. These include the patterned expression of the basal cell **keratins** (K5, K14), suprabasally expressed keratins (K1, K10) and **involucrin**, a precursor of the cornified cell envelope (Dale et al, 1985; Holbrook, 1991). Late differentiation markers such as **filaggrin** and **transglutaminase** appear in the epidermis just prior to the onset of **keratinization** (cornification) of the interfollicular epidermis (Holbrook, 1991; Polakowska et al, 1994). At 20–24 weeks gestation, granular cells and terminally differentiated **stratum corneum** cells (corneocytes) appear. The final remnants of the fetal-specific incompletely keratinized intermediate layers and periderm are deleted by apoptosis (Polakowska et al, 1994), and lost. Epidermal strata between the basal and granular layers are now referred to as **spinous cell layers** and the fetal epidermis closely resembles the epidermis of the neonate (Figure 12.3b). There is evidence, however, that the barrier function of the fetal epidermis is not completely operative.

CLASSES OF MALFORMATION AFFECTING THE SKIN

Skin diseases are usually classified on the basis of the primary skin lesions: macules (flat lesions), papules (raised lesions), nodules (lesions beneath the skin), and blisters and ulcerations (interruption of skin integrity). This classification is of most use to those conversant and comfortable with the nomenclature of skin disease and is the method of classification found in most standard dermatological textbooks. The chapter by Atherton (1992) in *The Rook–Wilkinson–Ebling Textbook of Dermatology* is comprehensive and has many pertinent references to individual diseases. (Ectodermal dysplasia is frequently used in a very broad generic sense in the clinical literature and the original case descriptions should be interpreted carefully.)

Here we propose a clinical classification (Table 12.1) that may be helpful in the development of an aetiological approach to skin congenital malformations. This classification is based on the major tissue or cell type involved, the extent of involvement of the skin and the association of the skin defects with defects in other organ systems, and conforms somewhat to the categories of developmental mechanisms that are discussed below. We concentrate on those diseases which are often present at birth, or occur during the first year of life, in which the aetiology is still under study and which appear to be caused by defects in early skin morphogenesis. Several skin diseases are, however, caused by mutations in structural proteins associated with terminal differentiation of the skin. For example, abnormalities of the keratins, intracellular molecules of the epidermis, are known. Mutations in K1 and K10 cause epidermolytic hyperkeratosis, and K5 and K14 mutations underlie epidermolysis bullosa simplex. Abnormalities of type VII collagen are associated with fragility of the dermal–epidermal interface in the autosomal recessive and dominant forms of epidermolysis bullosa, and abnormalities of laminin 5 (epiligrin, kalinin, nicein), with the junctional form of epidermolysis bullosa. These diseases and their defects have been reviewed extensively elsewhere (Goldsmith, 1993) and so are not listed in the classifi-

Table 12.1   Developmental disorders of the skin

A. Disease phenotypically limited to one skin component

1. *Local*
   (a) Epidermis and epidermal appendages
           Naevus sebaceous
           Woolly hair naevus
   (b) Melanocyte
           Melanocytic naevus
           Naevus depigmentosus
           Naevus of Ota/Ito
           Piebaldism*
           Poliosis
   (c) Basement membrane zone
           Bart syndrome
   (d) Dermis
           Connective tissue naevus
           Dermoid cyst
           Haemangioma
           Lymphangioma circumscriptum
           Naevus anaemicus
           Solitary mastocytoma
   (e) Subcutaneous tissue
           Naevus lipomatosus

2. *Generalized*
   (a) Epidermis
           Epidermal naevi*
           Pachyonychia congenita
   (b) Epidermal appendages
           Monilethrix
           Pili torti
   (c) Melanocyte
           Bathing trunk naevi
           Mongolian spot
           Naevi
           Piebaldism*
   (d) Basement membrane zone
   (e) Dermis
           Urticaria pigmentosa (mast cell disease)
   (f) Subcutaneous tissue
           Naevus lipomatosus

3. *Generalized with Blaschko line patterns*
           Epidermal naevi*

B. Disease involving more than one skin component

1. *Local*
           Congenital scalp defect

2. *Generalized*
           Anhidrotic ectodermal dysplasia
           Bathing trunk naevi
           Hidrotic ectodermal dysplasia

Table 12.1 *Continued*

C. Diseases obviously involving more than skin

1. *Local*

   Nail–patella syndrome*

2. *Generalized*

   Aplasia cutis congenita with spiral alopecia*
   Anhidrotic ectodermal dysplasia*
   Conradi's disease
   Focal dermal hypoplasia*
   Incontinentia pigmenti*
   McCune–Albright syndrome
   Trichothiodystrophy
   Waardenburg syndrome*
   Dyskeratosis congenita*
   Restrictive dermopathy*
   Hypodontia–nail dysplasia syndrome*
   Ankyloblepharon–ectodermal dysplasia–clefting syndrome*
   Basal cell naevus syndrome*

---

* These disorders are presented in more detail elsewhere in this chapter.

cation. Table 12.1 is not intended to be complete but to emphasize some of the diseases and to propose one approach that might usefully be employed when attempting to identify the underlying mechanisms. Diseases may appear in more than one category.

CELLULAR AND MOLECULAR MECHANISMS CONTROLLING SKIN DEVELOPMENT

CHROMOSOMAL MOSAICISM

The skin can be a highly informative structure for the medical geneticist. As an organ with a naturally occurring highly visible and variable marker (pigmentation), the skin can provide strong clues as to the chromosomal mechanism underlying a defect involving the skin alone or as part of a syndrome. Many skin defects with a mosaic distribution follow Blaschko's lines (Happle, 1985; Bolognia et al, 1994) and are often recognized as linear streaks or patches of differentially pigmented skin, reminiscent of the well-known banding of allophenic mice (Mintz, 1970). The **mosaicism** manifested in Blaschko's lines can arise by several different mechanisms. Two distinct clones of cells (for example, with different pigmentation or growth potential) may arise early in embryogenesis by X-chromosome inactivation, somatic mutation, gametic half-chromatid mutation, or true chimerism that arises by the fertilization of an egg and its polar body by two sperm or by the fusion of two embryos (reviewed by Hall, 1988; Bolognia et al, 1994). Female carriers of X-linked dominant or recessive mutations that affect pigmentation or structural aspects of the skin demonstrate a mosaic phenotype that is heritable and often lethal in males. Sporadic occurrences of malformations affecting the skin, not exhibiting Mendelian inheritance, can indicate chromosomal mosaicism arising from a somatic mutation early in embryogenesis or from a half-chromatid mutation in one of the gametes before fertilization. The type and extent of abnormality that result depend on many factors including the time of development, the nature of the mutation and whether the cells affected are migratory or stationary (Hall, 1988). Sporadic disorders tend to affect males and females equally, and the anomalies are distributed in scattered and asymmetrical patterns, often following Blaschko's lines in the skin. Although the mutations must occur very early in development, the lack of genetic transmission has been taken as evidence that many represent dominant lethal mutations that survive in the affected individual by mosaicism (Happle, 1987). Within the skin, survival of cells carrying the mutation may occur through cell–cell interactions mediated by growth factors produced by normal cells (Stosiek et al, 1994).

Sporadic disorders due to somatic mosaicism have been documented in **epidermal** and **sebaceous naevi** (Bolognia et al, 1994; Stosiek et al, 1994; see Table 12.2 and Figure 12.4). For example, chromosomal mosaicism has been shown in **epidermal verrucous naevus**, where a translocation of chromosome 1 was present in two unrelated patients in lesional skin but not normal skin or lymphocytes. Interestingly, several genes associated with epidermal terminal differentiation map to this chromosome 1 site including those coding for profilaggrin, involucrin, loricrin, trichohyalin, CRABPI and II (Stosiek et al,

Table 12.2 Epidermal naevus

Cutaneous:	Epidermal naevus
	Naevus sebaceous going down forehead
	Multiple histopathological patterns occur, mostly papillomatous hyperplasia
	Abnormally shaped hair follicles
	Abnormal dermis in most cases
	Haemangiomas (37%)
	Dermatomegaly (15%) – increased skin thickness, warmth, hairiness
	Nail matrix may be deformed
	Often absent hair over scalp lesion at birth
Skeletal (50%):	Abnormal skull shape
	Kyphosis/scoliosis
Nervous system:	Seizures (70%)
	Mental retardation (50%)
	Cerebral haemangiomas
Ocular:	Lipodermoid (20%)
	Coloboma (12%)
Other:	15% hemihypertrophy
	Systemic tumours including Wilms' in some patients
Genetics:	Male = female incidence
	80% before the age of 15

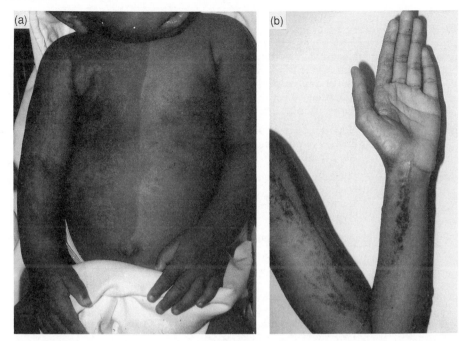

Figure 12.4 (a) Epidermal naevus predominantly affecting the right side of the body. A pattern following Blaschko's lines can be seen on the right upper arm. There are scattered small papules on the right side of the chest. (b) Linear hyperpigmented and hyperkeratotic lesions with a distribution along Blaschko's lines

1994). A rare subgroup of epidermal naevi with histopathological features typical of **epidermolytic hyperkeratosis** has recently been correlated with mutations in the K10 gene in lesional skin (Paller et al, 1994).

Examples of two X-linked disorders that exhibit skin defects following Blaschko's lines are dominantly inherited **incontinentia pigmenti** (IP) and X-linked recessive **anhidrotic (hypohidrotic) ectodermal dysplasia** (EDA) (see Tables 12.3 and 12.4). IP occurs predominantly in females, perhaps indicative of a lethal phenotype in the non-mosaic state. Linear skin defects are present at birth and there may be other affected tissues of neuroectodermal origin including the teeth, eyes and the CNS. Two IP loci have been mapped to Xp11.21 and Xq28, although the genes have not yet been identified (reviewed by Gorski and Burright, 1993). The occurrence of mosaic IP in a few cases of males with a normal karyotype suggests that IP may result from an unstable pre-mutation of a gene on the X-chromosome that is normally silenced in males (Traupe and Vehring, 1994). In EDA, the clinical manifestations of the disorder are usually apparent in males, although female carriers can exhibit a range of disorder due to variation in X-inactivation. EDA is characterized by abnormal morphogenesis of three structures: the hair follicles, eccrine sweat glands and teeth. The tendency of skin defects to follow Blaschko's lines in this disorder can be a helpful diagnostic tool for the identification of female carriers. For example,

Table 12.3   Incontinentia pigmenti

Cutaneous:	Neonatal linear red blisters (95%) Linear verrucous papules Linear and swirl-like hyperpigmentation Alopecia (40%) Partial or total absence of nails (7%)
Dental (65%):	Hypodontia or anodontia Enamel hypoplasia Abnormally shaped teeth
Nervous system:	Microcephaly and mental retardation (16%) Hydrocephalus Seizures Hypotonia
Ocular (35%):	Neovascularization Cataracts Glaucoma Strabismus
Genetics:	55% positive family history Mutation rate $0.6-2.0 \times 10^{-5}$ Male lethality with affected males 47,XXY or mosaics Two X loci: IP1 Xp11.21; IP2 Xq28
Animal homologue (mouse):	*Tattered* (*Td*; streaked scarring and alopecia) centromeric region of X may be homologous to *IP1 Striated* (*Str*) linked to *HPRT* and may be linked to *IP2*

Table 12.4   Anhidrotic epidermal dysplasia

Cutaneous:	Extensive peeling at birth Abnormal hair patterning Decreased sweating and hyperthermia Hypoplastic nipples Atopic dermatitis frequent Alopecia, variable
Oral cavity:	Underdeveloped maxillary and mandibular alveolar processes Dental anomalies from anodontia to peg-shaped incisors and canines
Facial:	Frontal bossing Prominent supraorbital ridges Saddle nose Ears small and anteriorly displaced
Genetics:	Xq12–13.1 by flanking markers Female carriers frequently have mosaic manifestations of trait
Animal homologue (mouse):	*Tabby* (*Ta*)

sweat tests that reveal the pattern of eccrine glands in the skin may show a whorled pattern representing alternating regions of functional and non-functional glands in the female carrier (Zonana, 1993 and references therein).

The distribution of skin defects along Blaschko's lines may be a clue for the genetic basis of uncharacterized disorders. **Aplasia cutis congenita** is a heterogeneous group of disorders characterized by localized or widespread absence of skin and can be divided into at least nine subtypes (Frieden, 1986). The aetiology in most types is unknown. The presence of congenital symmetrical abdominal skin defects and spiral alopecia in one case has been taken as evidence of somatic mosaicism rather than X-chromosome inactivation, because the only X-linked disorder with associated aplasia cutis congenita, focal dermal hypoplasia, is clearly distinct (Hennekam, 1992).

DEVELOPMENTAL FIELDS AND EPIDERMAL–DERMAL INTERACTIONS

The concept of the **developmental field**, long operational in developmental biology but not often given due consideration in medical genetics (reviewed by Opitz, 1985), has implications for understanding both normal and abnormal skin development. The emphasis of Opitz (1985) is not to review molecular mechanisms underlying morphogenesis in fields but rather to frame the developmental field concept formulated by early German embryologists in the context of normal vertebrate development and human clinical genetics. Opitz defines a field as 'that part of an embryo that reacts as a temporally and spatially coordinated, epimorphically hierarchical unit to normal localized forces of organization and differentiation'. Some of the consequences of the existence of developmental fields are that anatomically distinct structures are developmentally interrelated, their development is co-ordinated and that, because there is a tremendous amount of gene interaction within the field, a set of embryonic primordia can react identically to different dysmorphogenetic causes (Opitz, 1985). Consideration of skin development within this context may then help to provide insights into some of the characteristics of skin birth defects including the occurrence of skin defects within multi-organ syndromes and the heterogeneity of chromosomal defects linked to disorders with similar clinical presentations.

For example, the midline has been proposed as a developmental field (Opitz and Gilbert, 1982). The malformation syndrome known as **G syndrome** or **Opitz–G syndrome** is thought to arise from defective midline development and affects a number of diverse midline structures (Opitz, 1987). In one case report, the authors have proposed that posterior scalp defects associated with Opitz syndrome (Fryns et al, 1992) reflect another manifestation of a midline defect. Interestingly, the authors point out that other syndromes with defective midline development as a key feature, e.g. trisomy 13 and 4p deletion, are also associated with scalp defects (Fryns et al, 1992). A defective gene may affect early midline morphogenetic processes such as segmentation, fusion and cell death (Opitz, 1987) and have pleiotropic effects including dysmorphogenesis of the skin.

Can the skin itself be considered a developmental field? Pattern formation, particularly of the epidermal appendages, is probably an outcome of establishment of fields within the developing skin and involves local epidermal–dermal interactions. Individual epimorphic units, such as the hair follicles or nails, are formed in distinct spatial and temporal patterns and these are superimposed on other patterns. In the case of the nail field, the size and shape of the field appears to be related to the underlying bone of the digit. Accordingly, an increase in the size of the digit such as occurs on broad fingers (Johnson, 1966) causes a parallel increase in the size of the nail field and resultant nail. A small nail field in EDA results in the formation of a small, but normally differentiated nail (Telfer, 1991). Likewise, a disruption in the nail field may account for the nail disorders that are seen after maternal exposure to hydantoin and related anticonvulsant drugs (Pappert et al, 1991).

Another important aspect of the field concept is the fact that it encompasses phylogenetic relatedness. There is similar structure and function of related developmental units among different species, yet the final forms, such as feathers in birds and hairs in mammals, diversify during progressive stages of development. There must then be at least two different kinds of developmental instructions, those that are phylogenetically general and those that are species-specific (Opitz, 1987). This idea has been borne out in studies of normal skin development through classical tissue recombination experiments. Interspecific epidermal–dermal recombinants between mouse and chick have shown that the dermis provides cues to the epidermis to form appendages in a pattern and type that are regionally specific. The early dermal cues can cross species and this indicates that the induction probably involves the action of highly conserved signalling molecules (see Chapter 1). The final response of the epidermis to these cues is restricted by class, however. For example, chick dorsal dermis instructs mouse epidermis to form skin appendages in a chick-specific hexagonal pattern, but these appendages are mammalian hair follicles rather than avian feathers (reviewed by Sawyer, 1983; Hardy, 1992).

Involvement of certain organs together in human congenital malformations suggests that they have co-ordinated development and may result from mutations that function early in developmental fields. The **ectodermal dysplasias** (reviewed by Solomon et al, 1987; Holbrook, 1988), a heterogeneous group of disorders, primarily involving structures of ectodermal (or neuroectodermal) origin, may be good examples of such malformations. The hair follicles, eccrine glands and teeth affected in EDA have in common a developmental programme directed by reciprocal epithelial–mesenchymal interactions, although the mesenchyme of the hair follicles and sweat glands is primarily of mesodermal origin and the mesenchyme of the teeth is derived from neural crest. The genetic heterogeneity even within EDA (there have been reports of both X-linked recessive and autosomal recessive inheritance) may reflect the fact that the development of these fields involves complex multi-gene interactions. Disorders with defects in structures that may have co-ordinated development include many with both skin and eye malformations such as IP and **hypodontia–nail dysplasia syndrome**, which affects both teeth and nails (Murdoch-Kinch et al, 1993).

The importance of epidermal–dermal interactions in morphogenesis and differentiation of the skin may be well illustrated by two human genodermatoses: restrictive dermopathy and focal dermal hypoplasia. Although skin disorders are rare among the early lethal diseases, autosomal recessive **restrictive dermopathy** results in late fetal death or stillbirth (Verloes et al, 1992). The taut skin characteristic of this disorder results from a hypoplastic dermis and associated histological abnormalities of the epidermis. It has been suggested that the defect involves a regulatory factor of epidermal–dermal interactions (Holbrook et al, 1987) with pleiotropic effects resulting in dysplasia of other ectodermal derivatives and bone (Verloes et al, 1992). **Focal dermal hypoplasia** (Solomon et al, 1987), characterized by localized ectodermal/mesodermal dysplasia and hypoplasia of the epidermal derivatives (see Table 12.5) is perhaps another example of defective epithelial–mesenchymal interactions.

PROGRAMMED CELL DEATH

One of the most exciting 'new' concepts in skin biology, which will probably impact on medical genetics, is that of **programmed cell death** or **apoptosis** (reviewed, with emphasis on skin, by Haake and Polakowska, 1993; Paus et al, 1993; Polakowska and Haake, 1994). Naturally occurring cell death during

Table 12.5   Focal dermal hypoplasia (Goltz syndrome)

Cutaneous:	Atrophic macules, sometimes eroded Linearly arranged following Blaschko's lines Soft fatty herniations on limbs Perioral or perianal reddish mulberry papules Marked epidermal thinness Distorted or absent nail plate
Skeletal:	Linear striations in metaphyses of long bones (osteopathia striata), also present in carriers Skeletal hypoplasia, aplasia and syndactyly
Dental (40%):	Enamel defect, hypoplasia or anodontia
Ocular (20%):	Microphthalmus, coloboma, strabismus
Gastrointestinal/ respiratory:	Hernia and exomphalos Laryngeal and oesophageal papillomas
Intelligence:	Often normal
Genetics:	88% females ?9q32–qter Rare familial incidence ?X-chromosome mosaicism
Differential diagnosis:	Xp22.2 deletion has microphthalmus, acute weeping linear skin lesions and neck lesions that heal with hyperpigmentation
Pathophysiology:	Decreased growth potential of fibroblasts Defective collagen fibril formation

embryogenesis has long been recognized and, in fact, Glucksmann (1951) described and emphasized the significance of more than 50 individual instances of apoptosis among almost all organs and tissues in vertebrate embryos. What is relatively new is the recognition that this gene-directed, active process functions not only in embryogenesis but also in teratogenesis, homeostasis of adult tissues, elimination of damaged, deleterious cells, formation and prevention of neoplasias, and in the immune response. Accordingly, the field of apoptosis has gained renewed interest, resulting in an explosion of research into the cellular and molecular mechanisms controlling physiological cell death.

With regard to the skin, little is known about control of apoptosis but much can be inferred from consideration of the many studies on skin development and differentiation (Polakowska and Haake, 1994). Control of apoptosis in toad epidermis has been studied extensively (Budtz, 1994). These studies showed that apoptosis removes excess epidermal cells that are created by a rate of proliferation exceeding the needs of the differentiating cell pool. In the toad, control of this process appears to depend on pituitary hormones, whereas the endogenous regulatory signals in developing human skin are not known. However, we do know, from studying the distribution of apoptotic cells in human fetal skin (Polakowska et al, 1994), that apoptosis functions in the deletion of stage-specific epidermal cells such as the periderm, and in remodelling of the appendages.

There are many good molecular candidates for control of apoptosis during skin development. Retinoic acid (RA) and homeobox genes have been linked to the regulation of apoptosis in one of the classic programmed cell death examples, the interdigital mesenchyme of the limb (Zakeri et al, 1994). RA treatment can induce apoptosis and partially correct the defect of decreased interdigital apoptosis in the *Hammer toe* mutant (Zakeri and Ahuja, 1994), a mouse defect mapped to chromosome 5 (Martin et al, 1990; Zakeri et al, 1994). Interestingly, a human disease, **complex bilateral polysyndactyly**, has recently been mapped to chromosome 7, homologous to mouse chromosome 5, and the locus is near known homeobox genes (Tsukurov et al, 1994). Syndactyly in this disorder, and in other human birth defects and syndromes, may therefore result from lack of apoptosis normally controlled by RA and/or homeobox genes. An interesting human disorder with syndactyly is **ankyloblepharon–ectodermal dysplasia– clefting syndrome** (Solomon et al, 1987), where there is associated fusion of eyelids at birth and cleft lip or palate, both defects that may be mechanistically linked to apoptosis.

Dysregulation of apoptosis may also lead to hypoplasia of the skin. A disorder of fibroblasts, characterized by dead and degenerating cells in the dermis, has been reported to be the primary cause of the arrest of dermal development that occurs in restrictive dermopathy (Paige et al, 1992).

Some genodermatoses are associated with a predisposition to malignancy, in addition to defects present at birth, perhaps another clue that a gene associated with the cell death pathway is defective. Homeostasis of the skin requires constant balance between cell birth and cell death. Studies of the regulatory molecules that control normal epidermal differentiation and apoptosis suggest that these two processes are closely related (Haake and Polakowska, 1993;

Polakowska and Haake, 1994) and that **skin neoplasias** can result from dysregulation of the apoptotic pathway. For example, most squamous cell carcinomas that have been studied have mutations in the tumour suppressor gene, *p53* (Brash et al, 1991), which functions by arrest of the cell cycle to permit repair after DNA damage and can also initiate the apoptotic pathway in cells with extensive damage (Lane et al, 1992). Loss of *p53* function leads to fixation of mutation and eventual cellular transformation (Kaufmann and Kaufman, 1993). Similarly, aberrant expression of *bcl-2*, the proto-oncogene involved in suppression of the cell death pathway, is believed to lead to formation of malignancies such as some melanomas (Duval et al, 1994). **Dyskeratosis congenita**, mapped to Xq28 (Arngrimsson et al, 1993), is a condition character-ized by reticulate skin pigmentation, nail abnormalities, hyperplasia of the lacrimal duct and a predisposition to malignancies (Davidson and Connor, 1988), and may represent a defect in a gene that functions in cell death.

In an exciting recent discovery, **basal cell naevus syndrome** (naevoid basal cell carcinoma syndrome or Gorlin syndrome), characterized by multiple developmental anomalies and a predisposition to basal cell carcinoma, has been mapped to the *patched* (*ptc*) gene (Hahn et al, 1996; Johnson et al, 1996). *ptc* codes for a transmembrane protein with putative tumour suppressor activity. Although cellular processes controlled by *ptc* have not yet been identified, association of anomalies such as syndactyly in some individuals with basal cell naevus syndrome suggests that apoptosis may be affected.

Considering the widespread occurrence of apoptosis in development, the known roles of apoptosis in human fetal skin, and the plethora of initiators and inhibitors of this process, it is easy to speculate that some human birth defects will be linked to control of the apoptotic pathway.

MIGRATION AND PROLIFERATION OF IMMIGRANT CELL POPULATIONS

Another major developmental process that affects the skin is the migration and associated survival, proliferation and differentiation of the immigrant cells of the epidermis. We focus only on the neural crest-derived **melanocytes** because control of neural crest migration has been studied in some detail and because there are numerous skin defects revealed by aberrant pigmentation. Neural crest migration is discussed elsewhere (see Chapters 8, 9, 10 and 11) so what follows is only a generalized discussion. The migration of neural crest cells appears to be controlled by the extracellular environment (reviewed by Gilbert, 1994) and the expression of adhesion molecules such as N-cadherin on the surface of neural crest cells. The regionally specific composition of the extracellular matrix, containing a diversity of molecules such as fibronectin, tenascin, laminin and proteoglycans together with crest cell expression of receptors for these molecules (integrins), has a major influence on the directionality of migration and indeed on the ability of neural crest cells to migrate (Bronner-Fraser, 1993). In the developing human epidermis, keratinocyte–melanocyte interactions determine both the number of melanocytes and their epidermal distribution (Haake and Scott, 1991; Scott and Haake, 1991).

Studies of mice with altered skin and hair pigmentation patterns have led to the discovery of several genes controlling the proliferation, survival and differentiation of melanocytes and in parallel have contributed to the identification of the defect underlying several human pigment disorders. **Piebaldism**, characterized by a white forelock in humans and white spotting in mice, results from a reduction in numbers of melanocytes and is determined during embryogenesis (reviewed by Halaban and Moellmann, 1993; see Table 12.6). Two mouse mutants representing piebaldism, *Steel* (*Sl*) and *White spotting* (*W*), have been characterized at the molecular level. *W* is a mutation in the c-*kit* proto-oncogene, which codes for a membrane receptor tyrosine kinase. The *Sl* locus codes for the kit ligand, also known as Steel factor, stem cell factor or mast cell growth factor (reviewed by Halaban and Moellmann, 1993. c-*kit* function is required for melanocyte survival and migration into hair follicles and into the epidermal layer during embryogenesis (Nishikawa et al, 1991; Okura et al, 1995). Cells secreting stem cell factor are located along the migratory pathways of melanoblasts (Matsui et al, 1990) and the effect of functional kit signal transduction on normal human melanocytes is primarily to promote their proliferation (Spritz et al, 1994). Mutations in c-*kit* have also been demonstrated for human piebaldism (Tomita, 1994) but whether any cases are caused by *Sl* mutations remains to be seen. **Waardenburg syndrome** is a dominantly inherited condition (see Table 12.7). There are at least three subtypes of this disorder but primary features include deafness, a white forelock and differently coloured eyes (heterochromia irides). Again, study of a mouse mutant, in this case *Splotch*, has been critical in the identification of defective genes (see Chapter 8).

Table 12.6   Piebaldism

Cutaneous:	White forelock (80–90%):
	Bilateral hypopigmentation on limbs and trunk
Genetics:	Autosomal dominant at 4q12
Molecular basis:	Mutation in *KIT* proto-oncogene, a cell-surface receptor tyrosine kinase
Animal homologue (mouse):	*White spotting* (*W*) locus for c-*kit* oncogene and *Steel* (*Sl*) locus for kit ligand (mast cell growth factor or stem cell factor)

Table 12.7   Waardenburg syndrome

Cutaneous:	White forelock (40%)
	Fusion of the eyebrows (45%)
Facial:	Lateral displacement of medial canthi (99%)
	Prominent broad root of nose (78%)
Nervous system:	Heterochromia iridis (21%)
	Congenital deafness (20%)
Genetics:	Autosomal dominant

Pax-3 (in mice) and *PAX3* (*HuP2*, in humans), expressed early in development in the dorsal neural tube, are paired-box genes coding for DNA-binding proteins that are probably transcription factors (reviewed by Gruss and Walther, 1992). *Splotch* results from defective *Pax-3* and mutations in *PAX3* recently have been shown in Waardenburg syndrome (Tassabehji et al, 1993).

MOLECULAR MECHANISMS: CONSERVED GENETIC PATHWAYS MAY DIRECT SKIN DEVELOPMENT

One important concept that has recently emerged is that relatively few pathways have evolved to direct the wide variety of inductive interactions in both invertebrate and vertebrate embryos (e.g. Feitz et al, 1994). Practical application of this knowledge has led to a particularly powerful experimental approach – the search for vertebrate homologues of signalling molecules first identified in distantly related species with simpler developmental programmes and well-defined genetics (see Chapter 1). This has been spectacularly successful. Genes identified and studied in flies, worms, fish and amphibians thus have contributed significantly to the understanding of the molecular mechanisms directing mammalian development. The genes that have been implicated in these early events are highly conserved molecules that function in many species and in many different cell types. For example, primary embryonic inductions responsible for the formation of the dorsal mesoderm, neural tube and other tissues have been linked to the action of peptide growth factors, highly conserved molecules that have remarkable functional similarities across species (see Gilbert, 1994).

It is clear that progressive inductions linked by a cascade of conserved gene expression direct the morphogenetic movements leading to the establishment of the primary germ layers and that a major consequence is that tissues are brought into proximity allowing the secondary inductions involved in organogenesis. The secondary inductions involved in the specialized organogenesis of the skin and its appendages, the epithelial–mesenchymal (epidermal–dermal) inter-actions, are not completely understood at a molecular level. We know that activity of the genes involved function downstream in a pathway of progressive embryonic inductions and may therefore be affected by normal or mutant forms of genes expressed at earlier stages, such as gastrulation. In other words, the developmental history of cells participating in skin morphogenesis determines their response to secondary inductive signals.

Dysmorphogenesis of some or all of the appendages is one of the most common of the birth defects involving the skin, for example in the ectodermal dysplasias. What are some of the potential candidate genes that, when defective, could result in these phenotypes? One of the earliest events, occurring prior to the morphological appearance of skin appendages, may be the establishment of the overall pattern of the appendage fields by specification of positional information in the skin. Within multicellular systems cell fate is thought to be directed by the acquisition of positional information through the action of morphogens (Wolpert, 1994). Strong candidates for morphogens that function in establishment of the skin fields (such as the hair follicle and nail field) are the *sonic hedgehog* (*shh*) genes, retinoic acid and its receptors, and again, homeobox genes. The evidence implicating these molecules comes from studies of systems with well-defined programmes of pattern formation including the CNS, the axial skeleton and the limb bud. *shh* has been implicated as the morphogen functioning in two well-defined paradigms of embryonic induction: the neural floor plate and the limb bud (Echelard et al, 1993; Riddle et al, 1993). Evidence suggests that the shh protein acts in a concentration-dependent manner, consistent with the definition of a classic morphogen, and that *shh* functions upstream of homeobox genes in a complex regulatory network in these tissues. One current hypothesis is that RA, once considered as the morphogen in the limb bud (Eichele, 1990), can affect pattern by influencing the expression of *shh* (Riddle et al, 1993) (see Chapter 7).

There is some evidence for similar activity in the skin including *shh* expression predominantly in the epithelia of developing whisker, hair and tooth (Bitgood and McMahon, 1995; Iseki et al, 1996). Expression at the earliest stages of morphogenesis suggests that shh is an essential epithelial signalling molecule functioning in epithelial–mesenchymal interactions. There is patterned expression of homeoproteins in developing chick feathers (Chuong et al, 1990) and mouse hair follicles (Bieberich et al, 1991). A gradient in the skin of mouse *Hoxc-8* (formerly *Hox 3.1*) expression, a gene that earlier shows region-specific expression in the ectodermal and mesodermal tissues that give rise to skin, was localized to the dermal papilla of the hair bulb (Bieberich et al, 1991) and transgenic mice containing *Hoxb-4* regulatory regions show activity in the epidermal placode of the early hair germ (Whiting et al, 1991), suggesting that Hox genes function in patterning and specification of hair follicle type. *MSX2* and *HOXD1*, two other homeobox genes, recently have been shown to be expressed in the germinative epidermal cells of the hair follicle matrix (Reynolds et al, 1994). RA can affect appendage morphogenesis and cell-type specificity in the developing skin. In chick embryos, RA administration causes feather formation in presumptive scale forming skin (Dhouailly and Hardy, 1978). In the mouse, vibrissal follicles undergo transdifferentiation to form mucous-secreting glands when exposed to a high concentration of RA and the morphogenesis of some of the pelage follicles is inhibited (Hardy, 1968, 1992). Interestingly, the dermis of the vibrissal follicle is derived from neural crest. Neural crest is also the origin of the major tissues that are sensitive to RA-induced teratogenesis, which appears to occur through retinoic acid receptor-β (RAR-β) mediated pathways (Mendelsohn et al, 1991; Soprano et al, 1994). The effect on vibrissal follicles involves induction of RAR-β in the dermis (Viallet et al, 1991) so that RA-induced transdifferentiation may be specific to the hair follicles with neural crest-derived mesenchyme (Viallet and Dhouailly, 1994). We may take this one step further and suggest that dorsal lip follicles may be aberrant in humans exposed to RA in utero although this has not been documented, perhaps because attention has been drawn to the more prominent and severe facial deformities. The studies in mice also illustrate the fact that there is heterogeneity among hair follicles and this may account for the differences in involvement between body sites in some of the human skin disorders involving appendages.

MORE GENES INVOLVED IN HAIR FOLLICLE MORPHOGENESIS: INSIGHTS FROM NORMAL AND MUTANT MICE

Studies of normal and mutant (both naturally occurring and genetically engineered) mice have proven to be valuable in elucidating molecular mechanisms that direct skin morphogenesis and, again, the hair follicle stands as a most informative structure. Hardy (1992) has summarized the nature of the reciprocal epidermal–dermal interactions in the normal developing hair follicle and speculated on some of the regulatory signalling molecules. The distributions of many of the growth factors and their receptors, cell adhesion molecules and extracellular matrix molecules have already been described in the developing hair follicle of mouse and human (reviewed by Holbrook et al, 1993). Proteoglycans are differentially expressed in the dermal papilla during development and hair cycling (Couchman, 1993). From experimental studies it is known that administration of either **epidermal growth factor** (EGF) or **transforming growth factor-α** (TGF-α) (Wynn et al, 1989; Hardy, 1992) can inhibit hair development, and transgenic mouse studies of autocrine and paracrine growth factors expressed in the skin have provided some mechanistic insights into their roles.

Keratinocyte growth factor (KGF), a member of the fibroblast growth factor (FGF) family, is expressed by dermal fibroblasts and acts as a mitogen for keratinocytes (Rubin et al, 1989). Secretion of this paracrine growth factor can then affect the proliferation of competent epidermal cells, that is, those expressing the K isoform of the FGFR2 receptor, which binds KGF; this includes cells within the developing follicle (Peters et al, 1992). Ectopic expression of KGF in the developing epidermis of transgenic mice, driven by the K14 promoter, resulted in a very interesting phenotype (Guo et al, 1993). In addition to epidermal thickening, affected regions of the skin were devoid of hair follicles. It appeared that pluripotent embryonic basal cells had entered the epidermal lineage rather than participated in hair follicle morphogenesis. Taken together with the fact that there is a transient loss of receptors for EGF in the basal cells of embryonic appendage primordia, Guo et al (1993) speculate that downregulation of growth is critical to appendage morphogenesis. Similar results were obtained by over-expression of the parathyroid hormone-related peptide (Wysolmerski et al, 1994), another factor related to growth regulation. Over-expression of TGF-α, the autocrine growth factor that modulates keratinocyte growth via EGF receptors, has less profound effects on hair follicle morphogenesis. The only significant effect of TGF-α over-expression was found to be a delay in the first hair cycle (Vassar and Fuchs, 1991). A regulatory role of TGF-α in hair development was demonstrated in mice with a null mutation of the TGF-α gene and a phenotype of wavy hair and curly whiskers (Mann et al, 1993).

Members of the **transforming growth factor-β** (TGF-β) family also have been implicated in control of the proximate tissue interaction in the hair follicle. **Bone morphogenetic proteins**, BMP-2 and BMP-4, expressed in mutually exclusive patterns in the follicle (Jahoda and Reynolds, 1993), and in similar or adjacent cell populations as shh is expressed, can affect hair follicle morphogenesis when ectopically expressed in transgenic mice (Blessing et al, 1993). The mouse *notch* gene product has been linked to onset of different cell fates in the hair bulb matrix (Kopan and Weintraub, 1993). *Bmp-2* (Blessing et al, 1993) and *skn-1* (Andersen et al, 1993) are expressed in the differentiating hair. **Involucrin** is expressed in the inner and outer root sheath cells of the follicle, and over-expression of human involucrin in transgenic mice results in an abnormal hair morphology that resembles diffuse alopecia in humans (Crish et al, 1993), suggesting that precise regulation of even late differentiation markers is crucial for normal hair development. Our laboratory has shown that the *bcl-2* oncogene product is highly expressed in the dermal papilla and within the matrix and bulge region of the developing human follicle, suggesting that this cell-death related gene functions in hair follicle morphogenesis (Polakowska et al, 1994).

Figure 12.5 summarizes many of the known genes and gene products that function in hair follicle morphogenesis and shows the general sites of their actions. As discussed earlier, the genes encoding many of these molecules may be considered as strong candidate genes for human disorders involving appendage morphogenesis such as the alopecias and many of the ectodermal dysplasias.

INTERFOLLICULAR EPIDERMIS: REGULATION OF PROLIFERATION AND DIFFERENTIATION

The structure and function of the interfollicular epidermis depend on several processes that must be initiated during development and continue throughout

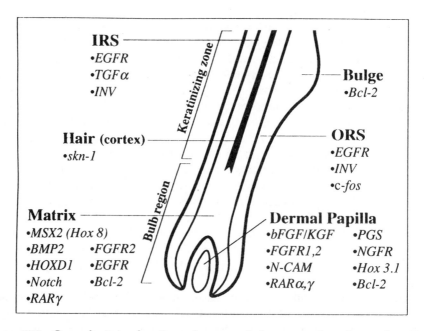

Figure 12.5 General sites of action of many of the genes thought to function in development of the hair follicle. The precise temporal and spatial activities of these genes are not implied here. IRS, inner root sheath; ORS, outer root sheath

life, because the epidermis is a continually renewing tissue. These processes include: establishment and maintenance of relatively constant cell numbers; interactions between keratinocytes and immigrant cells; adhesion between neighbouring keratinocytes, between basal keratinocytes, the basal lamina and the underlying dermis; and terminal differentiation to produce functional corneocytes. Tissue culture studies of human and mouse epidermal cells, in-vivo animal studies and, more recently, transgenic and gene-targeting studies in mice have elucidated many of the genes and regulatory pathways involved in the normal skin. Proliferation, confined predominantly to the basal cell layer, is regulated via growth factors such as TGF-α and KGF, as well as the proto-oncogene, c-*myc* (Pietenpol et al, 1990), and hyperplastic skin disorders, such as **psoriasis**, have been linked to an over-expression of TGF-α (Elder et al, 1991). RA and calcium can both modulate the response of keratinocytes to these mitogens. The RAR-γ1 is the major isoform of receptor in the epidermis and mediates the effects of RA, such as the regulation of the number of EGF receptors on some types of keratinocytes (Zheng et al, 1992). Proliferative basal keratinocytes eventually become post-mitotic and enter the differentiation pathway. The 'decision' to begin to differentiate and move up into the suprabasal layer is partially regulated by differential adhesion to the basal lamina, consisting of molecules such as type IV collagen and laminin, and anchored to the underlying dermis by type VII collagen filaments, and is mediated by integrins (Watt et al, 1988). Factors that cause withdrawal from the cell cycle, such as TGF-β and the tumour suppressor p53, may also function in the onset of differentiation (reviewed by Polakowska and Haake, 1994).

PTC, mapped to 9q22.3, and identified as the gene defective in autosomal dominant basal cell naevus syndrome (Hahn et al, 1996; Johnson et al, 1996), is a good example of a gene that functions in conserved developmental pathways. In the epidermis the PTC gene product appears to function as a tumour suppressor, regulating keratinocyte proliferation. Sporadic loss of the normal allele in progenitor cells during development is thought to give rise to the multiple anomalies whereas allelic loss during adult life leads to the formation of basal cell carcinomas.

Epidermal keratinocytes in different epidermal strata, representing progressive stages of differentiation, can be recognized on the basis of their characteristic keratin intermediate filament expression patterns. Pairs of acid and basic keratins, such as K5 and K14 in basal keratinocytes, and K1 and K10 in suprabasal, differentiating keratinocytes (reviewed by Fuchs, 1990), are responsible for the structural integrity of the keratinocyte. Keratins associate with another terminal differentiation marker, **filaggrin**, that packages the keratin filaments and contributes to the corneocyte phenotype. An insoluble cell envelope is formed beneath the cell membrane in late stages of keratinocyte differentiation. The envelope is formed by transglutaminase-mediated cross-linking of proteins such as **involucrin** and **loricrin** (reviewed by Polakowska and Goldsmith, 1991). The formation of lamellar bodies and the constitution of lipids between differentiated corneocytes are also important to the function of the epidermis as an impermeable barrier (see Williams, 1992).

It is thus evident that terminal differentiation of the epidermis in the fetus and as a continual process throughout life is complex and requires integration of many genes and their products. As would be predicted, many of the birth defects involving the skin implicate these critical processes.

Identification of mutations in genes coding for the keratin intermediate filaments has contributed greatly to the understanding of the molecular basis of several human genodermatoses as well as helped to elucidate the important normal function of keratins in the maintenance of epidermal integrity. Point mutations in the basal-cell specific K5 and K14 cause **epidermolysis bullosa simplex** (EBS), a severe congenital blistering disorder characterized by cytolysis within the basal cell layer (Bonifas et al, 1991; Coulombe et al, 1991; Lane et al, 1992). The suprabasally expressed K1 and K10 are mutated in **epidermolytic hyperkeratosis** (EH), characterized by generalized erythema and blistering after birth, and keratoses in childhood (Cheng et al, 1992; Chipev et al, 1992; Compton et al, 1992; Rothnagel et al, 1992). More recently, K9, almost exclusively synthesized in palms and soles, has been linked to another disorder, **epidermolytic palmoplantar keratoderma** (EPPK) (Reis et al, 1994). The point mutations in these keratins and resultant amino-acid changes affect the rod domain, thought to be important in the heterodimerization of the keratins. The specific phenotypes of EBS, EH and EPPK then reflect the regional and cell-layer specific expression of the affected keratins (Reis et al, 1994). Genes coding for products with late-acting function in epidermal differentiation have also been associated with human genodermatoses. For example, **X-linked ichthyosis** has deficient steroid sulphatase, an enzyme involved in formation of the interepidermal lipids in the stratum corneum (reviewed by Williams, 1992). Lamellar ichthyosis, an inherited autosomal recessive disorder of cornification, results, in some cases, from deleterious mutations in the transglutaminase 1 (TGM1) gene on chromosome 14 (Huber et al, 1995; Russel et al, 1995). This disease is hererogeneous, however, as some families show absence of linkage with TGM1 but a second disease-causing gene on chromosome 2, and additional pedigrees suggest the existance of at least a third disease-causing gene (Parmentier et al, 1996).

Abnormalities in the connective tissue components of the skin have also been linked with human genodermatoses that present at birth. Mutations in collagen genes or genes associated with collagen metabolism have been identified in several of the major subgroups of **Ehlers–Danlos syndrome** (reviewed by Yeowell and Pinnell, 1993). **Marfan syndrome** has been mapped to the *fibrillin* gene on chromosome 15 (Tsipouras and Devereux, 1993).

PERSPECTIVES AND AGENDA FOR THE FUTURE

In summary, genes whose mutations affect the morphogenesis of the skin may be quite diverse, depending on the timing and site of their action since the nature of inductive interactions and the architecture of the skin is continually changing during development. Mutations in regulatory genes that are active very early in development may be lethal or affect a number of organ systems (such as those derived from ectoderm and/or neuroectoderm). Later-acting genes may affect only the morphogenesis of a specific skin-related structure that is not closely related to the viability of the organism (such as hair follicles). Mutations in genes that code for structural proteins such as those expressed during epidermal histogenesis are not likely to be lethal to the embryo but severely compromise the well-being of the newborn. Highly conserved genes that belong to signalling pathways which function in diverse cell types, and at different developmental stages, may be good candidates for the molecular defects underlying some of the multi-organ syndromes. The precise molecular defects may be difficult to predict and will vary, depending upon the transcriptional factors, membrane receptors for growth factors, receptors for matrix molecules and growth factors involved.

Defining the known congenital disorders on a molecular basis is a major priority and progress will undoubtedly come from several complementary lines of research. The current gene targeting studies in mice of genes known to function in human skin have been fruitful, as have been gene mapping studies in human disorders where inheritance is evident and large families are available for study. Clearly, molecular definition of the known animal mutations that model skin disease (Sundberg, 1994) will be important. New avenues of skin research will undoubtedly emerge with the search for gene homologues in those animal model systems where there is a strong experimental genetics dimension, such as flies and worms. The identification of homologues, demonstration of their expression in specific cell populations and at important stages of skin morphogenesis, and eventual gene targeting studies of these genes in mice, promise to elucidate many of the genes responsible for skin defects in humans.

ACKNOWLEDGEMENTS

The authors would like to thank Vincent Falciano for illustrations and Karen Anvelt for preparation of the manuscript.

REFERENCES

Andersen, B., Schonemann, M.D., Flynn, S.E. et al (1993) Skn-1a and Skn-1i: two functionally distinct Oct-2-related factors expressed in epidermis. *Science* 260, 78–81.

Arngrimsson, R., Dokal, I., Luzzatto, L. and Connor, J.M. (1993) Dyskeratosis congenita: three additional families show linkage to a locus in Xq28. *J. Med. Genet.* 30, 618–619.

Atherton, D.J. (1992) Naevi and other developmental defects. In *The Rook–Wilkinson–Ebling Textbook of Dermatology* (Eds: R.H. Champion, J.L. Burton and F.J.G. Ebling), 5th edn, pp. 445–526. Blackwell Scientific: Oxford.

Bieberich, C.J., Ruddle, F.H. and Stenn, K.S. (1991) Differential expression of the *Hox 3.1* gene in adult mouse skin. In *The Molecular and Structural Biology of the Hair* (Eds: K.S. Stenn, A.G. Messenger and H.P. Baden). Annals of the New York Academy of Sciences, vol. 642, pp. 346–354. New York Academy of Sciences: New York.

Bitgood, M.J. and McMahon, A.P. (1995) Hedgehog and Bmp genes are coexpressed at many diverse sites of cell–cell interaction in the mouse embryo. *Dev. Biol.* 172, 126–138.

Blessing, M., Nanney, L.B., King, L.E., Jones, C.M. and Hogan, B.L.M. (1993) Transgenic mice as a model to study the role of TGFβ-gal related molecules in hair follicles. *Genes Dev.* **7**, 204–215.

Bolognia, J.L., Orlow, S.J. and Glick, S.A. (1994) Lines of Blaschko. *J. Am. Acad. Dermatol.* **31**, 157–190.

Bonifas, J.M., Rothman, A.L. and Epstein, E.H. (1991) Epidermolysis bullosa simplex: evidence in two families for keratin gene abnormalities. *Science* **254**, 1202–1205.

Brash, D.E., Rudolph, J.A., Simon, J.A. et al (1991) A role for sunlight in skin cancer: UV-induced *p53* mutations in squamous cell carcinoma. *Proc. Natl Acad. Sci. USA* **88**, 10124–10128.

Bronner-Fraser, M. (1993) Mechanisms of neural crest cell migration. *BioEssays* **15**, 221–230.

Budtz, P.E. (1994) Epidermal homeostasis: a new model that includes apoptosis. In *Apoptosis II: The Molecular Basis of Apoptosis in Disease* (Eds: L.D. Tomei and F.O. Cope), pp. 165–183. Cold Spring Harbor Laboratory Press: Cold Spring Harbor, NY.

Cheng, J., Syder, A.J., Yu, Q.C. et al (1992) The genetic basis of epidermolytic hyperkeratosis: a disorder of differentiation-specific epidermal keratin gene. *Cell* **70**, 811–819.

Chipev, C.C., Korge, B.D., Markova, N. et al (1992) A leucine–proline mutation in the H1 subdomain of keratin 1 causes epidermolytic hyperkeratosis. *Cell* **70**, 821–828.

Chuong, C.M., Oliver, G., Ting, S.A. et al (1990) Gradient of homeoproteins in developing feather buds. *Development* **110**, 1021–1030.

Compton, J.G., DiGiovanna, J.J., Santucci, S.K. et al (1992) Linkage of epidermolytic hyperkeratosis to the type II keratin gene cluster on chromosome 12q. *Nature Genetics* **1**, 301–305.

Cotsarelis, G., Sun, T.T. and Lavker, R.M. (1990) Label-retaining cells reside in the bulge area of pilosebaceous unit: implications for follicular stem cells, hair cycle, and skin carcinogenesis. *Cell* **61**, 1329–1337.

Couchman, J.R. (1993) Hair follicle proteoglycans. *J. Invest. Dermatol.* **101**, Suppl., 60S–64S.

Coulombe, P.A., Hutton, M.E., Letai, A. et al (1991) Point mutations in human keratin 14 genes of epidermolysis bullosa simplex patients: genetic and functional analyses. *Cell* **66**, 1301–1311.

Crish, J.F., Howard, J.M., Zaim, T.M., Murthy, S. and Eckert, R.L. (1993) Tissue-specific and differentiation-appropriate expression of the human involucrin gene in transgenic mice: an abnormal epidermal phenotype. *Differentiation* **53**, 191–200.

Dale, B.A., Holbrook, K.A., Kimball, J.R., Hoff, M. and Sun, T.T. (1985) Expression of epidermal keratins and filaggrin during human fetal skin development. *J. Cell Biol.* **101**, 1257–1269.

Davidson, R. and Connor, J.M. (1988) Dyskeratosis congenita. *J. Med. Genet.* **25**, 843–846.

Dhouailly, D. and Hardy, M.H. (1978) Retinoic acid causes the development of feathers in the scale-forming integument of the chick embryo. *Roux's Arch.* **185**, 195–200.

Duval, J., Malhotra, R., Savas, W.K., Kumar, W. and Woda, B. (1994) *Bcl-2* and *p53* expression in malignant melanoma. Society for Investigative Dermatology Meeting Program 40. (Abstract.)

Echelard, Y., Epstein, D.J., St-Jacques, B. et al (1993) Sonic hedgehog, a member of a family of putative signaling molecules, is implicated in the regulation of CNS polarity. *Cell* **75**, 1417–1430.

Eichele, G. (1990) Pattern formation in vertebrate limbs. *Curr. Opin. Cell Biol.* **2**, 975–980.

Elder, J.T., Fisher, G.J., Duell, E.A., Kragbelle, K. and Voorhees, J.J. (1991) Regulation of keratinocyte growth and differentiation: interactive signal pathways. In *Physiology, Biochemistry and Molecular Biology of the Skin* (Ed.: L.A. Goldsmith), pp. 266–313. Oxford University Press: New York.

Feitz, M.J., Concordet, J.-P., Barbosa, R. et al (1994) The hedgehog gene family in *Drosophila* and vertebrate development. *Development* Suppl., 43–51.

Frieden, I.J. (1986) Aplasia cutis congenita: a clinical review and proposal for classification. *J. Am. Acad. Dermatol.* **14**, 646–660.

Fryns, J.P., Delooz, J. and Van den Berghe, H. (1992) Posterior scalp defects in Opitz syndrome, another symptom related to a defect in midline development. *Clin. Genet.* **42**, 314–316.

Fuchs, E. (1990) Epidermal differentiation: the bare essentials. *J. Cell Biol.* **111**, 2807–2814.

Gilbert, S.F. (1994) *Developmental Biology*, 4th edn. Sinauer: Sunderland, MA.

Glucksmann, A. (1951) Cell deaths in normal vertebrate ontogeny. *Biol. Rev.* **26**, 59–86.

Goldsmith, L.A. (Ed.) (1993) *Seminars in Dermatology: Molecular Biology of the Skin.* W.B. Saunders: Philadelphia, PA.

Gorski, J.L. and Burright, E.N. (1993) The molecular genetics of incontinentia pigmenti. *Sem. Dermatol.* **12**, 255–265.

Guo, L., Yu, Q.C. and Fuchs, E. (1993) Targeting expression of keratinocyte growth factor to keratinocytes elicits striking changes in epithelial differentiation in transgenic mice. *EMBO J.* **12**, 973–986.

Gruss, P. and Walther, C. (1992) *Pax* in development. *Cell* **69**, 719–722.

Haake, A.R. and Polakowska, R.R. (1993) Cell death by apoptosis in epidermal biology. *J. Invest. Dermatol.* **101**, 107–112.

Haake, A.R. and Scott, G.A. (1991) Physiologic distribution and differentiation of melanocytes in human fetal and neonatal skin equivalents. *J. Invest. Dermatol.* **96**, 71–77.

Hahn, H., Wicking, C., Zaphiropoulos, P.G. et al (1996) Mutations of the human homolog of Drosophila patched in the nevoid basal cell carcinoma syndrome. *Cell* **85**, 841–851.

Halaban, R. and Moellmann, G. (1993) White mutants in mice shedding light on humans. *J. Invest. Dermatol.* **100**, Suppl., 176S–185S.

Hall, J.G. (1988) Review and hypotheses. Somatic mosaicism: observations related to clinical genetics. *Am. J. Hum. Genet.* **43**, 355–363.

Happle, R. (1985) Lyonization and the lines of Blaschko. *Hum. Genet.* **70**, 200–206.

Happle, R. (1987) Lethal genes surviving by mosaicism: a possible explanation for sporadic birth defects involving the skin. *J. Am. Acad. Dermatol.* **16**, 899–906.

Hardy, M.H. (1968) Glandular metaplasia of hair follicles and other responses to vitamin A excess in cultures of rodent skin. *J. Embryol. Exp. Morphol.* **19**, 157–180.

Hardy, M.H. (1992) The secret life of the hair follicle. *Trends Gene.* **8**, 55–61.

Hashimoto, K. (1972) The ultrastructure of the skin of human embryos. X. Merkel tactile cells in the finger and nail. *J. Anat.* **3**, 99–120.

Hennekam, R.C. (1992) Aplasia cutis congenita reminiscent of the lines of Blaschko. *Hum. Genet.* **90**, 469–471.

Holbrook, K.A. (1988) Structural abnormalities of the epidermally derived appendages in skin from patients with ectodermal dysplasia: insight into developmental errors. *Birth Def.* **24**, 15–44.

Holbrook, K.A. (1991) Structure and function of the developing human skin. In *Physiology, Biochemistry and Molecular Biology of the Skin* (Ed.: L.A. Goldsmith), pp. 63–110. Oxford University Press: New York.

Holbrook, K.A., Dale, B.A., Witt, D.R., Hayden, M.R. and Toriello, H.V. (1987) Arrested epidermal morphogenesis in three newborn infants with a fatal genetic disorder (restrictive dermopathy). *J. Invest. Dermatol.* **88**, 330–339.

Holbrook, K.A., Smith, L.T., Kaplan, E.D. et al (1993) Expression of morphogens during human follicle development in vivo and a model for studying follicle morphogenesis in vitro. *J. Invest. Dermatol.* **101**, Suppl., 39S–49S.

Huber, M., Rettler, I., Bernasconi, K. et al (1995) Mutations of keratinocyte transglutaminase in lamellar ichthyosis. *Science* **267**, 525–528.

Iseki, S., Araga, A., Ohuchi, H. et al (1996) Sonic hedgehog is expressed in epithelial cells during development of whisker, hair, and tooth. *Biochem. Biophys. Res. Comm.* **218**, 688–693.

Jahoda, C.A.B. and Reynolds, A.J. (1993) Dermal–epidermal interactions: follicle-derived cell populations in the study of hair-growth mechanisms. *J. Invest. Dermatol.* **101**, Suppl., 33S–38S.

Johnson, C.F. (1966) Broad thumbs and broad great toes with facial abnormalities and mental retardation. *J. Pediatr.* **68**, 942–951.

Johnson, R.L., Rothman, A.L., Xie, J. et al (1996) Human homolog of patched, a candidate gene for the basal cell nevus syndrome. *Science* **272**, 1668–1671.

Kaufmann, W.K. and Kaufman, D.G. (1993) Cell cycle control, DNA repair and initiation of carcinogenesis. *FASEB J.* **7**, 1188–1191.

Kopan, R. and Weintraub, H. (1993) Mouse notch: expression in hair follicles correlates with cell fate determination. *J. Cell Biol.* **121**, 631–641.

Lane, A.T., Negi, M. and Goldsmith, L.A. (1987) Human periderm: a monoclonal antibody marker. *Curr. Probl. Dermatol.* **16**, 83–93.

Lane, E.B., Rugg, E.L., Navsaria, H. et al (1992) A mutation in the conserved helix termination peptide of keratin 5 in hereditary skin blistering. *Nature* **356**, 244–246.

Larsen, W.J. (1993) *Human Embryology*. Churchill Livingstone: New York.

Lyon, M.F. (1961) Gene action in the X chromosome of the mouse (*Mus musculus* L.). *Nature* **190**, 372–373.

Mann, G.B., Fowler, K.J., Gabriel, A. et al (1993) Mice with a null mutation of the *TGFα* gene have abnormal skin architecture, wavy hair, and curly whiskers and often develop corneal inflammation. *Cell* **73**, 249–261.

Martin, G.R., Richman, M., Reinsch, S., Nadeau, J.H. and Joyner, A. (1990) Mapping of the two mouse engrailed-like genes: close linkage of *En-1* to dominant hemimelia (Dh) on chromosome 1 and of *En-2* to hemimelic extra-toes (Hx) on chromosome 5. *Genomics* **6**, 302–308.

Matsui, Y., Zsebo, K.M. and Hogan, B.L.M. (1990) Embryonic expression of a haematopoietic growth factor encoded by the *Sl* locus and the ligand for c-kit. *Nature* **347**, 667–669.

Mendelsohn, C., Ruberte, E., LeMeur, M., Morris-Kay, G. and Chambon, P. (1991) Developmental analysis of the retinoic acid-inducible RAR-β2 promoter in transgenic animals. *Development* **113**, 723–734.

Mintz, B. (1970) Clonal expression in allophenic mice. *Symp. Int. Soc. Cell Biol.* **9**, 15.

Moll, I., Moll, R. and Franke, W.W. (1986) Formation of epidermal and dermal Merkel cells during human fetal skin development. *J. Invest. Dermatol.* **87**, 779–787.

Moll, I., Lane, A.T., Franke, W.W. and Moll, R. (1990) Intradermal formation of Merkel cells during human fetal skin development. *J. Invest. Dermatol.* **94**, 359–364.

Munger, B.L. (1965) The intraepidermal innervation of the snout skin of the opossum: a light and electron microscope study, with observations of Merkel's Tastzellen. *J. Cell Biol.* **26**, 79–97.

Murdoch-Kinch, C.A., Miles, D.A. and Poon, C.-K. (1993) Hypodontia and nail dysplasia syndrome. *Oral Surg. Oral Med. Oral Path.* **75**, 403–406.

Nishikawa, S., Kusakabe, M., Yoshinaga, K. et al (1991) In utero manipulation of coat color formation by a monoclonal anti-c-kit antibody: two distinct waves of c-kit dependency during melanocyte development. *EMBO J.* **10**, 2111–2118.

Okura, M., Maeda, H., Nishikawa, S. and Mizoguchi, M. (1995) Effects of monoclonal anti-c-kit antibody (ACK2) on melanocytes in newborn mice. *J. Invest. Dermatol.* **105**, 332–328.

Opitz, J.M. (1985) Editorial comment. The developmental field concept. *Am. J. Med. Genet.* **21**, 1–11.

Opitz, J.M. (1987) Editorial comment. G syndrome (hypertelorism with esophageal abnormality and hypospadias, or hypospadias–dysphagia, or 'Optiz–Frias' or 'Opitz-G' syndrome): perspective in 1987 and bibliography. *Am. J. Med. Genet.* **28**, 275–285.

Opitz, J.M. and Gilbert, E.F. (1982) Editorial comment. CNS anomalies and the midline as a 'development field'. *Am. J. Med. Genet.* **12**, 443–455.

Paige, D.G., Lake, B.D., Bailey, A.J., Ramani, P. and Harper, J.I. (1992) Restrictive dermopathy: a disorder of fibroblasts. *Br. J. Dermatol.* **127**, 630–634.

Paller, A.S., Syder, A.J., Chan, Y.-M. et al (1994) Genetic and clinical mosaicism in a type of epidermal nevus. *New. Engl. J. Med.* **331**, 1408–1415.

Pappert, A.S., Scher, R.K. and Cohen, J.L. (1991) Nail disorders in children. *Pediatr. Dermatol.* **38**, 921–940.

Parmentier, L., Lakhdar, H., Blanchet-Bardon, C. et al (1996) Mapping of a second locus for lamellar ichthyosis to chromosome 2q33-35. *Human Molecular Genetics* **5**, 555–559.

Paus, R., Rosenbach, T., Haas, N. and Czarnetzki, B.M. (1993) Patterns of cell death: the significance of apoptosis for dermatology. *Exp. Dermatol.* **2**, 3–11.

Peters, K.G., Werner, S., Chen, G. and Williams, L.T. (1992) Two FGF receptor genes are differentially expressed in epithelial and mesenchymal tissues during limb formation and organogenesis in the mouse. *Development* **114**, 233–243.

Pietenpol, J.A., Holt, J.T., Stein, R.W. and Moses, H.L. (1990) Transforming growth factor β1 suppression of *c-myc* gene transcription: role in inhibition of keratinocyte proliferation. *Proc. Natl Acad. Sci. USA* **87**, 3758–3762.

Polakowska, R.R. and Goldsmith, L.A. (1991) The cell envelope and transglutaminases. In *Physiology, Biochemistry and Molecular Biology of the Skin* (Ed.: L.A. Goldsmith), pp. 168–201. Oxford University Press: New York.

Polakowska, R.R. and Haake, A.R. (1994) Apoptosis: the skin from a new perspective. *Cell Death Differ.* **1**, 19–31.

Polakowska, R.R., Piacentini, M., Bartlett, R., Goldsmith, L.A. and Haake, A.R. (1994) Apoptosis in human skin development: morphogenesis, periderm and stem cells. *Dev. Dyn.* **199**, 176–188.

Rawles, M.E. (1963) Tissue interactions in scale and feather development as studied in dermal–epidermal recombinations. *J. Embryol. Exp. Morphol.* **11**, 765–789.

Reis, A., Hennies, H.C., Langbein, L. et al (1994) *Keratin 9* gene mutations in epidermolytic palmoplantar keratoderma (EPPK). *Nature Genetics.* **6**, 174–179.

Reynolds, A.J., Lawrence, C.M. and Jahoda, C.A.B. (1994) Hair follicle and fibre reconstruction. International Research Workshop on Alopecia Areata. Bethesda, MD.

Riddle, R.D., Johnson, R.L., Laufer, E. and Tabin, C. (1993) Sonic hedgehog mediates the polarizing activity of the ZPA. *Cell* **75**, 1401–1416.

Rothnagel, J.A., Dominey, A.M., Dempsey, L.D. et al (1992) Mutations in the rod domain of keratins 1 and 10 in epidermolytic hyperkeratoses. *Science* **257**, 1128–1130.

Rubin, J.S., Osada, H., Finch, P.W. et al (1989) Purification and characterization of a newly identified growth factor specific for epithelial cells. *Proc. Natl Acad. Sci. USA* **86**, 802–806.

Russell, L.J., DiGiovanna, J.J., Rogers, G.R. et al (1995) Mutations in the gene for transglutaminase 1 in autosomal recessive lamellar ichthyosis. *Nature Genetics* **9**, 279–283.

Sawyer, R.H. (1983) The role of epithelial–mesenchymal interactions in regulating gene expression during avian scale morphogenesis. In *Epithelial–Mesenchymal Interactions in Development* (Eds: R.H. Sawyer and J.F. Fallon), pp. 115–146. Praeger: New York.

Scott, G.A. and Haake, A.R. (1991) Keratinocytes regulate melanocyte number in human fetal and neonatal skin equivalents. *J. Invest. Dermatol.* **97**, 776–781.

Sengel, P. (1976) *Morphogenesis of Skin*. Cambridge University Press: Cambridge.

Solomon, L.M., Cook, B. and Klipfel, W. (1987) The ectodermal dysplasias. *Dermatol. Clinics* **5**, 231–237.

Soprano, D.R., Gyda, M., Jiang, H. et al (1994) A sustained elevation in retinoic acid receptor-β2 mRNA and protein occurs during retinoic acid-induced fetal dysmorphogenesis. *Mech. Dev.* **45**, 243–253.

Spritz, R.A., Ho, L. and Strunk, K.M. (1994) Inhibition of proliferation of human melanocytes by a *KIT* antisense oligodeoxynucleotide: implications for human piebaldism and mouse dominant white spotting (*W*). *J. Invest. Dermatol.* **103**, 148–150.

Stosiek, N., Ulmer, R., von den Driesch, P. et al (1994) Chromosomal mosaicism in two patients with epidermal verrucous nevus. *J. Am. Acad. Dermatol.* **30**, 622–625.

Sun, T.T., Cotsarelis, G. and Lavker, R.M. (1991) Hair follicle stem cells: the bulge-activation hypothesis. *J. Invest. Dermatol.* **96**, Suppl., 77S–78S.

Sundberg, J.P. (1994) *Handbook of Mouse Mutations with Skin and Hair Abnormalities*. CRC Press.: Boca Raton, Florida.

Tassabehji, M., Read, A.P., Newton, V.E. et al (1993) Mutations in the *PAX3* gene causing Waardenburg syndrome type 1 and type 2. *Nature Genetics* **3**, 26–30.

Telfer, N.R. (1991) Congenital and hereditary nail disorders. *Sem. Dermatol.* **10**, 2–6.

Tomita, Y. (1994) The molecular genetics of albinism and piebaldism. *Arch. Dermatol.* **130**, 355–358.

Traupe, H. and Vehring, K.H. (1994) Unstable pre-mutation may explain mosaic disease expression of incontinentia pigmenti in males. *Am. J. Med. Genet.* **49**, 397–398.

Tsipouras, P. and Devereux, R.B. (1993) Marfan syndrome: genetic basis and clinical manifestations. *Sem. Dermatol.* **12**, 219–228.

Tsukurov, O., Boehmer, A., Flynn, J. et al (1994) A complex bilateral polysyndactyly disease locus maps to chromosome 7q36. *Nature Genetics* **6**, 282–286.

Vassar, R. and Fuchs, E. (1991) Transgenic mice provide new insights into the role of TGF-α during epidermal development and differentiation. *Genes Dev.* **5**, 714–727.

Verloes, A., Mulliez, N., Gonzales, M. et al (1992) Restrictive dermopathy, a lethal form of arthrogryposis multiplex with skin and bone dysplasias: three new cases and review of the literature. *Am. J. Med. Genet.* **43**, 539–547.

Viallet, J.P. and Dhouailly, D. (1994) Retinoic acid and mouse skin morphogenesis. I. Expression pattern of retinoic acid receptor genes during hair vibrissa follicle, plantar, and nasal gland development. *J. Invest. Dermatol.* **103**, 116–121.

Viallet, J.P., Ruberte, E., du Manoir, S. et al (1991) Retinoic acid-induced glandular metaplasia in mouse skin is linked to the dermal expression of retinoic acid receptor β mRNA. *Dev. Biol.* **144**, 424–428.

Watt, F.M., Jordan, P.W. and O'Neill, C.H. (1988) Cell shape controls terminal differentation of human epidermal keratinocytes. *Proc. Natl Acad. Sci. USA* **85**, 5576–5580.

Whiting, J., Marshall, H., Cook, M. et al (1991) Multiple spatially specific enhancers are required to reconstruct the pattern of *Hox 2.6* gene expression. *Genes Dev.* **5**, 2048–2059.

Williams, M.L. (1992) Ichthyosis: mechanisms of disease. *Pediatr. Dermatol.* **9**, 365–368.

Wolpert, L. (1994) Do we understand development? *Science* **266**, 571–572.

Wynn, P.C., Maddocks, I.G., Moore, G.P.M. et al (1989) Characterization and localization of receptors for epidermal growth factor in ovine skin. *J. Endocrinol.* **121**, 81–90.

Wysolmerski, J.J., Broadus, A.E., Zhou, J. et al (1994) Over-expression of parathyroid hormone-related protein in the skin of transgenic mice interferes with hair follicle development. *Proc. Natl Acad. Sci. USA* **91**, 1133–1137.

Yeowell, H.N. and Pinnell, S.R. (1993) The Ehlers–Danlos syndromes. In *Seminars in Dermatology: Molecular Biology of the Skin* (Ed.: L.A. Goldsmith), pp. 239–240. W.B. Saunders: Philadelphia, PA.

Zakeri, Z.F. and Ahuja, H.S. (1994) Apoptotic cell death in the limb and its relationship to pattern formation. *Biochem. Cell Biol.* **72**, 603–613.

Zakeri, Z., Quaglino, D. and Ahuja, H.S. (1994) Apoptotic cell death in the mouse limb and its suppression in the *hammertoe* mutant. *Dev. Biol.* **165**, 294–297.

Zheng, Z.-S. and Goldsmith, L.A. (1990) Modulation of epidermal growth factor receptors by retinoic acid in ME180 cells. *Cancer Res.* **50**, 1201–1205.

Zheng, Z.S., Polakowska, R., Johnson, A. and Goldsmith, L.A. (1992) Transcriptional control of epidermal growth factor receptor by retinoic acid. *Cell Growth & Differentiation* **3**, 225–232.

Zonana, J. (1993) Hypohidrotic (anhidrotic) ectodermal dysplasia: molecular genetic research and its clinical applications. In *Seminars in Dermatology: Molecular Biology of the Skin* (Ed.: L.A. Goldsmith). W.B. Saunders: Philadelphia, PA.

13 The Vertebral Column

SUSANNE DIETRICH[1] and MICHAEL KESSEL[2]

[1] Department of Developmental Neurobiology, UMDS Guy's Hospital, London, UK and
[2] Max-Planck-Institut für biophysikalische Chemie, Abteilung Molekulare Zellbiologie, Göttingen, Germany

The vertebral column represents the central, and characteristic, skeletal structure of vertebrates, giving rise to the name of the entire subphylum. Vertebrae confer optimal mechanical features for numerous functions, from flexibility to stabilization to protection. Thus, the replacement of the notochord by the vertebral column can be considered a breakthrough during the evolution of chordates. It is all the more remarkable how severe vertebral malformations are tolerable and compatible with life. Defects include abnormality of intervertebral discs, misshapen, fused, split or transformed vertebrae, but also chaotic vertebral patterns or complete agenesis of the lumbar and caudal part. The spectrum of birth defects affecting the human vertebral column is mostly known from X-ray analyses or from anatomical collections. Some are diagnosed at birth; many become apparent only much later, due to specific dysfunctions; but often irregularities of the vertebral column never cause symptoms, and are only detected by chance. On the other hand, recent progress in prenatal diagnostics allows the detection of vertebral malformations as early as chondrogenesis and initial bone formation. In most cases the cause of vertebral defects is unclear, except for those patients where an inherited syndrome can be recognized, or where a teratogenic insult during pregnancy is documented. Thus, in order to understand congenital defect and to develop appropriate preventive and corrective strategies, an understanding of vertebral column formation during embryogenesis becomes increasingly important.

DEVELOPMENTAL ANATOMY OF THE VERTEBRAL COLUMN

The elucidation of the developmental steps involved in the generation of a structurally normal vertebral column has proceeded steadily since the last century (reviewed by Christ and Wilting, 1992). Significant advances have been achieved using model systems, mainly mice, chicken and frogs, and applying embryological and modern molecular techniques; this has enabled us to identify key players in these complex morphogenetic events. Attention is focused on the early embryo, when the rostrocaudal body axis becomes organized during gastrulation and the events of prevertebrae formation take place.

Embryos, Genes and Birth Defects. Edited by P. Thorogood.
© 1997 John Wiley & Sons Ltd.

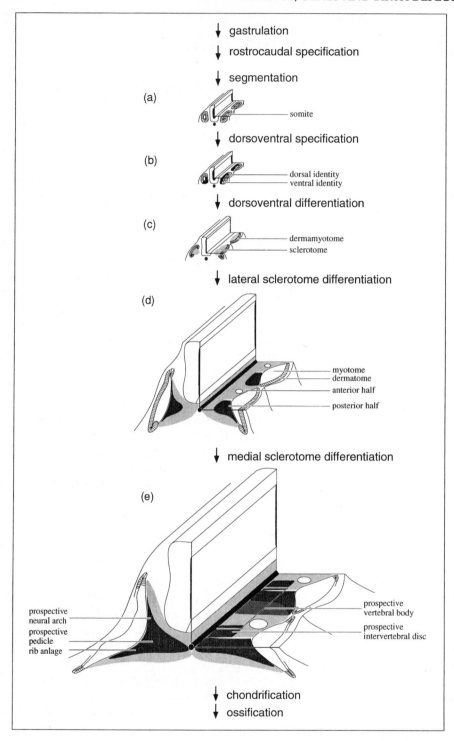

The normal human vertebral column consists of seven cervical, twelve thoracic, five lumbar, five sacral and four or five caudal (coccygeal) vertebrae, each vertebra displaying a unique morphology. While almost all mammals develop seven cervical vertebrae, the overall number, particularly of caudal vertebrae, varies considerably. Within the vertebrate subphylum, the number, shape and articulation of vertebrae differ even more obviously. However, the principles of vertebral column formation are the same in all vertebrate species.

The formation of the rostrocaudal body axis begins with the onset of gastrulation. In higher vertebrates, cells from the epiblast internalize or ingress through the so-called primitive streak, and spread internally to form initially definitive endoderm, and then mesoderm: in particular the midline mesoderm (notochord) and the paraxial mesoderm (reviewed by Stern, 1992). The latter, also called presomitic mesoderm or **segmental plate**, will develop into somites and finally vertebrae. While at its caudal end new cells are constantly added by ingression from the primitive streak, more rostrally presomitic cells increase mutual adhesion and segment as discrete, epithelial spheres called **somites** (Figure 13.1a), each sphere enclosing some mesenchymal cells in its interior – the **somitocoel**. Thus, **somitogenesis** for the first time applies a segmental organization to the rostrocaudal body axis (reviewed by Keynes and Stern, 1988).

Although the somites display a uniform morphology differing only in size, they are not interchangeable: when shifted along the rostrocaudal axis, they develop according to their original axial level. Thus, in classical experiments thoracic somites or presomitic mesoderm transplanted into the cervical region still formed ribs in their new, ectopic location. Such results suggest that the positional information along the rostrocaudal axis is laid down earlier during gastrulation (Chevallier, 1975; Chevallier et al, 1977). Since somite reversal leads to reversed orientation of its descendants, then we can assume that anteroposterior values within a segment are determined very early as well (Aoyoma and Asamoto, 1988).

The **sclerotome**, which provides exclusively vertebral column material, arises upon dorsoventral differentiation of the somite: within each somite, only cells of the ventromedial epithelium and somitocoel (Huang et al, 1994) adopt a sclerotomal fate. They emerge from the somite by de-epithelialization, while the dorsolateral **dermomyotome** destined to give rise to dermis and musculature still retains its epithelial characteristics. Later, **dermatome** and **myotome** (giving rise to smooth muscle of dermis and striated trunk musculature respectively) separate dorsomedially, and myogenic cells leave the dorsolateral sector and colonize the body wall and presumptive limb field (Figure 13.1b,c,d; reviewed by Keynes and Stern, 1988; Töndury and Theiler, 1990; Christ and Wilting, 1992).

In contrast to the specification of the anteroposterior pattern, the dorsoventral values are not intrinsic to the somites: thus, in dorsoventrally rotated somites,

---

Figure 13.1 Development of the vertebral column in mammals and birds. The dark shading in (b) represents the ventrally specified somite sector that gives rise to the sclerotome. The dark shading in (d) and (e) represents the condensed areas of the sclerotome that develop into neural arch, parts of the vertebral body, intervertebral disc and rib anlagen. Note that two somites contribute to a single vertebral body

the sclerotomes still develop in the ventromedial position while the dermomyotomes reside dorsolaterally (Aoyoma and Asamoto, 1988). A dorsally implanted floor plate or notochord represses dermomyotome formation and induces sclerotome formation instead (Pourquié et al, 1993; Goulding et al, 1994). Notochord ablation on the other hand prevents sclerotome formation (e.g. Kitchin, 1949; Teillet and Le Douarin, 1983). Molecular markers that indicate the specification of the ventromedial somite prior to sclerotome formation (Figure 13.1c) do not appear without notochordal activity (e.g. Brand-Saberi et al, 1993; Dietrich et al, 1993). Thus, the dorsoventral values of the paraxial mesoderm depend on the appositional, instructive induction by the notochord.

During sclerotome formation, the morphologically visible segmental borders disappear. However, cells from adjacent somites do not mix (Bagnall et al, 1989), suggesting that the segmental identity is maintained. A morphologically defined segmentation reappears when the sclerotome differentiates. First, cells within the posterior half of the lateral sclerotome accumulate due to accelerated proliferation (Wilting et al, 1994; Figure 13.1d). These cells are destined to form the **neural arch** anlage, while the less cell-dense anterior somite half will promote neural outgrowth, thereby applying a segmental organization to the spinal cord (reviewed by Christ and Wilting, 1992). Slightly later, cell condensation can be observed also in the ventromedial (perichordal) portion of the sclerotome (Figure 13.1e): the lateral band of condensed tissue expands towards the midline. Anteriorly, a new condensation independently arises, encompassing the posterior aspect of the anterior sclerotomal sector. While the densely packed cells will later give rise to the **intervertebral disc**, the anlage of the **vertebral body** is formed by the less cell-dense areas between the intervertebral disc anlagen. However, as the less cell-dense zones expand by relative and absolute means, the developing vertebral bodies are thought to incorporate the borders of the condensed tissue including the ventral neural arch elongation (Figure 13.1e; Gasser, 1979; Dalgleish, 1985; Bagnall and Sanders, 1989). This interpretation is supported by a specific type of birth defect: in the mouse mutant *undulated*, the medial sclerotome condensation is impaired at the lumbosacral level, preventing the formation of intervertebral discs and vertebral bodies (Grüneberg, 1963; Wallin et al, 1994; Dietrich and Gruss, 1995). Note that there is no simple one-to-one ratio between somites and vertebrae: labelling and transplantation experiments of half-somites have repeatedly demonstrated that one somite always contributes to two adjacent vertebral bodies (Bagnall et al, 1989; Bagnall, 1992; Ewan and Everett, 1992; Goldstein and Kalcheim, 1992). The only deviation from this rule are the occipital somites, which do not give rise to discrete vertebrae, but unite to form the base of the skull (e.g. Couly et al, 1993).

After sclerotome condensation, the shape of the future vertebral column is determined: each vertebra is represented by a mesenchymal progenitor or prevertebra. Thus, pattern formation is finished, and the conversion of prevertebrae into cartilage and bone begins. **Chondrogenesis** starts in the prospective vertebral bodies and progresses dorsally and ventrally to encompass neural arch and rib anlagen (Figure 13.2a). The first signs of **ossification** are found in the vertebral body and bilaterally in the neural arches, where chondroclasts remove the hypertrophied cartilage and osteoblasts replace the cartilage by endochondral ossification. Secondarily, further ossification centres appear in the vertebral epiphyses. Finally, the ossification centres unite to form the adult shape of the vertebrae. In humans, most ossification centres within the neural arches unite postnatally within the first year. However, the ossification of sacrum and coccyx continues until the 20–35th year of life.

In summary, the development of the vertebral column during embryogenesis can be subdivided into two phases. In the first, the pattern of the future vertebral column is generated: during gastrulation the rostrocaudal axis is established, and becomes segmented during somitogenesis. Sclerotome formation then establishes the skeletogenic tissue, which differentiates to give rise to the individual vertebral components. In the second phase, continuing even into adulthood, the prevertebrae are progressively converted into cartilage and bone.

CLASSIFICATION OF VERTEBRAL COLUMN DEFECTS

As vertebral column formation is evolutionary conserved, most if not all of the vertebral malformations seen in humans can also be found in other mammals. In fact, almost one century of mouse genetics has led to an impressive collection of vertebral column mutants that probably represents all types of possible vertebral disorders (reviewed by Grüneberg, 1963; Lyon and Searle, 1989). Most of the mouse mutants have originally been identified because of their short or kinky tail phenotype visible after birth, but careful anatomical studies reveal primary defects during embryogenesis that similarly affect the trunk (Table 13.1).

Table 13.1 Classification of vertebral column defects, murine mutants and involved genes

Process	Phenotype	Murine mutant	Gene
Gastrulation	Complex phenotype including vertebral agenesis	*Brachyury curtailed*	*T*
Dorsoventral specification	Vertebral agenesis	*truncate* *Danforth's short tail* *Pintail* $shh^{-/-}$	? ? ? *shh*
Somitogenesis	Half- and block vertebrae	*pudgy*	?
Sclerotome condensation	Agenesis or malformation of corresponding elements	*undulated*	*Pax-1*
Neural tube closure	Agenesis of dorsal neural arch	*Splotch*	*Pax-3*
Axial specification	Homeotic transformation	*rachiterata* Hox mutants	? Hox genes
Mesenchyme condensation, bone fracture repair	Complex phenotype	*short ear*	*Bmp-5*

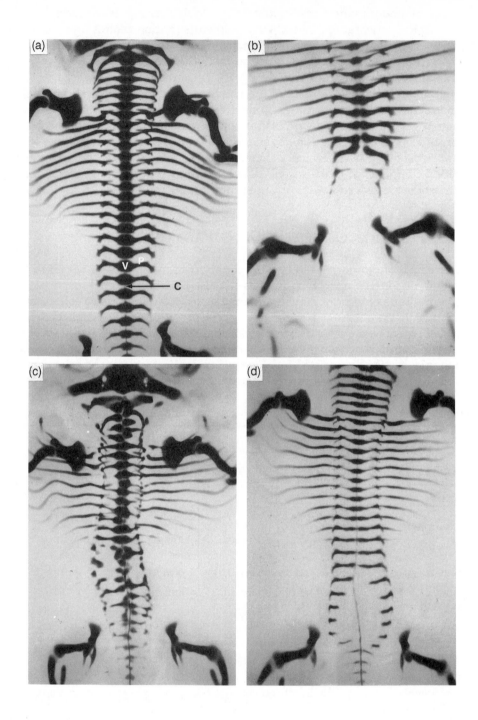

In many of these murine mutants, vertebral malformations can be traced back to the prechondral phase of vertebral column formation, indicating that early patterning events are compromised. In general, the earlier development deviates from normal, the more severe will be the effect on the phenotype. Thus, disorders of gastrulation that disrupt the normal allocation of cells to the mesodermal germ layer will block vertebral column formation. However, as all three germ layers are generated during this process, these animals usually develop more complex phenotypes: for instance, in homozygous *Brachyury* (*T*/*T*) embryos and embryos obtained from *T*/*T* embryonic stem cells, nascent mesodermal cells fail to leave the primitive streak and gastrulation comes to a halt (Beddington et al 1992). In the allele *curtailed* (T^c/T^c), the embryos rostrally fail to develop a notochord, externally visible somites or a closed neural tube (Searle, 1966). Due to the defective mesodermal pattern, molecular markers of sclerotome induction appear only in small, disorganized patches (Dietrich et al, 1993), and regions caudal to the level of the forelimbs are not formed at all (Searle, 1966). Since the embryos also lack an allantois, they fail to establish a proper placental relationship with the maternal blood circulation and do not survive beyond mid-gestation.

In contrast, **vertebral agenesis** caused by disorders during sclerotome formation may be compatible with life, as typically only parts of the rostrocaudal axis are affected. However, severe truncation of the vertebral column often coincides with urogenital defects and atresia ani, and the animals do not survive postnatally. Since sclerotome formation depends on the inductive activity of the notochord, it is mainly notochord mutants that are found within this category (reviewed by Grüneberg, 1963). In animals heterozygous for the *Brachyury curtailed* mutation (T^c/+), the tail somites are present while neither the caudal notochord nor neural tube develops (Searle, 1966). Molecular markers that indicate induction of the sclerotomal pathway within the somites are never activated, even when the ventral paraxial mesoderm appears mesenchymal and hence sclerotome-like (Dietrich et al, 1993). Instead, markers specific for dermomyotome remain expressed throughout the somite. Being misspecified, these cells degenerate, and no caudal vertebral column is formed, leading to essentially tail-less animals (Searle, 1966). This phenomenon, however, is not restricted to the caudal extreme of the body. In *truncate* (*tc*/*tc*) mice, notochord formation may terminate at any axial position. In the affected region, somite ventralization is hindered, and the corresponding vertebrae appear to be deleted

---

Figure 13.2 Vertebral columns of murine wildtype and mutant embryos. Skeletons of mouse embryos at day 13.5 post-coitum. Stained for cartilage with Alcian blue. (See also Table 13.1.) (a) Wild-type animal. The ventral half of the vertebral column is already preformed in cartilage. Vertebral body (V), pedicle of the neural arch (P) and notochord (c) are indicated. (b) Homozygous *Danforth's short tail* mouse. In the posterior body regions, the notochord degeneration prevents the dorsoventral specification of the somites and hence the formation of vertebrae. (c) In *pudgy* homozygotes, defective somitogenesis leads to a disorganized array of half- and block vertebrae. (d) In *undulated extensive* homozygotes, the retarded lumbosacral sclerotome condensation prevents the formation of complete vertebral bodies

(Theiler, 1959; Dietrich et al, 1993). Premature termination of the vertebral column is also typical of mouse mutants in which the notochord is formed but subsequently degenerates. In *Danforth's short tail* (*Sd/Sd*) mice, this process lasts about 4 days until the dissolution of the notochord is complete (Gluecksohn-Schoenheimer, 1945; Paavola et al, 1980). In rostral regions where the notochord degeneration takes place after the dorsoventral patterning, development of the vertebral column appears unaltered. However, caudally, the notochord is lost even before somitogenesis, completely preventing somite ventralization and vertebral column formation. In the lumbar region, the disintegrating notochord encounters differentiating somites. At these levels the ventralized tissues again become dorsalized, and express dermomyotomal markers at the expense of sclerotomal, demonstrating once again that the notochord is required also to maintain the dorsoventral specification of the paraxial mesoderm (Gluecksohn-Schoenheimer, 1945; Dietrich et al, 1993; Koseki et al, 1993). The more complete the notochordal resorption, the more vertebral components fail to develop (Figure 13.2b). Thus, in *Pintail* (*Pt/Pt*) mice, where the notochord slowly disappears due to low mitotic rates, the sclerotome and vertebral column develop both in the trunk and the upper caudal region. Here, only the formation of the nuclei pulposi is compromised, leading to accelerated ageing of the intervertebral discs (Berry, 1960; Dietrich et al, 1993).

While disorders of gastrulation and, more specifically of sclerotome formation, lead to absence, truncation or interruption of the vertebral column, disorders of somitogenesis are compatible with sclerotome, and hence vertebral column, development. However, multiple vertebral column components can be lacking or fused, along the entire rostrocaudal axis leading to **half-** and **'block' vertebrae**, together with various dyssymphyses. In *pudgy* (*pu/pu*) mice only a rudimentary segmentation takes place: somites appear late, irregularly shaped and improperly separated (reviewed by Grüneberg, 1963). Sclerotomal markers that usually show a segmented pattern are expressed in broad stripes laterally flanking notochord and neural tube. Some latent segmentation can be detected, when the sclerotome differentiates. However, the anlagen of the vertebral components, and similarly the expression domains of relevant molecular markers, remain improperly delineated, fused or lacking, thus anticipating the chaotic state of the chondral and bony vertebral column (Grüneberg, 1963; S. Dietrich and P. Gruss, unpublished observations; Figure 13.2c). This phenotype suggests that somitogenesis is an intrinsic programme of the paraxial mesoderm which, independent from dorsoventral pattern specification, defines segmental borders and establishes anteroposterior values within a segment, both of which are crucial for the delimitation of individual vertebrae.

In contrast to those disorders of segmentation that cause multiple malformations of all vertebral elements, specific vertebral column components can be lacking or malformed, when the sclerotome condensation is compromised. A delay of this process has been observed, for example, in the allelic series of undulated mutants, *undulated* (*un*), *undulated extensive* (*un^{ex}*) and *undulated short tail* (*un^{s}*). In these animals, the ventromedial condensations are particularly retarded. At lumbosacral levels, they appear with a developmental delay of about 2 days, and never reach normal size and shape. As a consequence, both intervertebral discs and vertebral bodies fail to develop (Figure 13.2d; Grüneberg, 1963; Wallin et al, 1994, Dietrich and Gruss, 1995). Where somites and vertebrae are smaller, the sclerotomal condensations may reach the critical threshold and chondrify, leading to reduced vertebral bodies.

Disorders of the dorsal vertebral column components frequently coincide with **neural tube defects** (see Chapter 8): the mutant *Splotch* (*Sp/Sp*) is characterized by a lumbosacral spina bifida and neural overgrowth. In the affected region the neural arches fail to meet dorsally and, instead, fuse with the adjacent rudiments (Auerbach, 1954), suggesting that an open neural tube provides a barrier for the sclerotomal cells to reach the dorsal midline. However, there are reports that neural crest cells, which do not develop normally in these mice, contribute to the spinous processes in wild-type embryos (Takahashi et al, 1992). Thus, the neural tube defects may directly interfere with vertebral column formation.

The birth defects described so far are characterized by the agenesis of vertebrae or vertebral elements. These defects result from disturbed patterning processes that usually take place along the entire rostrocaudal axis. However, in all vertebrates the anatomy of individual vertebrae exactly correlates with their axial position. Mis-specification of the axial identity therefore leads to **homeotic transformations**: all vertebral components develop, but with shape characteristic of another, usually adjacent, vertebra. For instance, *rachiterata* (*rh/rh*) mice show a transformation of the last cervical vertebra into a thoracic type, thereby generating 14 pairs of ribs (Theiler et al, 1974). However, the *rh* mutation may not only affect the axial specification; somitogenesis is also disturbed, leading to irregularly shaped somites. As a consequence, malformed and fused vertebrae develop, although to a lesser extent than in *pudgy* mice. In contrast, homeotic transformations alone have been obtained by modulating the function of Hox genes, and this will be discussed subsequently.

While disorders in pattern formation result in specific prevertebral phenotypes, general disorders of metabolism, mesenchyme condensation, cartilage and bone formation affect the composition, and therefore secondarily the morphology, of the skeleton including the vertebral column. In the mouse mutant *short ear* (*se/se*), which is a mutation of the *Bmp-5* gene, the formation of many of the mesenchymal skeletal anlagen is retarded, leading to reduction or elimination of various skeletal elements in the axial and appendicular skeleton. In these mice, bone fractures are repaired with delay, illustrating the role of the gene for both skeletal growth and maintenance (Kingsley, 1994).

GENES INVOLVED IN VERTEBRAL COLUMN DEVELOPMENT

The classical approach to studying development on a molecular level starts with the recognition of a mutant phenotype and tries to proceed to the responsible gene. Although some successful examples are available for mice, e.g. the *Brachyury* or *T* gene (Herrmann et al, 1990), this approach is by no means standard. Thus, while murine mutants had been helpful to analyse the cell biology of vertebral column development, they mostly failed to reveal the underlying genes. Genetic approaches, however, have been successfully applied to isolate developmental control genes from *Drosophila melanogaster* (Ingham, 1988). By screening genomic or cDNA libraries from vertebrates with probes obtained from such *Drosophila* genes, the vertebrate homologues were identified (reviewed by Kessel and Gruss, 1990). This was possible as small regions of the fly genes encoding functional units like DNA-binding domains are highly conserved within the animal kingdom. Evidence is increasing that these basic molecular functions have been 'invented' only a few times, and evolutionary pressure has led to a modular use of these existing elements rather than the formation of new ones (see Chapter 1).

Among the genes isolated by cross-species hybridization, many were found to be expressed during development, some in the prevertebral column. To study their function, mutants have been generated by transgenic techniques, especially by ectopic expression or inactivation via homologous recombination, techniques that are discussed elsewhere in this volume (see Chapter 4). However, not all of these passed the test of reverse genetics: alteration or abolition of expression does not necessarily result in an altered vertebral morphology. Functional redundancy or feedback control by regulatory networks may play more important roles in higher animals than previously thought. Nevertheless, in some instances the application of reversed genetics did generate birth defects of the vertebral column and these examples will be briefly reviewed.

HOX GENES: THE CONTROL OF ROSTROCAUDAL SPECIFICATION

A particularly useful element for the isolation of developmental control genes proved to be the **homeobox**, a 183-bp DNA sequence that encodes a DNA-binding domain as part of a 'homeo protein' (McGinnis et al, 1984; Scott and Weiner, 1984). In vertebrates like mice and humans, more than 100 homeobox-containing genes are present, possibly up to 1000 (Kappen et al, 1993; Schubert et al, 1993). Many of them seem to play multiple roles in processes of pattern formation and cell specification (reviewed by Stein et al, 1996).

A subgroup of this gene family are the **Hox genes**, in vertebrates consisting of 39 highly conserved genes, located in four gene clusters on different chromosomes, the Hox A, B, C and D clusters (reviewed McGinnis and Krumlauf, 1992; Zeltser et al, 1996). Hox genes are expressed in cells of mesodermal and ectodermal origin along the body axis. Distinct anterior boundaries of expression are characteristic for each gene, defining the beginning of a caudally extending expression domain. Genes from more 5' locations in the Hox clusters are expressed earlier and, with the exception of the second genes of a cluster, always occupy more anterior expression domains. Thus, a temporal and structural co-linearity exists between the position of a gene in a cluster and its expression pattern. The expression patterns of Hox genes in the paraxial mesoderm, mostly in prevertebrae, are summarized from many separate publications in Figure 13.3 (Kessel, 1992). The specific combination of Hox genes expressed in a paraxial

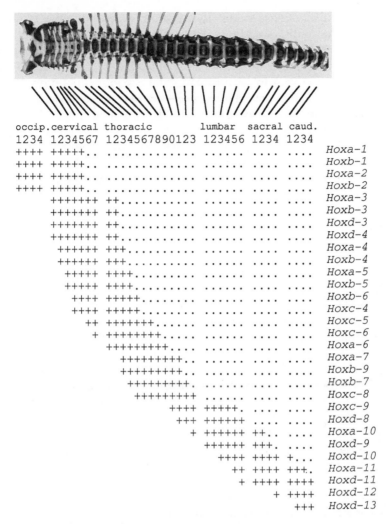

Figure 13.3 Prevertebral Hox codes. The vertebral column of a newborn mouse is displayed horizontally at the top; rostral/anterior is to the left. Expression domains of specific Hox genes are indicated by a horizontal series of plus signs. Note, that anterior boundaries of expression are significant, while the posterior boundaries are much less well defined. A vertically aligned series of plus signs indicates the combination of expressed Hox genes characteristic for one prevertebra, i.e. its Hox code. References for the original in-situ analyses can be found in Kessel and Gruss (1991) and Kessel (1992)

segment has been defined as its 'Hox code' (Kessel and Gruss, 1991; and see Chapters 7 and 10 for details of Hox codes in other organ systems). Evidence is accumulating that a specific Hox code is indeed involved in the rostrocaudal specification of a mesodermal segment and in the determination of vertebral identities, and becomes translated into a specific vertebral anatomy (reviewed by Haack and Kessel, 1994).

The first line of evidence came from ectopic expression studies. Transgenic mice were created with an additional *Hoxa-7* gene driven by an actin promoter (Balling et al, 1989; Kessel et al, 1990). They ubiquitously expressed the transgene and, with respect to the rostrocaudal axis, *Hoxa-7* was thereby activated earlier and, significantly, rostral to its normal expression domain (Figure 13.3). As a consequence, the craniocervical axial skeleton developed posterior properties: instead of contributing to the base of the skull, the last occipital somites gave rise to a vertebra, a 'pro-atlas' (Figure 13.4 a,b). Moreover, the first cervical vertebra, the atlas, formed a vertebral body, while in wild-type mice this material associates with the second vertebra to form the dens axis. The observed mutant phenotype constituted a **posterior transformation**, in that one metameric unit or segment, had assumed the 'identity' of another, in this experiment a more posterior segment. Meanwhile, similar actin–Hox constructs were used to study *Hoxb-7*, the paralogous gene of *Hoxa-7*, and *Hoxb-6* (McLain et al, 1992). A strikingly similar phenotype was observed and may indicate functional overlap of these highly conserved proteins (McLain et al, 1992).

A more restricted mis-expression using a *Hoxa-1* promoter driving the *Hoxd-4* gene was described by Lufkin et al (1992). As expected from the normal *Hoxa-1* pattern, the transgenic mice had extended the *Hoxd-4* expression domain rostrally into the occipital region. While the first cervical vertebra, the atlas, which normally expresses *Hoxa-4*, appeared normal, the directly adjacent exoccipital bone was split into two or more bony structures, equivalent to extra neural arches.

While a rostrally expanded expression domain causes posterior transformation, the prolonged caudal expression of Hox genes may result in **anterior transformations**. When multiple copies of the *Hoxc-6* gene controlled by its own promoter were introduced into mice, only the anterior boundary of expression was maintained (Jegalian and De Robertis, 1992). Thus, a gene typical for the thoracic region was active in lumbar prevertebrae, leading to an additional, 14th rib. Similarly, a lumbar rib was obtained by expanding the *Hoxc-8* expression domain using the *Hoxa-4* promoter (Pollock, 1992).

The second line of evidence supporting the concept of a 'Hox-code' underlying the specification of vertebral phenotype was obtained by inactivation of Hox genes via homologous recombination, leading to deficiencies or anterior transformations. Inactivation of the *Hoxa-1* gene resulted in a deformation of the basioccipital bone, the somite derivative rostral to the vertebral column (Lufkin et al, 1991; Chisaka et al, 1992). Mice lacking a functional *Hoxb-4* gene showed an anterior homeotic transformation of the axis, which now resembled the atlas both with respect to a broad neural arch and an anterior tubercle (Ramirez-Solis, 1993). Associated with its vertebral body was, however, still the typical body of the dens axis. Note that the Hox code for C2 generated in *Hoxb-4* null mutants predicts exactly a chimera between C1 and C2 (Figure 13.3). Furthermore, inactivation of the *Hoxc-8* gene caused homeotic transformations of the eighth thoracic vertebra (sternal rib) and of the first lumbar (14th rib) (Le Mouellic et al, 1992).

However, not all inactivation experiments resulted in an altered vertebral identity. Null mutants of the *Hoxa-3* gene lacked a skeletal phenotype, although the gene is normally expressed in the atlas anlage and more caudal vertebrae (Chisaka and Capecchi, 1991). Nevertheless, this mutant was strongly affected in those neural crest derivatives corresponding to the anterior expression domain in the neuroectoderm. A paralogous gene of *Hoxa-3*, *Hoxd-3*, displays a similar expression pattern, but here inactivation resulted in a significant vertebral phenotype. Atlas and axis underwent anterior transformations (Condie and Capecchi, 1993). Generation of homozygous *Hoxa-3/Hoxd-3* double-mutants indicated a synergistic interaction of the two genes: these mutants did not generate an atlas at all (Condie and Capecchi, 1994). Thus, even if the inactivation of *Hoxa-3* alone did not reveal an essential function in atlas specification, the double knockout supports the idea of Hox genes specifying axial positions in a combinatorial manner.

RETINOIC ACID AND RETINOIC-ACID BINDING PROTEINS: REGULATORS OF HOX GENE EXPRESSION

Retinoic acid (RA) is well known as a potent teratogen, influencing in particular the correct formation of embryonic patterns, in both animals and humans (Lammer et al, 1985) (see Chapter 5). Exposure of embryos leads to a wide spectrum of defects including spina bifida, and craniofacial and vertebral malformations, depending on duration, dose and embryonic stage. On the other hand, RA and other retinoids, as well as the RA binding proteins and receptors, are present in embryos throughout post-implantation embryogenesis, suggesting that RA intoxication interferes with its normal function as a signal molecule (see also Chapter 7).

Upon RA application, the expression patterns of Hox genes appear to be specifically altered. In tissue culture systems they are sequentially activated following the 3' to 5' order on the chromosome (Simeone et al, 1990). The 3' genes require the lowest concentration and are the first to be activated. In contrast, some 5' genes cannot be activated by RA or may even be down-regulated. Experiments with frog embryos, with chick embryos in culture or with mouse embryos in utero, have recently indicated that RA similarly influences Hox gene expression in vivo, leading to specific morphological changes (Sive et al, 1990; Kessel and Gruss, 1991; Kessel, 1992, 1993; Sundin and Eichele, 1992).

The effect of RA on the development of the vertebral column was systematically studied in mice, and correlated with changes of the Hox code (Kessel and Gruss, 1991; Kessel, 1992). The type and axial level of the vertebral alterations depended on the timepoint of RA application. The most anterior effect was seen after exposure at mid-gastrulation, briefly before the primitive streak has reached the tip of the egg cylinder: the embryos activated their Hox genes earlier, and with respect to the normal rostrocaudal axis, more rostrally. Thus, in contrast to the mis-expression studies, the entire set of Hox genes was involved, leading to an anterior shift of all the positional values along the rostrocaudal axis. Consequently, posterior homeotic transformations were found throughout the vertebral column, encompassing the destruction of the basisphenoid bone,

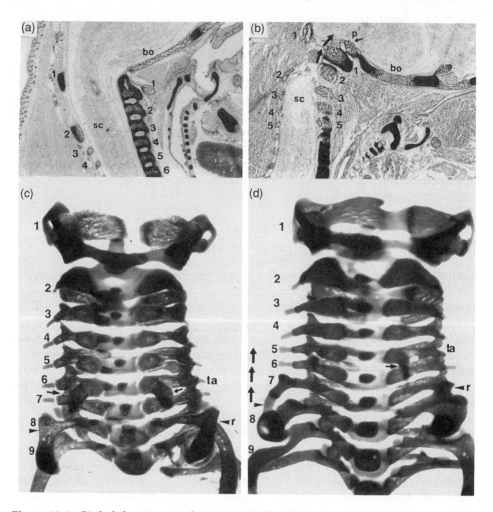

Figure 13.4 Birth defects in mice due to misregulated Hox genes.

(a,b) Sagittal sections of a newborn wild-type mouse (a), or of a transgenic mouse ectopically expressing the *Hoxa-7* gene (b) (Kessel et al, 1990; and see text). Ventral (right) and dorsal (left) parts of cervical vertebrae are numbered; bo, basioccipital bone. (a) Note the absence of a vertebral body from the atlas (1), the corresponding vertebral body (body of the dens axis, d) is associated with the second vertebra, the axis (2). (b) Two posterior homeotic transformations (arrows) have occurred at the craniocervical transition. Note association of the atlas with a vertebral body; therefore there is no formation of a dens axis. The formation of an additional vertebral body, a pro-atlas (p), is associated with the basioccipital bone (bo), at the base of the skull.

(c,d) Cervical vertebral columns from a newborn wild-type mouse (c) and from a mouse that had been exposed to retinoic acid (RA) during embryogenesis (d) (Kessel, 1992; and see text). (c) Note the presence of tuberculi anterior (ta, arrow) on vertebra 6, and the presence of the first rib (r, arrowhead) on vertebra 8 in the wild-type column. (d) Vertebral identities are homeotically transformed at the cervicothoracic transition (vertical arrows). Note the presence of a tuberculum anterior (ta, arrow) on vertebra 5, and the first rib (r, arrowhead) on vertebra 7 after RA exposure.

the partial formation of a pro-atlas, generation of tuberculi anterior on the fifth vertebra, cervical ribs on C6, and a rostral shift of the sacrum (Figure 13.4c,d).

If mouse embryos were exposed one day later (day 8.5 post-coitum), their body axis had properly formed up to the mid-thorax. RA exposure now led to anterior transformations, detectable within or caudal from the mid-thoracic region. They included the formation of eight sternal ribs, a total of 14–15 ribs and a posterior shift of the sacral bone. In-situ analysis revealed a delayed activation of 5' Hox genes, and their expression domains were shifted caudally. Higher RA doses even inhibited the expression of 5' Hox genes. In this case, agenesis of the vertebral column, beginning from the axial level specified at the time of RA exposure, was observed (Kessel and Gruss, 1991; Kessel, 1992).

The establishment of the intricate Hox gene expression patterns requires additional genes that function as mediators of the RA signal. In recent years, three **retinoic acid receptor** (RAR) genes, *RAR-α*, *-β* and *-γ*, were isolated, which bind to transcriptionally regulatory sites of genes, including the Hox genes (Langston and Gudas, 1992; Leid et al, 1992). While *RAR-α* is expressed ubiquitously in post-implantation mouse embryos, the γ-receptor seems to be restricted to structures developing into bones, i.e. the anlagen for the vertebral column, the skull and the limbs (Ruberte et al, 1990, 1991). Inactivation of the *RAR-γ* gene resulted in anterior homeotic transformations of vertebrae, including a partial axis to atlas conversion, and a C7 to C6 transformation (Lohnes et al, 1993). Furthermore, these mutants were resistant to the teratogenic effects of high RA doses during gastrulation. These findings demonstrate the importance of a complex molecular machinery underlying the specification of the rostrocaudal body axis.

EVOLUTIONARY CONSERVED REGULATORS OF HOX GENES: LESSONS FROM *POLYCOMB* GROUP AND *CAUDAL* GENES

In *Drosophila*, the active and repressed state of Hox genes is maintained by members of the *trithorax* group and the *polycomb* group (reviewed by Paro, 1990). Murine cognates of the *polycomb* group genes *posterior sex combs* and *suppressor two of zeste*, the proto-oncogene *bmi-1* and the tumour suppressor gene *mel-18* have been isolated, all of them containing the putative DNA binding RING-finger domain (Tagawa et al, 1990; Freemont et al, 1991; van Lohuizen et al, 1991). Transrepression of Hox genes via direct DNA binding has been demonstrated for *mel-18* as well as *Drosophila polycomb* group proteins (Kanno et al, 1995; Müller, 1995). As expected from the phenotypes displayed by flies lacking functional *polycomb* group genes, murine loss-of-function mutants for both *mel-18* and *bmi-1* similarly exhibit posterior transformation of vertebrae along the entire axis, concomitant with an anterior extension of Hox gene expression domains (Simon et al, 1992; van der Lugt et al, 1994; Akasaka et al, 1996). The opposite phenotype is observed when *bmi-1* is over-expressed, resulting in a dose-dependent anterior transformation of vertebrae and the posterior shift of the anterior expression boundary of *Hoxc-5* (Alkema et al, 1995). These findings suggest a conserved structure and function of *polycomb* group genes, acting as transcriptional repressor of Hox genes both in insects and vertebrates.

Further evidence for a conserved regulatory network controlling segment identity is derived from functional analyses of *caudal* genes. The *Drosophila* homeobox gene *caudal* is a determinant for the posterior pole of the fly embryo (Macdonald and Struhl, 1986). Mutation in the *C. elegans caudal* homologue *ceh-3* leads to an anterior homeotic transformation via misregulation of the Hox gene *mab-5* (Kenyon, 1986). Similarly, targeted disruption of the mouse *caudal* homologue *Cdx-1* results in a posterior shift of the expression domains of *Hoxd-3, Hoxc-5, Hoxc-6, Hoxa-7* and *Hoxc-8*, and the anterior homeotic transformation of vertebrae (Subramanian et al, 1995). In the control region of mouse Hox genes, putative *Cdx-1* binding sites have been identified. In vitro, the gene is able to transactivate *Hoxa-7*, suggesting that in contrast to *polycomb* group genes *caudal* homologues act as activators of Hox genes specifying segment identity.

SONIC HEDGEHOG: CONTROL OF DORSOVENTRAL SPECIFICATION

While the role of Hox genes in the establishment of positional information along the rostrocaudal axis is quite well understood, we know much less about the processes that lead to prevertebrae formation. However, many laboratories are searching for signalling molecules that are released from the notochord to ventralize the neural tube and somite, thereby inducing sclerotome formation. One candidate is the **sonic hedgehog** protein, a potentially secreted factor that initially has been identified by a cross-species approach using parts of the *Drosophila hedgehog* gene as a probe. In vertebrates, besides other expression domains, the gene is active both in the notochord and the floor plate of the neural tube (see Chapter 8) and, when ectopically expressed, enhances sclerotome formation and retards the formation of the dermomyotome (Echelard et al, 1993; Krauss et al, 1993; Riddle et al, 1993; Fan and Tessier-Lavigne, 1994; Johnson et al, 1994; Roelink et al, 1994). However, mice carrying a targeted disruption of the *shh* gene still express the sclerotomal marker *Pax-1* at low levels, and some lateral sclerotomal derivatives such as ribs are formed (Chiang et al, 1996). This suggests that additional factors released by the notochord and floor plate contribute to the induction of sclerotome formation.

PAX GENES: CONTROL OF SCLEROTOME CONDENSATION

The nine **Pax** genes belonging to the paired box containing gene family have been identified by homology screens, using the *Drosophila* gene *gooseberry* as a probe (Deutsch et al, 1988; Wallin et al, 1993). Like the homeobox, the paired box encodes a DNA-binding domain, and some Pax genes possess a homeobox in addition. While most of these genes show a predominant expression within the CNS (reviewed by Tremblay et al, 1995), the *Pax-1* gene is active during sclerotome formation and differentiation. Upon somite ventralization, transcription starts within the ventromedial sector of the somite, persisting in the sclerotome after de-epithelialization; the signal enhances when the lateral sclerotome condenses to form the neural arch anlage. Similarly, elevated levels of *Pax-1* expression are found during medial sclerotome condensation; the gene is repressed again when chondrogenesis begins (Deutsch et al, 1988; Dietrich et al, 1993; Wallin et al, 1994; Dietrich and Gruss, 1995).

Based on chromosomal co-localization, *Pax-1* was identified as the affected gene in the murine mutant *undulated*, of which three alleles had been independently isolated, all exhibiting *Pax-1* mutations (Balling et al, 1988; Dietrich and Gruss, 1995). In all alleles, the loss of vertebral components, in particular of vertebral bodies and intervertebral discs, could be traced back to delayed sclerotome condensation, suggesting that this process is a *Pax-1*-dependent, intrinsic programme of the sclerotome. However, as additional sclerotome mutants become available, *Pax-1* might not be the only factor governing sclerotome condensation. In addition, as with many other vertebrate regulatory genes, a paralogue, *Pax-9*, is present in the genome and may provide redundant information or act in concert with *Pax-1* (Wallin et al, 1993). Therefore, it will be of interest to study double-mutant mice that lack both of these structurally highly related genes.

MSX GENES: MEDIATORS OF NEURAL TUBE–VERTEBRAL COLUMN INTERACTION?

As in several mouse mutants the dorsal dyssymphysis of the neural arches results from, or at least coincides with, neural tube defects, increasing attention is focused on the role of the neuroectoderm during vertebral column formation. The *Msx-2* homeobox gene (formerly Hox-8) has been found to be preferentially expressed in dorsal structures, including the roof plate of the neural tube, its overlying ectoderm and the intervening mesenchyme. In the trunk this mesenchyme forms the dorsal-most part of the neural arch, the spinous process (Takahashi and Le Douarin, 1990; Takahashi et al, 1992). Ectopic expression of *Msx-2* induced ectopic cartilage, and no spinous process formed in the absence of *Msx-2* expression. Thus, the gene appears to be involved in the patterning of vertebrae, dependent on a cascade of tissue interactions between the dorsal neural tube and overlying ectoderm.

AN AGENDA FOR THE FUTURE

Anatomical studies, embryological techniques and molecular analyses have produced significant insights into the development of both normal and pathological vertebral columns. In particular, the mechanisms leading to the specification of the rostrocaudal axis are already quite well understood. On the other hand, our knowledge about the formation of the mesenchymal vertebral anlagen is mainly descriptive. Only a few candidate genes that may regulate these processes have been identified, although the number of mouse mutants showing disorders during this phase of vertebral column formation suggests that a variety of genes are required to control these processes. However, it can be expected that the integrated application of old and new techniques will generate novel approaches to identifying these developmental control genes. Missing components of the regulatory network underlying vertebral column formation are likely be identified and this will allow us to understand more fully the development of the axial skeleton at the genetic level.

REFERENCES

Akasaka, T., Kanno, M., Balling, R. et al (1996) The role for *mel-18*, a *Polycomb* group-related vertebrate gene, during the anteroposterior specification of the axial skeleton. *Development* **122**, 1513–1522.

Alkema, M.J., van der Lugt, N.M., Bobeldijk, R.C., Berns, A. and van Lohuizen, M. (1995) Transformation of axial skeleton due to overexpression of *bmi-1* in transgenic mice. *Nature* **374**, 724–727.

Aoyoma, H. and Asamoto, K. (1988) Determination of somite cells: independence of cell differentiation and morphogenesis. *Development* **104**, 15–28.

Auerbach, R. (1954) Analysis of the developmental effects of a lethal mutation in the house mouse. *J. Exp. Zool.* **127**, 305–329.

Bagnall, K.M. (1992) The migration and distribution of somite cells after labelling with the carbocyanine dye, DiI: the relationship of this distribution to segmentation in the vertebrate body. *Anat. Embryol.* **185**, 317–324.

Bagnall, K.M. and Sanders, E.J. (1989) The binding pattern of peanut lectin associated with sclerotome migration and the formation of the vertebral axis in the chick embryo. *Anat. Embryol.* **180**, 505–513.

Bagnall, K.M., Higgins, S. and Sanders, E.J. (1989) The contribution made by cells from a single somite to tissues within a body segment and assessment of their integration with similar cells from adjacent segments. *Development* **107**, 931–943.

Balling, R., Deutsch, U. and Gruss, P. (1988) *Undulated*, a mutation affecting the development of the mouse skeleton, has a point mutation in the paired box of *Pax-1*. *Cell* **55**, 531–535.

Balling, R., Mutter, G., Gruss, P. and Kessel, M. (1989) Craniofacial abnormalities induced by ectopic expression of the homeobox gene *Hox-1.1* in transgenic mice. *Cell* **58**, 337–347.

Beddington, R.S.P., Rashbass, P. and Wilson, V. (1992) *Brachyury* – a gene affecting mouse gastrulation and early organogenesis. *Development* Suppl., **16**, 157–165.

Berry, R.J. (1960) Genetic studies on the skeleton of the mouse. XXVI. *Pintail*. *Genet. Res.* **1**, 439–451.

Brand-Saberi, B., Ebensperger, C., Wilting, J., Balling, R. and Christ, B. (1993) The ventralizing effect of the notochord on somite differentiation in chick embryos. *Anat. Embryol.* **188**, 239–245.

Chevallier, A. (1975) Role du mesoderme somitique dans le developpement de la cage thoracique de l'embryon d'oiseau. *J. Embryol. Exp. Morphol.* **33**, 291–311.

Chevallier, A., Kieny, M., Mauger, A. and Sengel, P. (1977) Developmental fate of the somitic mesoderm in the chick embryo. In *Vertebrate Limb and Somite Morphogenesis* (Eds: D.A. Ede, J.R. Hinchliffe and M. Balls), pp. 421–432. Cambridge University Press: Cambridge.

Chiang, C., Litingtung, Y., Lee, E. et al (1996) Cyclopia and defective axial patterning in mice lacking *Sonic hedgehog* gene function. *Nature* **383**, 407–413.

Chisaka, O. and Capecchi, M.R. (1991) Regionally restricted developmental defects resulting from targeted disruption of the mouse homeobox gene *hox-1.5*. *Nature* **350**, 473–479.

Chisaka, O., Musci, T.S. and Capeccchi, M.R. (1992) Developmental defects of the ear, cranial nerves and hindbrain resulting from targeted disruption of the mouse homeobox gene *Hox-1.6*. *Nature* **355**, 516–520.

Christ, B. and Wilting, J. (1992) From somites to vertebral column. *Ann. Anat.* **174**, 23–32.

Condie, B.G. and Capecchi, M.R. (1993) Mice homozygous for a targeted disruption of *Hoxd-3* (Hox-4.1) exhibit anterior transformations of the first and second cervical vertebrae, the atlas and axis. *Development* **119**, 579–595.

Condie, B.G. and Capecchi, M.R. (1994) Mice with targeted disruptions in the paralogous genes of *hoxa-3* and *hoxd-3* reveal synergistic interactions. *Nature* **370**, 304–307.

Couly, G.F., Coltey, P.M. and Le Douarin, N.M. (1993) The triple origin of the skull in higher vertebrates: a study in quail–chick chimeras. *Development* **117**, 409–429.

Dalgleish, A.E. (1985) A study of the development of thoracic vertebrae in the mouse assisted by autoradiography. *Acta Anat.* **122**, 91–98.

Deutsch, U., Dressler, G.R. and Gruss, P. (1988) *Pax-1*, a member of a paired box homologous murine gene family, is expressed in segmented structures during development. *Cell* **53**, 617–625.

Dietrich, S. and Gruss, P. (1995) Undulated phenotypes suggest a role of *Pax-1* for the development of vertebral and extravertebral structures. *Dev. Biol.* **167**, 529–548.

Dietrich, S., Schubert, F.R. and Gruss, P. (1993) Altered Pax gene expression in notochord mutants of the mouse: the notochord is required for the dorsoventral patterning of the somite. *Mech. Dev.* **44**, 189–207.

Echelard, Y., Epstein, D.J., St-Jacques, B. et al (1993) Sonic hedgehog, a member of a family of putative signaling moleules, is implicated in the regulation of CNS polarity. *Cell* **75**, 1417–1430.

Ewan, K.B.R. and Everett, A.W. (1992) Evidence for resegmentation in the formation of the vertebral column using the novel approach of retroviral-mediated gene transfer. *Exp. Cell Res.* **198**, 315–320.

Fan, C.-M. and Tessier-Lavigne, M. (1994) Patterning of mammalian somites by surface ectoderm and notochord: evidence for sclerotome induction by a *hedgehog* homolog. *Cell* **79**, 1175–1186.

Freemont, P.S., Hanson, I.M. and Trowsdale, J. (1991) A novel cysteine-rich sequence motif. *Cell* **64**, 483–484.

Gasser, R.F. (1979) Evidence that sclerotomal cells do not migrate medially during embryonic development of the rat. *Am. J. Anat.* **154**, 509–524.

Glueeksohn-Schoenheimer, S. (1945) The embryonic development of mutants of the *Sd*-strain in mice. *Genetics* **30**, 29–38.

Goldstein, R.S. and Kalcheim, C. (1992) Determination of epithelial half-somites in skeletal morphogenesis. *Development* **116**, 441–445.

Goulding, M., Lumsden, A. and Paquette, A.J. (1994) Regulation of *Pax-3* expression in the dermomyotome and its role in muscle development. *Development* **120**, 957–971.

Grüneberg, H. (1963) *The Pathology of Development*. Blackwell Scientific: Oxford.

Haack, H. and Kessel, M. (1994) Homeobox genes and skeletal patterning. In *Bone* (Ed. B.K. Hall), vol. 9, pp. 119–144. CRC Press: Boca Raton.

Herrmann, B., Labeit, S., Poustka, A., King, T.R. and Lehrach, H. (1990) Cloning of the *T* gene required in mesoderm formation of the mouse. *Nature* **343**, 617–622.

Huang, R., Zhi, Q., Wilting, J. and Christ, B. (1994) The fate of somitocoele cells in avian embryos. *Anat. Embryol.* **190**, 243–250.

Ingham, P.W. (1988) The molecular genetics of embryonic pattern formation in Drosophila. *Nature* **335**, 25–34.

Jegalian, B.G. and De Robertis, E.M. (1992) Homeotic transformations in the mouse induced by overexpression of a human Hox-3.3 Transgene. *Cell* **71**, 901–910.

Johnson, R.L., Laufer, E., Riddle, R.D. and Tabin, C. (1994) Ectopic expression of *Sonic hedgehog* alters dorsal–ventral patterning of somites. *Cell* **79**, 1165–1173.

Kanno, M., Hasegawa, M., Ishida, A., Isono, K. and Taniguchi, M. (1995) *mel-18*, a *Polycomb* group-related mammalian gene, encodes a transcriptional negative regulator with tumour suppressive activity. *EMBO J.* **14**, 5672–5678.

Kappen, C., Schughart, K. and Ruddle, F.H. (1993) Early evolution of major homeo-domain sequence classes. *Genomics* **18**, 54–70.

Kenyon, C. (1986) A gene involved in the development of the posterior body region of *C. elegans*. *Cell* **46**, 477–487.

Kessel, M. (1992) Respecification of vertebral identities by retinoic acid. *Development* **115**, 487–501.

Kessel, M. (1993) Reversal of axonal pathways from rhombomere 3 correlates with extra Hox expression domains. *Neuron* **10**, 379–393.

Kessel, M. and Gruss, P. (1990) Murine developmental control genes. *Science* **249**, 374–379.

Kessel, M. and Gruss, P. (1991). Homeotic transformations of murine vertebrae and concomitant alteration of Hox codes induced by retinoic acid. *Cell* **67**, 89–104.

Kessel, M., Balling, R. and Gruss, P. (1990) Variations of cervical vertebrae after expression of a *Hox-1.1* transgene in mice. *Cell* **61**, 301–308.

Keynes, R.J. and Stern, C.D. (1988) Mechanisms of vertebrate segmentation. *Development* **103**, 413–429.

Kingsley, D.M. (1994) What do BMPs do in mammals? Clues from the mouse short-ear mutation. *Trends Genet.* **10**, 16–21.

Kitchin, I.C. (1949) The effects of notochordectomy in *Amblystoma mexicanum*. *J. Exp. Zool.* **112**, 393–415.

Koseki, H., Wallin, J., Wilting, J. et al (1993) A role for *Pax-1* as a mediator of notochordal signals during the dorsoventral specification of vertebrae. *Development* **119**, 649–660.

Krauss, S., Concordet, J.P. and Ingham, P.W. (1993) A functionally conserved homolog of the Drosophila segment polarity gene *hh* is expressed in tissues with polarizing activity in zebrafish embryos. *Cell* **75**, 1431–1444.

Lammer, E.J., Chen, D.T., Hoar, R.M. et al (1985) Retinoic acid embryopathy. *New Engl. J. Med.* **313**, 837–841.

Langston, A.W. and Gudas, L.J. (1992) Identification of a retinoic acid responsive enhancer 3 of the murine homeobox gene *Hox-1.6*. *Mech. Dev.* **38**, 217–228.

Le Mouellic, H., Lallemand, Y. and Brûlet, P. (1992) Homeosis in the mouse induced by a null mutation in the *Hox-3.1* gene. *Cell* **69**, 251–264.

Leid, M., Kastner, P. and Chambon, P. (1992) Multiplicity generates diversity in the retinoic acid signalling pathways. *Trends Biochem. Sci.* **17**, 427–433.

Lohnes, M., Kastner, P., Dierich, A. et al (1993) Function of retinoic acid receptor-γ in the mouse. *Cell* **73**, 643–658.

Lufkin, T., Dierich, A., LeMeur, M., Mark, M. and Chambon, P. (1991) Disruption of the *Hox-1.6* homeobox gene results in defects in a region corresponding to its rostral domain of expression. *Cell* **66**, 1105–1119.

Lufkin, T., Mark, M., Hart, C.P. et al (1992) Homeotic transformation of the occipital bones of the skull by ectopic expression of a homeobox gene. *Nature* **359**, 835–841.

Lyon, M.F. and Searle, A.G. (1989) *Genetic Variants and Strains of the Laboratory Mouse*. Oxford University Press: Oxford.

Macdonald, P.M. and Struhl, G. (1986) A molecular gradient in early *Drosophila* embryos and its role in specifying the body plan. *Nature* **324**, 537–545.

McGinnis, W. and Krumlauf, R. (1992) Homeobox genes and axial patterning. *Cell* **68**, 283–302.

McGinnis, W., Levine, M.S., Hafen, E., Kuroiwa, A. and Gehring, W.J. (1984) A conserved DNA sequence in homeotic genes of the *Drosophila* antennapedia and bithorax complexes. *Nature* **308**, 428–433.

McLain, K., Schreiner, C., Yager, K.L., Stock, J.L. and Potter, S.S. (1992) Ectopic expression of *Hox-2.3* induces craniofacial and skeletal malformations in transgenic mice. *Mech. Dev.* **39**, 3–16.

Müller, J. (1995) Transcriptional silencing by the *Polycomb* protein in *Drosophila* embryos. *EMBO J.* **14**, 1209–1220.

Paavola, L.G., Wilson, D.B. and Center, E.M. (1980) Histochemistry of the developing notochord, perichordal sheath and vertebrae in *Danforth's short-tail* (*Sd*) and normal C57BL/6 mice. *J. Embryol. Exp. Morph.* **55**, 227–245.

Paro, R. (1990) Imprinting a determined state into the chromatin of *Drosophila*. *Trends Genet.* **6**, 416–421.

Pollock, R.A. (1992) Altering the boundaries of *Hox-3.1* expression: evidence for antipodal gene regulation. *Cell* **71**, 911–923.

Pourquié, O., Coltey, M., Teillet, M.-A., Ordahl, C. and Le Douarin, N.M. (1993) Control of dorsoventral patterning of somitic derivatives by notochord and floorplate. *Proc. Natl Acad. Sci. USA* **90**, 5242–5246.

Ramirez-Solis, R. (1993) Hoxb-4 (Hox-2.6) Mutant mice show homeotic transformation of a cervical vertebra and defects in the closure of the sternal rudiments. *Cell* **73**, 279–294.

Riddle, H., Johnson, R.L., Laufer, E. and Tabin, C. (1993) Sonic hedgehog mediates the polarizing activity of the ZPA. *Cell* **75**, 1401–1416.

Roelink, H., Augsburger, A., Heemskerk, J. et al (1994) Floor plate and motor neuron induction by *vhh-1*, a vertebrate homolog of hedgehog expressed by the notochord. *Cell* **76**, 761–775.

Ruberte, E., Dollé, P., Krust, A. et al (1990) Specific spatial and temporal distribution of retinoic acid gamma transcripts during mouse embryogenesis. *Development* **108**, 213–222.

Ruberte, E., Dollé, P., Chambon, P. and Morriss-Kay, G. (1991) Retinoic acid receptors and cellular retinoid binding proteins. II. Their differential pattern of transcription during early morphogenesis in mouse embryos. *Development* **111**, 45–60.

Schubert, F.R., Nieselt-Struwe, K. and Gruss, P. (1993) The Antennapedia-type homeobox genes have evolved from three precursors separated early in metazoan evolution. *Proc. Natl Acad. Sci. USA* **90**, 143–147.

Scott, M.P. and Weiner, A.J. (1984) Structural relationships among genes that control development: sequence homology between the antennapedia, ultrabithorax and fushi tarazu loci of Drosophila. *Proc. Natl Acad. Sci. USA* **81**, 4115–4119.

Searle, A.G. (1966) *Curtailed*, a new dominant T-allele in the house mouse. *Genet. Res.* **7**, 86–95.

Simeone, A., Acampora, D., Arcioni, L. et al (1990) Sequential activation of Hox2 homeobox genes by retinoic acid in human embryonal carcinoma cells. *Nature* **346**, 736–766.

Simon, J., Chiang, A. and Bender, W. (1992) Ten different *Polycomb* group genes are required for spatial control of the *abdA* and *abdB* homeotic products. *Development* **114**, 493–505.

Sive, H.L., Draper, B.W., Harland, R.M. and Weintraub, H. (1990) Identification of a retinoic acid-sensitive period during primary axis formation in Xenopus laevis. *Genes Dev.* **4**, 932–942.

Stein, S., Fritsch, R., Lemaire, L. and Kessel, M. (1996) Checklist: vertebrate homeobox genes. *Mech. Dev.* **55**, 91–108.

Stern, C.D. (1992) Mesoderm induction and development of the embryonic axis in amniotes. *Trends Genet.* **8**, 158–163.

Subramanian, V., Meyer, B.I. and Gruss, P. (1995) Disruption of the murine homeobox gene *Cdx-1* affects axial skeletal identities by altering the mesodermal expression domains of Hox genes. *Cell* **83**, 641–653.

Sundin, O. and Eichele, G. (1992) An early marker of axial pattern in the chick embryo and its respecification by retinoic acid. *Development* **114**, 841–852.

Tagawa, M., Sakamoto, T., Shigemoto, K. et al (1990) Expression of novel DNA-binding protein with zinc-finger structure in various tumour cells. *J. Biol. Chem.* **265**, 20021–20026.

Takahashi, Y. and Le Douarin, N. (1990) cDNA cloning of a quail homeobox gene and its expression in neural crest-derived mesenchyme and lateral plate mesoderm. *Proc. Natl Acad. Sci. USA* **87**, 7482–7486.

Takahashi, Y., Monsoro-Burq, A.-H., Bontoux, M. and Le Douarin, N.M. (1992) A role for *Qhox-8* in the establishment of the dorsoventral pattern during vertebrate development. *Proc. Natl Acad. Sci. USA* **89**, 10237–10241.

Teillet, M.-A. and Le Douarin, N.M. (1983) Consequences of neural tube and notochord excision on the development of the peripheral nervous system in the chick embryo. *Dev. Biol.* **98**, 192–211.

Theiler, K. (1959) Anatomy and development of the '*truncate*' (boneless) mutation in the mouse. *Am. J. Anat.* **104**, 319–343.

Theiler, K., Varnum, D. and Stevens, L.C. (1974) Development of *rachiterata*, a mutation in the house mouse with 6 cervical vertebrae. *Zentralbl. Anat. Entwickl.* **145**, 81–85.

Töndury, G. and Theiler, K. (1990) *Entwicklungsgeschichte und Fehlbildungen der Wirbelsäule. Die Wirbelsäule in Forschung und Praxis.* Hippokrates Verlag: Stuttgart.

Tremblay, P., Dietrich, S., Stoykova, A., Stuart, E.T. and Gruss, P. (1995) Pax genes as pleiotropic regulators of embryonic development. In *Neural Cell Specification: Molecular Mechanisms and Neurotherapeutic Implications* (Eds: B.H. Juurlink et al). Plenum Press: New York.

van Lohuizen, M., Frasch, M., Wientjens, E. and Berns, A. (1991) Sequence similarity between the mammalian *bmi-1* proto-oncogene and the *Drosophila* regulatory genes *Psc* and *Su(z)2*. *Nature* **353**, 353–355.

van der Lugt, N.M.T., Domen, J., Linders, K. et al (1994) Posterior transformation, neurological abnormalities, and severe haematopoietic defects in mice with a targeted deletion of the *bmi-1* proto-oncogene. *Genes Dev.* **8**, 757–769.

Wallin, J., Mizutani, Y., Imai, K. et al (1993) A new Pax gene, *Pax-9*, maps to mouse chromosome 12. *Mammal. Genome* **4**, 354–358.

Wallin, J., Wilting, J., Koseki, H. et al (1994) The role of *Pax-1* in axial skeleton development. *Development* **120**, 1109–1121.

Wilting, J., Kurz, H., Brand-Saberi, B. et al. (1994) Kinetics and differentiation of somite cells forming the vertebral column: studies on human and chick embryos. *Anat. Embryol.* **190**, 573–581.

Zeltser, L., Desplan, C. and Heintz, N. (1996) *Hoxb-13*: a new Hox gene in a distant region of the HoxB cluster maintains colinearity. *Development* **122**, 2475–2484.

14 The Kidney

ADRIAN S. WOOLF

Developmental Biology Unit, Institute of Child Health, London, UK

THE ANATOMY OF NORMAL NEPHROGENESIS

Nephrogenesis is the term that is generally used to describe the development of the whole kidney although it more correctly refers to the differentiation of the nephron tubules alone. The description provided below is necessarily brief and further details are provided elsewhere (Grobstein, 1967; Saxen, 1987; Hardman et al, 1994a; Woolf, 1995). The **metanephros** is the direct precursor of the mammalian adult kidney and can first be identified in humans in the 6th week after fertilization and in mice at the 11th day of gestation. At this time many other organ systems are differentiating including the gonads which develop in close proximity to the kidneys. The bulk of the adult kidney is derived from two tissue compartments within the metanephros, namely the **nephrogenic mesenchymal cells** and the **ureteric bud epithelium**, itself a branch of the Wolffian or mesonephric duct. Epithelial cells are said to be polarized; they have an 'up' and a 'down' side which mediate specialized functions, including vectorial fluid transport between the lumen that they enclose and the rest of the body. In contrast, mesenchymal cells have no polarity and although they are less differentiated than epithelial cells, they have the potential to differentiate into specialized cells. In mammals, two other sets of kidney precursors, the pro- and mesonephros, degenerate as the metanephros grows and they will not be discussed further. In females the Wolffian duct also degenerates, but part of it remains as the vas deferens in males.

CELL INTERACTIONS IN NORMAL KIDNEY DEVELOPMENT

Two types of interaction between epithelial and mesenchymal cells occur during metanephric development (Figures 14.1 and 14.2). First, the differentiation and morphogenesis of the ureteric bud is dependent on the adjacent renal mesenchymal cells (Grobstein, 1955). **Epithelial branching morphogenesis** also occurs during the development of the lung, pancreas, thymus, liver, prostate, salivary and mammary glands and also requires the presence of mesenchymal cells or mesenchymal-derived factors (Grobstein, 1967). Only renal mesenchyme, however, can induce the ureteric bud to differentiate. Secondly, a **mesenchymal-to-epithelial conversion** occurs during the transition of renal mesenchyme into

Embryos, Genes and Birth Defects. Edited by P. Thorogood.
© 1997 John Wiley & Sons Ltd.

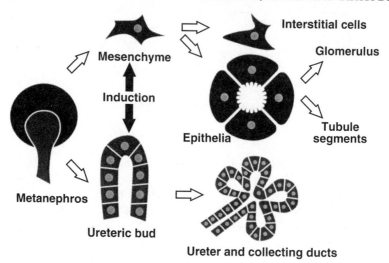

Figure 14.1 Cell lineage in nephrogenesis. Mutual inductions between the ureteric bud and the renal mesenchyme (stippled) cause the serial branching of the bud and the differentiation of mesenchyme into polarized epithelia and interstitial fibroblasts

nephron tubules. It is a major goal of developmental biology to identify the molecular mechanisms that mediate these tissue interactions (Birchmeier and Birchmeier, 1993).

CELL LINEAGES IN THE EARLY METANEPHROS

At the inception of the metanephros the ureteric bud contacts the nephrogenic mesenchyme and thereafter branches to form the arborial collecting duct system which drains urine from the nephron tubules into the ureter. The distal end of the ureteric bud and the mesonephric duct fuse with the developing urinary bladder to form the ureter and its valve-like insertion into the bladder. The bud cells express specific transcription factors, including *Pax-2* (Rothenpieler and Dressler, 1993; Winyard et al, 1996b) and *Hox 2.3* (Kress et al, 1990), and contain cytokeratin intermediate filament proteins that are characteristic of epithelial cells. The branching tips of the ureteric bud express receptor tyrosine kinases, including *met* (Sonnenberg et al, 1993; Woolf et al, 1995), *ros* (Sonnenberg et al, 1991) and *ret* (Pachnis et al, 1993), which are considered to transduce morphogenetic signals from the adjacent mesenchyme. The ligand for *met* is hepatocyte growth factor/scatter factor (HGF/SF; Stoker et al, 1987), the ligand for *ret* is glial cell line-derived neurotrophic factor (GDNF; Treanor et al, 1996) but the factor that binds *ros* is not yet identified.

Renal mesenchymal cells express vimentin intermediate filaments and are loosely embedded in a matrix of fibronectin and collagen I. They express growth factors including insulin-like growth factor II (IGF II) and HGF/SF (Woolf et al, 1995). After contact with the ureteric bud, renal mesenchymal cells become

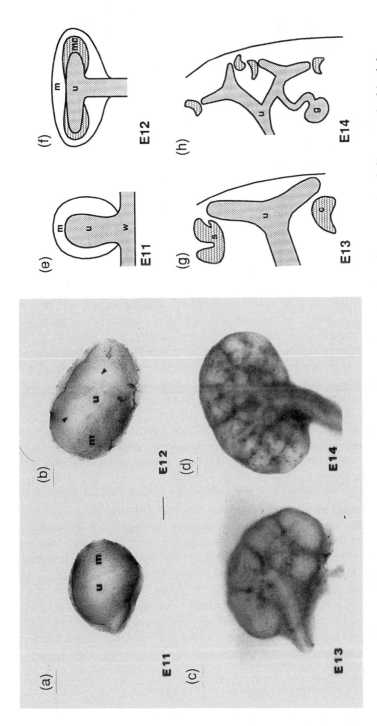

Figure 14.2 Early development of the metanephros. Stereomicroscopic images (a–d) and cross-sectional diagrams (e–h) of the mouse metanephros at E11 (a) and (e), E12 (b) and (f), E13 (c) and (g) and E14 (d) and (h). Note that the most primitive structures are located in the periphery of the E14 organ. Arrowheads in (b) indicate the first branch tips of the ureteric bud. u, ureteric bud; m, mesenchyme; w, Wolffian duct; mc, mesenchymal condensate; c and s, comma and S-shaped bodies; g, glomerulus. (a–d) Scale bar: 50 mm; (e–h): not to scale. (From Woolf et al 1995) (by copyright permission of the Rockefeller University Press)

induced to differentiate and undergo a burst of proliferation, up-regulating the expression of varied molecules including the WT1 transcription/splicing factor (Bard et al, 1993; Larsson et al, 1995), syndecan, a cell-surface proteoglycan (Vainio et al, 1989) and neural cell adhesion molecule (N-CAM). Cells that lie directly adjacent to the branching tips of the bud are programmed to differentiate into the nephron tubules while other mesenchymal cells differentiate into interstitial fibroblasts (Herzlinger et al, 1991; Weller et al, 1991) or die by **apoptosis**, or programmed cell death (Koseki et al, 1992; Coles et al, 1993; Winyard et al, 1996a). In the mature organ a subset of interstitial fibroblasts secrete erythropoietin, a hormone that stimulates the production of erythrocytes.

NEPHRON TUBULE FORMATION

The cells that are destined to convert into nephrons aggregate around the branching tips of the ureteric bud to form dense condensations which express the *Pax-2* transcription factor and uvomorulin (E-cadherin), a cell–cell adhesion molecule. The condensates then develop an apical and basolateral polarity to form immature epithelia, called **comma** and **S-shaped bodies**, and these subsequently differentiate into mature **nephrons**. During tubule formation the primitive epithelia express the laminin A chain, a molecule of the extracellular matrix, and its corresponding cell-surface integrin receptor (Klein et al, 1988). Most mature renal epithelial cells express cytokeratins, are joined by tight junctions and sit on a basement membrane composed of collagen IV, laminin, heparan sulphate and entactin/nidogen. The proximal ends of the nephron tubules later differentiate into the **podocyte layer**, which filters the plasma to form urine. These epithelial cells have a very different phenotype from epithelia in the rest of the nephron: they lack tight junctions between adjacent cells, they continue to express vimentin intermediate filaments rather than cytokeratins, and they express *WT1* into adulthood, whereas the expression of this gene is down-regulated as the rest of the nephron matures.

Throughout nephrogenesis, until 7 postnatal days in the mouse and 36 weeks gestation in humans, sequential layers of nephrons are born with the most immature elements located in the periphery. At the end of this process each human kidney contains about one million nephrons. In the human, however, the first vascularized glomeruli have formed by 10 weeks after fertilization and thus the metanephros starts to produce urine early in gestation. Even after this period of nephron formation the tubular cells continue to differentiate into the specialized epithelia of the **proximal and distal tubules** and **the loops of Henle**. Each tubule segment carries out specialized transport functions such as the reabsorption of sodium, bicarbonate, phosphate, amino acids and water, or the secretion of potassium and hydrogen ions.

BLOOD SUPPLY AND INNERVATION OF THE METANEPHROS

The mature kidney is a very vascular organ and receives 20% of the cardiac output. The high blood flow is a prerequisite to the generation of the urine ultrafiltrate, which amounts to 200 litres per day in normal adults. At the inception of nephrogenesis renal mesenchyme is surrounded by a rim of endothelial cells but no mature endothelia are seen within the metanephros (Loughna et al, 1996). Vessels appear in the loose interstitial tissue around the ureter and the primitive nephrons, and later capillaries can also be identified within the primitive glomeruli. In the metanephros, nephrons express vascular endothelial growth factor (VEGF), a mitogen and differentiation factor for endothelia and their precursors (Breier et al, 1992), and also platelet-derived growth factor (PDGF), a mitogen for mesangial cells (Alpers et al, 1992). Immature renal arterioles express renin, an enzyme that initiates the generation of angiotensin II, a powerful vasoconstrictor. In contrast, in the adult kidney, renin expression is confined to the afferent arteriole immediately proximal to the glomerulus. Within the glomerulus itself endothelia are in intimate contact with epithelial podocyte cells and both populations contribute to the first glomerular basement membrane, which acts as a filter to form an almost protein-free ultrafiltrate. Fibromuscular mesangial cells support the capillary loops and also perform a phagocytic function.

In the adult kidney the autonomic nervous system maintains vascular tone and affects the rate of glomerular blood flow and thus the rate of glomerular filtration. Nerves grow into the metanephros at a very early stage of development but little is known of their function during nephrogenesis. It is, however, of note that human renal malformations commonly coexist with major defects of development of the neural tube (Hulton et al, 1990).

CLINICAL IMPACT OF HUMAN KIDNEY MALFORMATIONS

In the context of this review, I use the term 'kidney malformation' to refer to any structural abnormality of the kidney, either macro- or microscopic, that causes disease. The most important macroscopic disorders are: (1) **renal dysplasias** (undifferentiated kidneys), (2) **renal agenesis** (absent kidneys) and (3) **polycystic kidney diseases**. I will also discuss the pathogenesis of structural diseases of the glomerulus that have a developmental basis, and these include the Denys–Drash syndrome (Coppes et al, 1993). Although the Wilms' tumour, a common childhood kidney neoplasm, can be considered an aberration of development, a full discussion of its pathogenesis is beyond the scope of this chapter. Human gene mutations also cause inherited disorders of tubule physiology, such as nephrogenic diabetes insipidus (failure of urine concentration) and hypophosphataemic rickets (failure of phosphate reabsorption and vitamin D metabolism). However, these diseases are not kidney malformations because organ structure is maintained even at the microscopic level.

RENAL DYSPLASIAS AND AGENESIS

Human kidney dysplasias and agenesis comprise a heterogeneous group of congenital disorders that represent major aberrations of renal development and the reader is referred to other reviews for their exhaustive classification and incidence (Hirata et al, 1990; Kaplan et al, 1991; Holliday et al, 1994; Woolf, 1995). A common example is the **multicystic dysplastic kidney**, which contains immature ducts surrounded by undifferentiated cells: in the metanephros, mesenchymal precursor cells fail to differentiate into nephrons and the ureteric bud fails to branch to form collecting ducts. These organs do not produce urine because they contain no mature glomeruli (Risdon, 1971; Potter, 1972). When followed with serial ultrasound scans before birth or during infancy, it can be seen that some of these organs involute, producing an aplastic phenotype (Mesrobian et al, 1993). Renal failure occurs when renal agenesis is bilateral (1 : 10 000 births) and the baby presents at birth with **Potter's sequence**. This term is used to describe the constellation of anuria, low volumes of amniotic fluid (oligohydramnios) and lung hypoplasia. The last is often considered to be secondary to the oligohydramnios. Kidney dysplasias are among the commonest diseases requiring dialysis and transplantation in the first years of life and constitute formidable therapeutic challenges (McEnery et al, 1992). Aplastic and multicystic dysplastic kidneys also occur unilaterally and the latter organs are often surgically removed because of a small but finite risk of malignancy or hypertension. In contrast, it is probable that no morbidity is generally associated with unilateral agenesis if the contralateral kidney is normal (Fotino, 1989; Woolf and Fine, 1991).

Although these disorders are usually sporadic, isolated (non-syndromal) renal malformations in first-degree relatives have been reported in 5–10% of index cases with bilateral disease, suggesting a genetic component and raising the possibility that some sporadic cases are due to new mutations (Kohn and Borns, 1973; Roodhooft et al, 1984; McPherson et al, 1987; Murugasu et al, 1991). It is striking that the severity of the malformation can vary between affected members. Moreover, individual members may have asymmetrical kidney disease, for example renal agenesis with a normal, dysplastic or absent contra-lateral kidney. Renal malformations also occur as part of defined syndromes that may occur sporadically or be inherited (Holliday et al, 1994). These include the X-linked **Kallmann syndrome**, where renal agenesis is associated with anosmia and infertility (Duke et al, 1995), and the autosomal dominant **branchio-oto-renal syndrome**, where the renal lesion occurs together with deafness and branchial fistulae. Human renal malformations are often associated with lesions of the lower urinary tract. For example, in males urethral valves often cause obstruction to flow of urine out of the bladder and therefore the urinary tract (urinary bladder, ureters and renal pelvis) becomes distended before birth. Another condition that commonly coexists with renal malformations is called **vesico-ureteric reflux**, where urine travels retrogradely up the ureter into the kidney each time the bladder muscles contract (Feather et al, 1996). This is sometimes inherited in an autosomal dominant manner and postnatally this disorder predisposes to recurrent bacterial infections of the kidney (**pyelonephritis**), which may cause scarring, high blood pressure and kidney failure. Recently *PAX2* mutations have been associated with the rare syndrome of optic nerve coloboma and vesico-ureteric reflux (Sanyanusin et al, 1995).

POLYCYSTIC KIDNEY DISEASES

Cysts are fluid-filled spaces surrounded by epithelial cells. A few cysts may be acquired as the normal kidney ages but these appear to be rare in childhood (Ravine et al, 1993). In the so-called polycystic kidney diseases the major anatomical steps of nephrogenesis are complete but there are more subtle abnormalities, discussed below, which suggest that the epithelial cells lining the cyst lumens are not fully differentiated. Readers are referred to recent reviews for the classification and discussion of the biology and clinical impact of these diseases (Kissane, 1990; Holliday et al, 1994; Woolf and Winyard, 1995).

Autosomal recessive polycystic kidney disease (ARPKD) is often a rapidly progressive disorder in which cyst formation from collecting ducts may be advanced before birth. This disease usually causes massively enlarged kidneys together with renal failure in infancy or childhood. ARPKD is relatively rare (1:5000 births) compared with the **autosomal dominant polycystic kidney disease** (ADPKD), which accounts for 5–10% of all end-stage kidney failure and is the commonest of inherited human diseases affecting 5 million people world-wide (1:500–1000 births). In this disorder, cysts arise from all segments of the nephron. Although small ADPKD cysts have been identified in autopsy material from terminations of pregnancy, cyst growth is generally slower than in ARPKD and therefore the disease usually does not cause kidney failure until adulthood. It is, however, increasingly recognized that this disease may present in the paediatric age-range and a recent analysis provides preliminary information that some ADPKD families show the phenomenon of anticipation, with earlier clinical presentations in successive generations (Fick et al, 1994). In **glomerulo-cystic disease**, glomerular cysts are inherited in an autosomal dominant manner, and this disorder is sometimes regarded as a variant of ADPKD (Kaplan et al, 1989). It should be noted that the polycystic kidney diseases are syndromes in which other organs are affected either by cysts, as in ADPKD, or by other pathologies (e.g. cerebral aneurysms in ADPKD and hepatic fibrosis in ARPKD).

Polycystic kidneys are also a feature of other disorders, two of which are inherited in an autosomal dominant manner: **von Hippel–Lindau syndrome** (with cerebellar haemangiomas and renal neoplasms) and **tuberous sclerosis** (with neuroectodermal lesions). In children and young adults, another cystic disorder called **medullary cystic disease** or **nephronophthisis** can also cause kidney failure and has variable modes of inheritance (Hildebrandt et al, 1994). In these disorders the renal cysts are microscopic and the kidneys do not become enlarged. Similarly, gross kidney morphology is preserved in the **medullary sponge kidney**. This entity anatomically resembles very mild ARPKD although cyst growth is not progressive and renal failure does not occur. Interestingly, multiple cysts may also arise in the kidneys of patients with chronic renal failure of any aetiology and sometimes regress after successful kidney transplantation. In the latter context the growth of renal cysts has been associated with the use of cyclosporin, a powerful immunosuppressive agent used to prevent organ rejection (Yeong-Hau et al, 1993).

CONGENITAL ABNORMALITIES OF GLOMERULAR AND VASCULAR DEVELOPMENT

In the **congenital nephrotic syndrome** there is a loss of size-selectivity in the glomerular filtration barrier and the infant presents with massive loss of protein into the urine (**proteinuria**), which leads to salt and water retention, oedema and malnutrition. This disorder probably represents a mixture of diseases including the **Finnish-type nephrotic syndrome** and a separate disease in which the mesangial area becomes fibrosed, called **mesangial sclerosis**. Both may be inherited and the latter phenotype also occurs in the **Denys–Drash syndrome** (Coppes et al, 1993) in which the glomerular disease is associated with ambiguous genitalia and bilateral Wilms' tumour, a renal neoplasm comprised of undifferentiated renal mesenchymal cells and primitive tubules. Another inherited disorder, **Alport syndrome**, affects the structure and function of the glomerular basement membrane and may cause leakage of blood and protein into the urine, culminating in renal failure either in childhood or adulthood. As classically described, the disease has X-linked recessive inheritance, but recently autosomal recessive forms have been recognized (Lemmink et al, 1994).

Renal artery stenosis is a common cause of systemic hypertension (high blood pressure) in children; in this disorder the major renal arteries and the intrarenal blood vessels are often narrowed by a condition called fibromuscular hyperplasia (Holliday et al, 1994). The pathogenesis may involve aberrant formation of blood vessels during development. The reduced renal blood flow increases renin secretion by renal arterioles distal to the stenosis and this protein initiates the production of angiotensin II which causes the hypertension. Usually, renal artery stenosis occurs in isolation but it may form part of a syndrome such as neurofibromatosis (von Recklinghausen's disease) and these patients also suffer from neuroectodermal lesions.

MOLECULAR MECHANISMS OF ABNORMAL NEPHROGENESIS: CLUES FROM ANIMAL STUDIES

IN-VITRO AND IN-VIVO MODELS OF DEVELOPMENTAL KIDNEY DISEASE

The mouse metanephros will undergo a remarkable degree of differentiation in organ culture and this technique has proved invaluable in understanding the mechanisms of nephrogenesis (Saxen, 1987). Grobstein (1955, 1967) demonstrated that neither the ureteric bud nor the renal mesenchyme differentiated when cultured in isolation but nephron formation and branching morphogenesis resumed when these tissues were recombined. Intriguingly it has been found that embryonic spinal cord can elicit nephron formation in isolated renal mesenchymes (Grobstein, 1955; Sariola et al, 1989) but the relevance of this observation to normal nephrogenesis is quite unclear. It is a major goal to identify the molecular mechanisms that mediate **tissue interactions** during normal nephrogenesis and, furthermore, defective signalling between nephro-genic cells is likely to be central to the pathogenesis of kidney malformations (Maizel and Simpson, 1983). More recently, the generation of transgenic mice in which genes are over-expressed or functionally ablated (see Chapter 4) has provided valuable insights into the molecular control of normal nephrogenesis and the pathogenesis of developmental kidney disorders. Tables 14.1 and 14.2 respectively detail the organ culture and transgenic experiments that are discussed below.

It is noteworthy that endothelia do not develop in metanephric organ culture (Bernstein et al, 1981) whereas, if the embryonic mouse kidney is transplanted

Table 14.1 Molecular inhibitors of kidney development in organ culture

Antibodies to GD_3 ganglioside
Antibodies to hepatocyte growth factor/scatter factor (HGF/SF)
Antibodies to insulin-like growth factors I and II (IGF I and II)
Antibodies to insulin-like growth factor I receptor
Leukaemia inhibition factor (LIF)
Antibodies to the laminin A chain
Lipopolysaccharide
Antibodies and antisense oligonucleotides to the low-affinity nerve growth factor (NGF)
  receptor
Antisense oligonucleotides to *Pax-2*
Antibodies to transforming growth factor-α (TGF-α)
Transforming growth factor-β (TGF-β)
Tumour necrosis factor-α (TNF-α)
Antisense oligonucleotides to WT1
β-D-xyloside

Table 14.2 Results of transgenic manipulation of genes implicated in kidney development

(1) **Transgenic mouse with null mutations, displaying a kidney phenotype**
  bcl-2
  fyn/yes double-mutants
  Platelet-derived growth factor-B (PDGF-B)
  Platelet-derived growth factor-β receptor
  ret and GDNF
  wt-1

(2) **Transgenic mouse with null mutations, without a kidney phenotype**
  Hepatocyte growth factor/scatter (HGF/SF)
  Insulin-like growth factor II (IGF II)
  Nerve growth factor (NGF) receptor (low affinity)

(3) **Transgenic mice that over-express genes, displaying an abnormal kidney phenotype**
  c-myc
  Growth hormone
  Insulin-like growth factor I (IGF I)
  Pax-2
  SV40 T antigen

on to avian chorioallantoic membrane, the organ becomes vascularized by host endothelia (Sariola et al, 1983). This ingrowth of capillaries is called **angio-genesis**. Other experiments, however, suggest that renal endothelia may alternatively arise from in-situ vessel formation by the process of **vasculo-genesis**. Thus, when mouse kidney rudiments were transplanted into the anterior chamber of the rat eye, intrarenal vessels originated from the donor tissue (Pinson et al, 1993). Furthermore, there is preliminary evidence that endothelial precursors can be isolated from the metanephric mesenchyme at a time when this tissue contains no mature blood vessels (Loughna et al, 1996): these cells express flk-1, a receptor tyrosine kinase for VEGF (Millauer et al, 1993). Similarly, the lineage of the mesangial cells, which support capillaries within the glomerulus, is currently unclear.

TRANSCRIPTION FACTORS

It is fashionable to view the cellular interactions that occur during development as resulting from a programme of stimulation and repression of gene expression which is itself controlled by master genes that code for transcription factors. These proteins have no direct effect on differentiation but instead are able to activate or repress the transcription of other genes which include those coding for growth factors or matrix molecules. Transcription factor genes form families that share common nucleotide sequences coding for characteristic DNA-binding domains, including the homeodomain (in Hox or homeobox transcription factors) and the paired domain (in Pax or paired-box transcription factors) (and see Chapters 7, 8, 10 and 13). I have already alluded to the expression of *Hox 2.3* (Kress et al, 1990) and *Pax-2* (Rothenpieler and Dressler, 1993) during normal nephrogenesis, although little is known of their target genes. Using antisense nucleotides to abolish *Pax-2* function in metanephric organ culture, it was recently demonstrated that this molecule is important for nephron formation. More striking was the demonstration that neonatal mice were born with a nephrotic syndrome when *Pax-2* was over-expressed in the kidney of transgenic mice (Dressler et al, 1993), further implicating the gene in the differentiation of renal epithelia.

Another important class of transcription factor genes encode proteins with DNA-binding zinc-fingers, and the *WT1* gene which is expressed in the renal mesenchyme belongs to this class (Bard et al, 1993; Larsson et al, 1995). Cell biology studies have shown that this protein binds to a consensus nucleotide sequence that is present in the regulatory promoter regions of many genes including those coding for IGF II (Drummond et al, 1991) and PDGF-A (Wang et al, 1992). In-vitro assays have demonstrated that the WT1 protein represses transcription of these growth factors. The complete story is, however, likely to be more complex because the *WT1* gene codes for multiple transcripts which may have different functions. In addition, certain WT1 isoforms may control nuclear RNA splicing (Larsson et al, 1995). In organ culture, disruption of *WT1* gene expression inhibits nephrogenesis (Rothenpieler, 1994) and mice engineered to have homozygous null mutations of the gene have a renal agenesis

(Kreidberg et al, 1993). More detailed analysis of these transgenic mice revealed that, in early development, the ureteric bud fails to contact the renal mesenchyme, which proceeds to die rather than differentiate into nephrons. In addition, these animals fail to develop gonads because the WT1 gene is also expressed early in the differentiation of these organs (Kreidberg et al, 1993).

GROWTH FACTORS THAT ENHANCE NEPHROGENESIS

The ability of the metanephros to grow in defined, serum-free media has allowed the roles of endogenously produced growth factors to be investigated. The strategy in these experiments has usually involved the functional blockade of the metanephric growth factor by **neutralizing antibodies** or perturbation of gene expression by **antisense oligonucleotides**. These studies have implicated IGF I and II (Rogers et al, 1991), HGF/SF (Woolf et al, 1995; see Figure 14.3), the low-affinity nerve growth factor (NGF) receptor (Sariola et al, 1991), transforming growth factor-α (TGF-α; Rogers et al, 1992) the embryonic homologue of epidermal growth factor (EGF), as factors that variously enhance cell survival, differentiation and morphogenesis during nephrogenesis. Homozygous null mutations for IGF II (De Chiara et al, 1990), low-affinity NGF receptor (Lee et al, 1992) and HGF/SF (Schmidt et al, 1995) have also been generated; in these mice, nephrogenesis has appeared grossly normal, although subtle anatomical or functional abnormalities are not excluded by these studies. The discrepancies between the in-vitro and in-vivo experiments may be explained as follows. First, some growth factors may be transferred from the mother to the fetus and this has been convincingly demonstrated for TGF-β. Mice with homozygous TGF-β null mutations are normal if born to a mother that expresses the protein, but mutant embryos develop severe heart defects if they gestate in a mutant female (Letterio et al, 1994). Secondly, the function of certain proteins may be replaced by similar molecules expressed in the same population of cells. Here a good example is provided by the intracellular tyrosine kinases *fyn* and *yes*. These genes are both expressed by many tissues but it seems that an animal can survive without one of them. When both genes are mutated, however, the animal develops severe immune-mediated glomerulonephritis in early adulthood (Stein et al, 1994). Although this lesion does not appear to be a birth defect, it clearly illustrates the potentially complex relationships between genes with similar functions.

Many growth factor receptors contain an intracellular tyrosine kinase domain that becomes phosphorylated when the ligand binds to the extracellular domain. One such receptor tyrosine kinase is called *ret*. This molecule was originally isolated as a transforming oncogene in human carcinomas and recently specific parts of the cellular proto-oncogene have been found to be mutated in four human diseases (Van Heyningen, 1994): (1) isolated medullary thyroid carcinomas, (2) multiple endocrine neoplasia (MEN) type 2A (medullary thyroid tumours and phaeochromocytomas), (3) MEN 2B (like MEN 2A, with ganglioneuromas) and (4) Hirschsprung's disease, a disorder of intestinal motility caused by congenital absence of parasympathetic nerves.

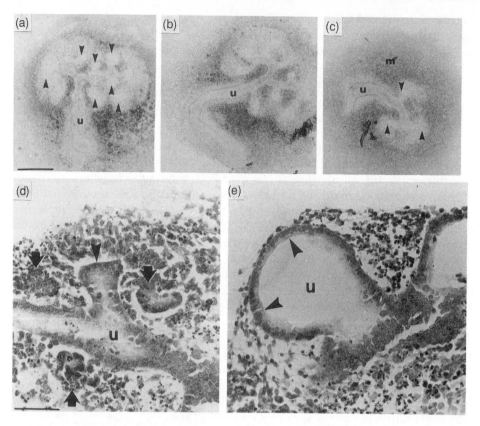

Figure 14.3 Blockade of hepatocyte growth factor/scatter factor (HGF/SF) in metanephric organ culture. Stereomicroscope images of E11 (a–c) rudiments after 3 days of culture in serum-free basal media alone (a), basal media and non-immune rabbit IgG Fab$_2$ (b) and basal media with rabbit anti-mouse HGF/SF IgG Fab$_2$ (c). Note that ureteric bud branching and nephron formation are limited in organs treated with anti-HGF/SF antibody. Photomicrographs of 10-μm paraffin sections stained with haematoxylin and eosin are shown for an E11 rudiment grown for 3 days in basal medium (d) and for the same period in the presence of anti-HGF/SF antibodies (e). Note the condensations of mesenchyme around the tips of the ureteric bud in (d) compared with the cystic dilatation of the bud surrounded by loose mesenchyme with pyknotic nuclei in (e). Arrowheads indicate the tips of the ureteric bud; arrows in (d) indicate mesenchymal condensates. u, ureteric bud or its derivatives; m, mesenchyme. Scale bars: 100 mm. (From Woolf et al (1995) by copyright permission of the Rockefeller University Press)

Mice that are genetically engineered so that both *ret* alleles are mutated have extraordinary kidney phenotypes, which range from absence of both kidneys and ureters to the presence of small, dysplastic kidneys (Schuchardt et al, 1994). As discussed above, during normal development *ret* is expressed in the branching tips of the ureteric bud where the receptor is presumed to transduce a morphogenetic signal from a GDNF produced by renal mesenchymal cells (Treanor et al, 1996).

The generation of mice with homozygous null mutations of PDGF-β, or its receptor tyrosine kinase (Leveen et al, 1994; Soriano, 1994), has convincingly demonstrated that this signalling system is necessary for the normal development of the mesangial cells of the glomerulus.

GROWTH FACTORS THAT INHIBIT NEPHROGENESIS

Finally there are other growth factors or cytokines that inhibit nephrogenesis in organ culture of the mouse metanephros. They include TGF-β (Rogers et al, 1993), leukaemia inhibitory factor (LIF; Bard and Ross, 1991) and tumour necrosis factor-α (TNF-α; Woolf et al, 1994). Interestingly, TGF-β also inhibits branching morphogenesis in other developing organs including the salivary gland (Hardman et al, 1994b). Perhaps some of these effects are mediated by interaction with other growth factors and, for example, TGF-β inhibits HGF/SF-induced branching morphogenesis in some in-vitro models (Santos and Nigam, 1993). TGF-β is expressed in the normal metanephros (Rogers et al, 1993) and in the adult kidney its expression is increased when the ureter is experimentally ligated (Koneto et al, 1993). It is therefore intriguing to speculate that levels of TGF-β, or of other molecules that inhibit nephrogenesis, may be increased in the presence of prenatal urinary tract obstruction caused, for example, by urethral valves. In this context it should be noted that TGF-β can induce apoptosis in epithelia in vitro (Oberhammer et al, 1993) and renal markers of programmed cell death are increased in the presence of postnatal experimental obstruction of the ureter (Connor et al, 1991).

CELL–CELL AND CELL–MATRIX ADHESION MOLECULES

Morphogenesis is a three-dimensional process and, for example, the branching ureteric bud is supported by renal mesenchyme, which contains both a cellular and an extracellular matrix component. Within the metanephros, matrices are composed of combinations of structural proteins such as collagens I and IV together with fibronectin, laminin, nidogen/entactin and also proteoglycans including heparan sulphate. Matrix molecules interact with each other and also with epithelial and mesenchymal cells via specific cell-surface molecules such as the integrins and proteoglycans. Experiments performed in vitro have shown that supporting material around branching epithelia need not contain living cells but that molecules of the extracellular matrix can suffice to support morphogenesis. For example, dispersed renal epithelial cells and also the ureteric bud can form branches when grown in collagen I gels and provided with appropriate growth factors (Taub et al, 1990; Montesano et al, 1991; Perantoni et al, 1991). Interestingly, embryonic kidneys from collagen-I deficient mice appear to develop normally in organ culture, possibly because increased quantities of collagens III and V may have substituted for collagen I (Kratochwil et al, 1986).

In metanephric organ culture, antibodies to the laminin A chain, or to its cell-surface integrin receptor, prevent the formation of polarized nephron tubules from the undifferentiated renal mesenchyme (Klein et al, 1988). Epimorphin is a 150-kD protein located on the surface of aggregated mesenchymal cells and the molecule is found in a wide variety of tissues that are undergoing organogenesis, including lung, kidney, intestine and skin (Hirai et al, 1992). In organ culture a monoclonal antibody to epimorphin perturbed epithelial development in the lung, and when epimorphin was expressed in an immortalized embryonic fibroblast cell line it acquired the ability to induce tubule formation when co-cultured with lung epithelial cells. Currently it is not clear whether the molecule has a specific function in kidney development. The addition of antibodies to GD_3 ganglioside will prevent branching of the ureteric bud in metanephric organ culture; this molecule is located on the surface of renal mesenchymal cells (Sariola et al, 1988). Finally, the chemical disruption of proteoglycans with β-D-xyloside has been reported to disrupt the branching of the ureteric bud (Platt et al, 1987).

INTRACELLULAR MOLECULES THAT CONTROL CELL PROLIFERATION AND DEATH

Transgenic mice (see Chapter 4) that over-express cellular and/or viral oncogenes commonly develop renal cysts. The products of these genes, such as c-myc protein (Trudel et al, 1991) and the SV40 simian virus T antigen (McKay et al, 1987), stimulate cell division, directly implicating excessive cell proliferation in renal cystic disease. These transgenic animals sometimes develop small renal epithelial neoplasms, a tendency shared with some patients with cystic kidneys. Further evidence supporting a primary role of proliferation in cyst formation comes from a mouse model that phenotypically resembles human ARPKD in that it develops polycystic kidneys and liver fibrosis (Moyer et al, 1994). Here the mutated gene has been defined and most likely codes for a protein with a role in cell division. Paradoxically, recent studies in mice have also directly implicated excessive cell death in the pathogenesis of cystic kidneys. bcl-2 is a gene that prevents apoptosis (programmed cell death), and genetically engineered mice that do not express functional bcl-2 protein have increased renal apoptosis, develop extensive renal cysts and subsequently die from kidney failure (Veis et al, 1994). Just how excessive cell death leads to cell proliferation and cyst formation remains a mystery. In this context it is of note that the over-expression of c-myc in cell lines in vitro can drive cells either into proliferation or apoptosis depending on the provision or absence of growth factors such as IGF I (Harrington et al, 1994).

DEVELOPMENTAL BIOLOGY OF HUMAN KIDNEY MALFORMATIONS

(The inheritance and chromosomal location of the diseases discussed in this section are given in Table 14.3.)

RENAL DYSPLASIAS AND AGENESIS

These malformations probably have varied aetiologies but **teratogens**, such as lead and glucose, have only rarely been implicated in their pathogenesis. Some

Table 14.3   Genetics of human kidney malformations

Renal dysplasias and agenesis
- Kallman syndrome: Recessive. Xp22.3. *KAL* gene. Matrix or cell adhesion molecule
- Coloboma, vesico-ureteric reflux and congenitally small kidneys: Autosomal dominant. *PAX2* mutation in chromosome 10
- Isolated renal disease: Autosomal dominant. Chromosome and gene unknown
- Branchio-oto-renal syndrome: Dominant. Chromosome 8. Gene unknown
- Isolated vesico-ureteric reflux: Autosomal dominant. Chromosome and gene unknown

Cystic kidney diseases
- Autosomal dominant polycystic kidney disease 1 (ADPKD1): 16p13.3. *PKD1* gene. Function unknown
- Autosomal dominant polycystic kidney disease 2 (ADPKD2): 4q13–q23. *PKD2* gene
- Juvenile nephronophthisis (medullary cystic disease): Recessive. 2q13. Gene unknown
- Tuberous sclerosis: Autosomal dominant. 16p13.3. *TSC2* gene. Tumour suppressor gene?
- von Hippel–Lindau disease: Autosomal dominant. 3p25–p26. Tumour suppressor gene?
- Autosomal recessive polycystic kidney disease (ARPKD): 6p21–cen. Gene unknown

Glomerular structural abnormalities
- Alport syndrome: X-linked. *Collagen IV* $\alpha5$. Basement membrane protein in glomerulus
- Alport syndrome: Autosomal recessive. *Collagen IV* $\alpha3$ and $\alpha4$. Basement membrane protein in glomerulus
- Congenital nephrotic syndrome (Finnish type): Autosomal recessive 19q12–13.1. Gene unknown
- Denys–Drash syndrome: Sporadic mutations. 11p13. *WT1* gene. Multiple functions including mesenchymal survival, glomerular epithelial cell function and tumour suppression

are associated with urethral obstruction and here the renal malformation might result from physical damage caused by an increased hydrostatic pressure within the urinary tract. In this context it is of note that when the mammalian renal tract is ligated during mid- to late-gestation it is possible to generate renal cysts and a mild kidney dysplasia (Gonzalez et al, 1990). In contrast, when the lower urinary tract of the chick kidney was experimentally obstructed at an even earlier stage of gestation it is not possible to perturb development of the metanephros (Berman and Maizels, 1982). It is difficult to reconcile the findings of these two studies. It should be noted that the ureter and its connection with the urinary bladder both have their developmental origins in the ureteric bud and mesonephric duct and it is possible that coexistent kidney, ureteric and bladder malformations have a common origin in aberrant embryology. Moreover, many other cases of renal dysplasias are not associated with an obstructed lower urinary tract and may result from an intrinsic disruption during early nephrogenesis.

Kidney malformations are commonly found in the presence of major chromosomal deletions or trisomies. Affected fetuses and neonates are usually not viable due to coexisting major malformations of the heart, brain and gut (Al-Khaldi et al,

1994). Renal agenesis and dysplasias can sometimes occur in kindreds suggesting that there is a genetic component to their pathogenesis; in such cases the renal disease may occur in isolation or form part of a syndrome such as the **branchio-oto-renal syndrome**. Renal agenesis, either uni- or bilateral, occurs in 30–50% of patients who suffer from the X-linked Kallmann syndrome (Hardelin et al, 1993). In this disorder, infertility and anosmia are classic clinical features. These are caused by the failure of migration of neurones from the olfactory placode into the brain during embryogenesis. Kallmann patients have a mutation of the *KAL* gene, which codes for a putative cell-surface or extracellular matrix protein that has homology with both N-CAM and fibronectin (Franco et al, 1991). In humans, *KAL* transcripts are expressed in the developing brain at 12 weeks of gestation and also in the meso- and metanephros at 6 weeks of gestation, critical times for organogenesis in these systems (Duke et al, 1995). These data strongly suggest that the KAL protein may be actively involved in nephrogenesis, although its exact role is not yet known. Based on this example, it is possible that mutations of other genes, including those which code for transcription and paracrine factors or their receptors, will also be implicated in the genesis of human renal malformations. For example, isolated **vesico-ureteric reflux**, a disorder that may coexist with renal dysplasia, is often inherited in an autosomal dominant manner but so far this gene has not been located (Feather et al, 1996). However, *PAX2* mutations are implicated in the rare coloboma–vesico-ureteric reflux syndrome (Sanyanusin et al, 1995). In the autosomal dominant branchio-oto-renal syndrome, kidney dysplasia may be a feature and the gene has been localized to chromosome 8.

POLYCYSTIC KIDNEY DISEASES

Genetic linkage of an ADPKD locus to the α-globin gene on chromosome 16 was reported in 1985. It is only recently, however, that the *PKD1* candidate gene has been isolated on 16p13.3 (European Polycystic Kidney Disease Consortium, 1994). Mutations of this gene may account for up to 90% of ADPKD cases, while another locus, on 4q13–q23, has been implicated in other patients. The normal function of the *PKD1* gene is unknown and is difficult to surmise since there is no significant homology of its predicted protein product with known proteins. In 1994, human ARPKD was mapped to chromosome 6p21–cen, although the specific mutation is not yet defined (Zerres et al, 1994). Both tuberous sclerosis and von Hippel–Lindau disease are inherited in an autosomal dominant fashion and may present with polycystic kidney disease. *TSC2*, a gene mutated in some patients with tuberous sclerosis, is expressed in a wide variety of tissues and its predicted protein product has homology to molecules implicated in the control of cell differentiation and proliferation. Interestingly, it is located very close to *PKD1* on chromosome 16 (European Chromosome 16 Tuberous Sclerosis Consortium, 1993). It has been postulated that the normal von Hippel–Lindau gene, located on chromosome 3p25–p26 (Latif et al, 1993), acts as a tumour suppressor in a similar fashion to the *WT1* transcription factor gene (Bard et al, 1993). From the above discussion it is apparent that human polycystic kidneys can be caused by mutations of diverse genes.

Cell biology of cyst formation

Given that the specific roles of many of these genes, either during or after renal development, remain undefined, can we learn anything useful about cyst pathogenesis from the investigation of kidney cells themselves? The mitotic rate of normal adult tubular epithelia is very low but, in a cystic kidney, epithelial cells must be continually born to provide a lining for enlarging cysts. Epithelial cells derived from renal cysts divide faster than their normal counterparts even when isolated in the test-tube (Woolf and Winyard, 1995). However, observations from our laboratory suggest that apoptosis is widespread in tissue between cysts in both multicystic dysplastic kidneys and in polycystic kidneys (Winyard et al, 1996a). Based on this evidence, excessive apoptosis would also explain the spontaneous involution seen in some cases of multicystic dysplastic kidneys, and may also contribute to the destruction of normal renal tissue in ARPKD and ADPKD. On the other hand, *PAX2*, a potential proto-oncogene, is over-expressed in cyst epithelia in multicystic dysplastic kidneys (Winyard et al, 1996b).

Mature kidney epithelial cells are said to be 'polarized'. They have an apical plasma membrane that faces the tubule lumen and a basal plasma membrane facing the interstitium. Each is distinct in its biochemistry and morphology. Subtle aberrations in the polarity of the renal epithelia have been detected in both human (Wilson et al, 1991) and animal polycystic kidney disease (Avner et al, 1992). Most notably, the Na^+-K^+-ATPase ion pump is found on the apical membrane of epithelial cells in polycystic disease, whereas it is normally situated in the basal membrane. This mislocalization could contribute to cyst expansion by the active secretion of ions into the lumen. Similarly, other studies have found that ADPKD cysts contain high concentrations of amino acids which are normally pumped out of the tubular lumen (Foxall et al, 1992). During nephron formation, the acquisition of polarity by nascent epithelia is directed by matrix proteins that envelop precursor mesenchymal cells. Although biochemical and structural abnormalities have been detected in the basement membranes of cystic epithelia, it is unknown whether such abnormalities are the prime movers or just epiphenomena of renal cyst formation. Renal cysts can be generated in the test-tube using immortalized epithelial cell lines. These models have implicated various ion pumps in cyst growth including Na^+-K^+-ATPase, Na^+-dependent H^+ and Ca^{2+} transport as well as Cl^-/HCO_3^- and Na^+/H^+ exchangers. Pharmacological blockade of these pumps with oubain, amiloride and cAMP inhibitors slow cyst growth in vitro (Macias et al, 1992).

ABNORMALITIES OF GLOMERULAR DEVELOPMENT

The **Denys–Drash syndrome** consists of nephrotic syndrome caused by mesangial sclerosis, together with bilateral Wilms' tumours and ambiguous genitalia. All affected children carry constitutional missense mutations of the *WT1* gene located on chromosome 11p13, usually in exons 8 or 9. The phenotype of the disease can be explained as follows. (1) Proteinuria and nephrotic syndrome result from abnormal biology of the podocyte epithelium, a site that expresses *WT1* into adulthood, (2) the ambiguous genitalia are caused by aberrant development of the gonads, a site of normal *WT1* expression and (3) the Wilms' tumours are due to mutations of *WT1*, which in this context functions as a tumour suppressor gene. The **Finnish-type nephrotic syndrome** is an autosomal recessive disease. Here the mutation has been localized to chromosome 19 but the precise gene mutation awaits discovery (Tryggvason et al, 1994). **Alport's syndrome** consists of X-linked inherited deafness with nephropathy due to structural abnormalities of the glomerulus. Some patients have mutations in the coding region of the *collagen IV α5* gene, which is expressed in the glomerular basement membrane. In addition, a very similar disease can occasionally be inherited in an autosomal recessive manner and in these cases the *collagen IV α3* or *α4* genes have been found to be mutated (Lemmink et al, 1994).

HOW MUCH HAVE ANIMAL MODELS OF DISEASE ILLUMINATED HUMAN DISORDERS?

When the reader compares the insights into nephrogenesis accrued from the animal models, reviewed above, with what is known about the molecular basis of human renal diseases, it can be seen that these two fields currently have little in common in terms of candidate genes. Perhaps the *WTI* and *PAX2* gene products are the only proteins which have clearly been implicated in the genesis of both human and mouse kidney birth defects. None of the loci implicated in inherited animal models of polycystic kidney disease are syntenic with the known human diseases. There are, however, more parallels when we consider broader biological concepts such as the control of cell death, proliferation and differentiation; this alone makes the existing animal models so important and these observations suggest directions for therapeutic intervention. In addition, comparatively little is known about the genes involved in the pathogenesis of human renal dysplasias and agenesis, and in due course some of these mutations may be found to be similar to those in animal models such as the *ret* or PDGF-β mutations discussed above.

NEW TREATMENTS FOR HUMAN KIDNEY MALFORMATIONS

The studies described above suggest aberrant biological processes in renal dysplasias and polycystic kidney diseases that might be targeted using specific therapies. The latter disorders could be the more easy to treat because the essential anatomy of the kidney is initially normal. Conventional treatment of human polycystic kidney disease has been based on more general strategies used for the amelioration of progressive renal failure. The large multicentre Modification of Diet in Renal Disease Study found no beneficial effects on the progression of renal cystic disease in ADPKD with either low-protein diets or blood pressure reduction (Klahr et al, 1993). Cyst decompression surgery has also been tried but has no significant effect in slowing long-term tissue destruction in ADPKD (Etsinga et al, 1992). Clinical trials in patients are hampered by the heterogeneity in presentation and the slowly progressive nature of many cystic kidney diseases. The ideal animal model with which to test potential anti-cyst therapies would be engineered to have the same gene defect as the human disease. Such a strategy has been used to produce a 'cystic fibrosis mouse' (Dorin et al, 1992) and could be developed for PKD1. In the mean time the nearest animal models are phenotypic, rather than genotypic, although some recent studies look promising.

Homozygous *cpk* knockout mice develop cystic kidneys and die from uraemia at 1 month of age in a disease that resembles early-onset human ARPKD (Woo et al, 1994). Treatment with Taxol prevents cyst formation in vitro and preserves renal function in vivo, prolonging life span beyond 6 months of age. Taxol stabilizes microtubules in the cell cytoskeleton; these structures have been implicated in the transport of newly synthesized proteins to the apical plasma membrane. Therefore, in the *cpk* cystic mice, Taxol may prevent the incorporation of Na^+-K^+-ATPase into the apical epithelial membrane and hence the abnormal movement of water and solutes into the lumen of the cysts. Taxol also inhibits cell proliferation by disrupting the function of mitotic spindles and it is possible that this action also contributes to the inhibition of growth of renal cysts.

Other drugs have been reported to be effective in slowing renal cystic diseases in animals, including corticosteroids (Barash et al, 1992) and EGF (Gattone and Lowden, 1992). The basis for the action of corticosteroids is currently unknown, whereas EGF is thought to drive the potentially cystic renal tubular epithelia into a more mature, less proliferative state. It is of note that EGF also prevents apoptosis in the embryonic kidney (Koseki et al, 1992; Coles et al, 1993), thus providing an alternative mechanism of action in view of the enhanced apoptosis that may occur in cystic renal diseases (Veis et al, 1994; Winyard et al, 1996a). Therefore, at least for certain strains of mice with cystic kidneys, medications appear promising. It now needs to be determined whether the therapies are effective in other animal models before these powerful drugs, with their potentially toxic side-effects, can be recommended for use in patients with cystic kidneys. It should also be remembered that human cystic kidneys often occur in the context of complex syndromes that affect multiple organs and we do not know whether the novel therapies that prevent the progression of renal cysts will also affect the natural history of associated conditions such as the intracranial aneurysms in ADPKD and hepatic fibrosis in ARPKD.

IS GENE THERAPY A FEASIBLE TREATMENT FOR RENAL MALFORMATIONS?

The alternative, long-term approach that must now be given serious consideration is renal gene therapy. The success of this strategy depends on defining all the genes that cause cystic renal disease and then refining the technology for gene transfer into the kidney. It is currently feasible to insert novel genes into the epithelia of postnatal kidneys, either by stem cell transfer (Woolf et al, 1990, 1993) or direct gene transduction (Moullier et al, 1994), but there are problems in achieving long-term gene expression in a biologically significant number of kidney cells. In addition, because many cystic kidney diseases progress in utero, the therapeutic window may only occur before birth, making the development of a technology for successful gene transfer even more of a challenge. However it is tantalizing to speculate that gene transfer could correct specific genetic defects leading to normal, cyst-free kidneys.

ACKNOWLEDGEMENTS

A.S.W. is supported by the National Kidney Research Fund and the Kidney Research Aid Fund.

REFERENCES

Al-Khaldi, N., Watson, A.R., Zucollo, J., Twining, P. and Rose, D.H. (1994) Outcome of antenatally detected cystic dysplastic kidney disease. *Arch. Dis. Child.* **70**, 520–522.

Alpers, C.E., Seifert, R.A., Hudkins, K.L., Johnson, R.J. and Bowen-Pope, D.R. (1992) Developmental patterns of platelet derived growth factor B-chain, PDGF receptor and α-actin expression in human glomerulogenesis. *Kidney Int.* **42**, 390–399.

Avner, E.D., Sweeney, W.E. and Nelson, W.J. (1992) Abnormal sodium pump distribution during renal tubulogenesis in congenital murine polycystic kidney disease. *Proc. Soc. Natl Acad. Sci. USA* **89**, 7447–7451.

Barash, B.D., Cowley, B.D., Takahashi, H. et al (1992) Glucocorticoid inhibition of renal cystic disease in two rodent models of inherited polycystic kidney disease. *J. Am. Soc. Nephrol.* **3**, 293.

Bard, J.B.H. and Ross, A.S.A. (1991) The ES-cell inhibition factor reversibly blocks nephrogenesis in cultured mouse kidney rudiments. *Development* **113**, 193–199.

Bard, J.B.H., Armstrong, J.F. and Bickmore, W.A. (1993) WT1, a Wilms' tumour gene. *Exp. Nephrol.* **1**, 218–233.

Berman, D. and Maizels, M. (1982) The role of urinary obstruction in the genesis of renal dysplasia. *J. Urol.* **128**, 1091–1097.

Bernstein, J., Cheng, F. and Roszka, J. (1981) Glomerular differentiation in metanephric culture. *Lab. Invest.* **45**, 183–193.

Birchmeier, C. and Birchmeier, W. (1993) Molecular aspects of mesenchymal–epithelial interactions. *Annu. Rev. Cell Biol.* **9**, 511–540.

Breier, G., Albrecht, U., Sterrer, S. and Risau, W. (1992) Expression of vascular endothelial growth factor during embryonic angiogenesis and endothelial cell differentiation. *Development* **114**, 521–532.

Coles, H.S.R., Burne, J.F. and Raff, M.C. (1993) Large-scale normal cell death in the developing rat kidney and its reduction by epidermal growth factor. *Development* **118**, 777–784.

Connor, J., Buttyan, R., Olsson, C.A. et al (1991) SGP-2 expression as a genetic marker of progressive cellular pathology in experimental hydronephrosis. *Kidney Int.* **39**, 1098–1103.

Coppes, M.J., Huff, V. and Pelletier, J. (1993) Denys–Drash syndrome: relating a clinical disorder to alterations in the tumor suppressor gene WT1. *J. Paediatr.* **123**, 673–678.

De Chiara, T.M., Efstratiadis, A. and Robertson, E.J. (1990) A growth-deficiency phenotype in heterozygous mice carrying an insulin-like growth factor II gene disrupted by targeting. *Nature* **345**, 78–80.

Dorin, J.R., Dickinson, P., Alton, E.W. et al (1992) Cystic fibrosis in the mouse by targeted insertional mutagenesis. *Nature* **359**, 211–215.

Dressler, G.R., Wilkinson, J.E., Rothenpieler, U.W. et al (1993) Deregulation of *Pax-2* expression in transgenic mice generates severe kidney abnormalities. *Nature* **362**, 65–67.

Drummond, I.A., Madden, S.L., Rohwer-Nutter, P. et al (1991) Repression of the insulin-like growth factor II gene by Wilms' tumor suppressor WT1. *Science* **257**, 674–677.

Duke, V.M., Winyard, P.J.D., Thorogood, P. et al (1995) *KAL*, a gene mutated in Kallmann's syndrome, is expressed in the first trimester of human development. *Mol. Cell. Endocrinol.* **110**, 73–79.

Etsinga, L.W., Barry, J.M., Torres, V.E. et al (1992) Cyst decompression surgery for autosomal dominant polycystic kidney disease. *J. Am. Soc. Nephrol.* **2**, 1219–1226.

European Chromosome 16 Tuberous Sclerosis Consortium (1993) Identification and characterisation of the tuberous sclerosis gene on chromosome 16. *Cell* **75**, 1305–1315.

European Polycystic Kidney Disease Consortium (1994) The polycystic kidney disease 1 gene encodes a 14 kb transcript and lies within a duplicated region on chromosome 16. *Cell* **77**, 881–894.

Feather, S., Woolf, A.S., Gordon, I., Risdon, R.A. and Verrier-Jones, K. (1996) Vesicoureteric reflux – is it all in the genes? *Lancet* **348**, 725–728.

Fick, G.M., Johnson, A.M. and Gabow, P.A. (1994) Is there evidence for anticipation in autosomal-dominant polycystic kidney disease? *Kidney Int.* **45**, 1153–1162.

Fotino, S. (1989) The solitary kidney: a model of chronic hyperfiltration. *Am. J. Kidney Dis.* **13**, 88–98.

Foxall, P.J.D., Price, R.G., Jones, J.K. et al (1992) High resolution proton magnetic resonance spectroscopy of cyst fluids from patients with polycystic kidney disease. *Biochem. Biophy. Acta* **1138**, 305–314.

Franco, B., Guioli, S., Pragliola, A. et al (1991) A gene deleted in Kallmann's syndrome shares homology with neural cell adhesion and axonal path-finding molecules. *Nature* **353**, 529–536.

Gattone, V.H. and Lowden, D.A. (1992) Epidermal growth factor ameliorates infantile polycystic kidney disease in mice. *J. Am. Soc. Nephrol.* **3**, 295.

Gonzalez, R., Reinberg, Y., Burke, B., Wells, T. and Vernier, R.L. (1990) Early bladder outlet obstruction in fetal lambs induces renal dysplasia and the prune-belly syndrome. *J. Pediatr. Surg.* **25**, 342–345.

Grobstein, C. (1955) Inductive interaction in the development of the mouse metanephros. *J. Exp. Zool.* **130**, 319–340.

Grobstein, C. (1967) Mechanisms of organotypic tissue interactions. *Nat. Cancer Inst. Monogr.* **26**, 279–299.

Hardelin, J.-P., Levilliers, J., Young, J. et al (1993) Xp22.3 deletions in isolated familial Kallmann's syndrome. *J. Clin. Endocrinol. Metab.* **76**, 827–831.

Hardman, P., Kolatsi, M., Winyard, P.J., Towers, P.R. and Woolf, A.S. (1994a) Branching out with the ureteric bud. *Exp. Nephrol.* **2**, 211–219.

Hardman, P., Landels, E., Woolf, A.S. and Spooner, B.S. (1994b) Transforming growth factor-β1 inhibits growth and branching morphogenesis in embryonic mouse submandibular and sublingual glands. *Dev. Growth Differ.* **36**, 567–577.

Harrington, E.A., Bennett, M.R., Fanidi, A. and Evan, G.I. (1994) c-Myc-induced apoptosis in fibroblasts is inhibited by specific cytokines. *EMBO J.* **13**, 3286–3295.

Herzlinger, D., Koseki, C., Mikawa, T. and Al-Awqati, Q. (1991) Metanephric mesenchyme contains multipotent stem cells whose fate is restricted after induction. *Development* **114**, 565–572.

Hildebrandt, F., Singh-Sawhney, I., Schnieders, B. et al (1994) Combined genetic and physical mapping to localise a gene for familial juvenile nephronophthisis (recessive medullary cystic disease). *J. Am. Soc. Nephrol.* **5**, 625.

Hirai, Y., Takebe, K., Takashina, M., Kobayashi, S. and Takeichi, M. (1992) Epimorphin: a mesenchymal protein essential for epithelial morphogenesis. *Cell* **69**, 471–481.

Hirata, G.I., Medearis, A.L. and Platt, L.D. (1990) Fetal abdominal abnormalities associated with genetic syndromes. *Clin. Perinatol.* **17**, 675–702.

Holliday, M.A., Barratt, T.M. and Avner, E. (1994) *Pediatric Nephrology*. Williams and Wilkins: Baltimore, MD.

Hulton, S.-A., Thomson, P.D., Milner, L.S., Isdale, J.M. and Ling, J. (1990) The pattern of congenital renal anomalies associated with neural tube defects. *Pediatr. Nephrol.* **4**, 491–492.

Kaplan, B.S., Gordon, I., Pincott, J. and Barratt, T.M. (1989) Familial hypoplastic glomerulocystic kidney disease. *Am. J. Med. Genet.* **34**, 569–573.

Kaplan, B.S., Kaplan, P. and Ruchelli, E. (1991) Inherited and congenital malformations of the kidneys in the neonatal period. *Clin. Perinatol.* **19**, 197–211.

Kissane, J.M. (1990) Renal cysts in pediatric patients: a classification and overview. *Pediatr. Nephrol.* **4**, 69–77.

Klahr, S., Beck, G., Breyer, G. et al (1993) Dietary protein restriction and reduced blood pressure goal in adults with polycystic kidney disease. *J. Am. Soc. Nephrol.* **4**, 263.

Klein, G., Langegger, M., Timpl, R. and Ekblom, P. (1988) Role of laminin A chain in the development of epithelial cell polarity. *Cell* **55**, 331–341.

Kohn, G. and Borns, P.F. (1973) The association of bilateral and unilateral renal aplasia in the same family. *J. Pediatr.* **83**, 95–100.

Koneto, H., Morrisey, J. and Klahr, S. (1993) Increased expression of TGF-β1 mRNA in the kidney of rats obstructed with unilateral ligation. *Kidney Int.* **44**, 313–321.

Koseki, C., Herzlinger, D. and Al-Awqati, Q. (1992) Apoptosis in metanephric development. *J. Cell Biol.* **119**, 1322–1333.

Kratochwil, K., Dziadek, M., Lohler, J., Harbers, K. and Jaenisch, R. (1986) Normal epithelial branching morphogenesis in the absence of collagen I. *Dev. Biol.* **117**, 596–606.

Kreidberg, J.A., Sariola, H., Loring, J.M. et al (1993) WT-1 is required for early kidney development. *Cell* **74**, 679–691.

Kress, C., Vogels, R., DeGraff, V. et al (1990) *Hox-2.3* upstream sequences mediate *lacZ* expression in intermediate mesoderm derivatives of transgenic mice. *Development* **109**, 775–786.

Larsson, S.H. Charlieu, J.-P., Miykawa, K. et al (1995) Subnuclear localisation of WT1 in splicing of transcription factor domains is regulated by alternative splicing. *Cell* **81**, 391–401.

Latif, F., Kalman, T., Gnarra, J. et al (1993) Identification of the von Hippel–Lindau disease tumor suppressor gene. *Science* **260**, 1317–1320.

Lee, K.-F., Li, E., Huber, J. et al (1992) Targeted mutation of the gene encoding the low affinity NGF receptor p75 leads to deficits in the peripheral sensory nervous system. *Cell* **69**, 733–749.

Lemmink, H.H., van den Heuvel, L., Mochizuki, T. et al (1994) Molecular and immunological studies in X-linked and autosomal recessive Alport's syndrome. *J. Am. Soc. Nephrol.* **5**, 629.

Letterio, J.J., Geiser, A.G., Kulkarni, A.B. et al (1994) Maternal rescue of TGF-β1 mice. *Science* **264**, 1936–1937.

Leveen, P., Pekney, M., Gebre-Medhin, S. et al (1994) Mice deficient in platelet derived growth factor B show cardiovascular and hematological abnormalities. *Genes Dev.* **8**, 1875–1887.

Loughna, S., Landels, E.C. and Woolf, A.S. (1996) Growth factor control of developing kidney endothelial cells. *Exp. Nephrol.* **4**, 112–116.

Macias, W.I., McAteer, J.A., Tanner, G.A., Fritz, A.I. and Armstrong, W.McD. (1992) NaCl transport by Madin Darby canine kidney cyst epithelial cells. *Kidney Int.* **42**, 308–319.

Maizel, M. and Simpson, S.B. (1983) Primitive ducts of renal dysplasia induced by culturing ureteral buds denuded of condensed renal mesenchyme. *Science* **219**, 509–510.

McEnery, P.T., Stablein, D.M., Arbus, G. and Tejani, A. (1992) Renal transplantation in children. *New Engl. J. Med.* **326**, 1727–1732.

McKay, K., Striker, L.J., Pinkert, C.A., Brinster, R.L. and Striker, G.E. (1987) Glomerulosclerosis and renal cysts in mice transgenic for the early region of SV40. *Kidney Int.* **32**, 827–837.

McPherson, E., Carey, J., Hall, J.G. et al (1987) Dominantly inherited renal adysplasia. *Am. J. Med. Genet.* **26**, 836–846.

Mesrobian, H.-G.J., Rushton, H.G. and Bulas, D. (1993) Unilateral renal agenesis may result from in utero regression of multicystic dysplasia. *J. Urol.* **150**, 793–794.

Millauer, B., Wizigmann-Voos, S., Schnürch, H. et al (1993) High affinity VEGF binding and developmental expression suggest flk-1 as a major regulator of vasculogenesis and angiogenesis. *Cell* **72**, 835–845.

Montesano, R., Matsumoto, K., Nakamura, T. and Orci, L. (1991) Identification of a fibroblast-derived epithelial morphogen as hepatocyte growth factor. *Cell* **67**, 901–908.

Moullier, P., Friedlander, G., Calise, D. et al (1994) Adenoviral-mediated gene transfer into renal tubular cells in vivo. *Kidney Int.* **45**, 1220–1225.

Moyer, J.H., Lee-Tischler, M.J., Kwon, H.-Y. et al (1994) Candidate gene associated with a mutation causing recessive polycystic kidney disease in mice. *Science* **264**, 1329–1333.

Murugasu, B., Cole, B.R., Hawkins, E.P. et al (1991) Familial renal adysplasia. *Am. J. Kidney Dis.* **18**, 490–495.

Oberhammer, F., Wilson, J.W., Dive, C. et al (1993) Apoptotic death in epithelial cells. *EMBO J.* **12**, 3679–3684.

Pachnis, V., Mankoo, B. and Constantini, F. (1993) Expression of the c-ret proto-oncogene during mouse development. *Development* **119**, 1005–1114.

Perantoni, A.O., Williams, C.L. and Lewellyn, A.L. (1991) Growth and branching morphogenesis of rat collecting duct anlagen in the absence of metanephrogenic mesenchyme. *Differentiation* **48**, 107–113.

Pinson, D.Y., St John, P.L., Tucker, D.C. and Abrahamson, D.R. (1993) Origin of glomerular microvasculature in kidneys developing *in oculo*. *J. Am. Soc. Nephrol.* **4**, 474.

Platt, J.L., Brown, D.M., Granlund, K., Oegema, T.R. and Klein, D.J. (1987) Proteoglycan metabolism associated with mouse metanephric development: morphologic and biochemical effects of b-D-xyloside. *Dev. Biol.* **123**, 293–306.

Potter, E.L. (1972) *Normal and Abnormal Development of the Kidney*. Year Book Medical: Chicago, IL.

Ravine, D., Gibson, R.N., Donlan, J. and Sheffield, L.J. (1993) An ultrasound renal cyst prevalence survey. *Am. J. Kidney Dis.* **22**, 6–11.

Risdon, R.A. (1971) Renal dysplasia. 1. A clinicopathological study of 76 cases. *J. Clin. Path.* **24**, 57–71.

Rogers, S.A., Ryan, G. and Hammerman, M.R. (1991) Insulin-like growth factors I and II are produced in the metanephros and are required for growth and development in vitro. *J. Cell Biol.* **113**, 1447–1453.

Rogers, S.A., Ryan, G. and Hammerman, M.R. (1992) Metanephric transforming growth factor-a is required for renal organogenesis in vitro. *Am. J. Physiol.* **262**, F533–F539.

Rogers, S.A., Ryan, G., Purchio, A.F. and Hammerman, M.R. (1993) Metanephric transforming growth factor-b1 regulates nephrogenesis in vitro. *Am. J. Physiol.* **264**, F996–F1002.

Roodhooft, A.M., Birnholz, J.C. and Holmes, L.B. (1984) Familial nature of congenital absence and severe dysgenesis of both kidneys. *New Engl. J. Med.* **310**, 1341–1345.

Rothenpieler, U.W. (1994) Antisense oligonucleotides directed against Wilms' tumor gene WT1 inhibit kidney differentiation and development. *J. Am. Soc. Nephrol.* **5**, 635.

Rothenpieler, U.W. and Dressler, G.R. (1993) *Pax-2* is required for mesenchyme-to-epithelium conversion during kidney development. *Development* **119**, 711–720.

Santos, O.F.P. and Nigam, S.K. (1993) HGF-induced tubulogenesis and branching of epithelial cells is modulated by extracellular matrix and TGF-β. *Dev. Biol.* **160**, 293–302.

Sanyanusin, P., Schimmenti, L.A., McNoe, L.A. et al (1995) Mutations of the PAX2 gene in a family with optic nerve colobomas, renal anomalies and vesico-ureteric reflux. *Nature Genetics* **9**, 358–364.

Sariola, H., Ekblom, P., Lehtonen, E. and Saxen, L. (1983) Differentiation and vascularisation of the metanephric kidney grafted on the chorioallantoic membrane. *Dev. Biol.* **96**, 427–437.

Sariola, H., Aufderheide, E., Bernhard, H. et al (1988) Antibodies to cell surface ganglioside GD$_3$ perturb inductive epithelial–mesenchymal interactions. *Cell* **54**, 235–245.

Sariola, H., Ekblom, P. and Henke-Fahle, S. (1989) Embryonic neurons as *in vitro* inducers of differentiation of nephrogenic mesenchyme. *Dev. Biol.* **132**, 271–281.

Sariola, H., Saarma, M., Sainio, K. et al (1991) Dependence of kidney morphogenesis on the expression of nerve growth factor receptor. *Science* **254**, 571–573.

Saxen, L. (1987) *Organogenesis of the Kidney.* Cambridge University Press: Cambridge.

Schmidt, C., Bladt, F., Goedecke, S. et al (1995) SF/HGF is essential for liver development. *Nature* **373**, 699–702.

Schuchardt, A., D'Agati, V., Larsson-Blomberg, L., Constantini, F. and Pachnis, V. (1994) Defects in kidney and enteric nervous system of mice lacking the tyrosine kinase receptor Ret. *Nature* **367**, 380–383.

Sonnenberg, E., Godecke, A., Walter, B., Bladt, F. and Birchmeier, C. (1991) Transient and locally restricted expression of the *ros 1* protooncogene during mouse development. *EMBO J.* **10**, 3693–3702.

Sonnenberg, E., Meyer, D., Weidner, K.M. and Birchmeier, C. (1993) Scatter factor/ hepatocyte growth factor and its receptor, the c-met tyrosine kinase, can mediate a signal exchange between mesenchyme and epithelia during mouse development. *J. Cell Biol.* **123**, 223–235.

Soriano, P. (1994) Abnormal kidney development and hematological disorders in platelet derived growth factor β-receptor mutant mice. *Genes Dev.* **8**, 1888–1896.

Stein, P.L., Vogel, H. and Soriano, P. (1994) Combined deficiencies of Src, Fyn and Yes tyrosine kinases in mutant mice. *Genes Dev.* **8**, 1999–2007.

Stoker, M., Gherardi, E., Perryman, M. and Gray, J. (1987) Scatter factor is a fibroblast-derived modulator of epithelial cell mobility. *Nature* **327**, 239–242.

Taub, M., Wang, Y., Szczesny, T.M. and Kleinman, H.K. (1990) Epidermal growth factor or transforming growth factor a is required for kidney tubulogenesis in matrigel cultures in serum-free medium. *Proc. Soc. Natl Acad. Sci. USA.* **87**, 4002–4006.

Treanor, J.J.S., Goodman, L., de Sauvage, F. et al (1996) Characterisation of a multicomponent receptor for GDNF. *Nature* **832**, 80–83.

Trudel, M., D'Agati, V. and Costantini, F. (1991) *c-myc* as an inducer of polycystic disease in transgenic mice. *Kidney Int.* **39**, 665–671.

Tryggvason, K., Kestila, M., Mannikko, M. et al (1994) Mapping of the locus for congenital nephrotic syndrome of the Finnish type to chromosome 19q. *J. Am. Soc. Nephrol.* **5**, 638.

Vainio, S., Jalkanen, M., Bernfield, M. and Saxen, L. (1989) Transient expression of syndecan in mesenchymal cell aggregates of the embryonic kidney. *Dev. Biol.* **152**, 221–232.

Van Heyningen, V. (1994) One gene – four syndromes. *Nature* **367**, 319–320.

Veis, D.J., Sorenson, C.M., Shutter, J.R. and Korsmeyer, S.J. (1994) Bcl-2-deficient mice demonstrate fulminant lymphoid apoptosis, polycystic kidneys and hypopigmented hair. *Cell* **75**, 229–240.

Wang, Z.Y., Madden, S.L., Devel, T.F. and Raucher III, F. (1992) The Wilms' tumor gene product, WT1, represses the transcription of the platelet derived growth factor A chain. *J. Biol. Chem.* **267**, 21999–22002.

Weller, A., Sorokin, L., Illegen, E.-M. and Ekblom, P. (1991) Development and growth of mouse embryonic kidney in organ culture and modulation of development by soluble growth factor. *Dev. Biol.* **144**, 248–261.

Wilson, P.D., Sherwood, A.C., Palla, Du J., Watson, R. and Norman, J.T. (1991) Reversed polarity of Na$^+$-K$^+$-ATPase: mislocalisation to apical plasma membranes in polycystic kidney disease epithelia. *Am. J. Physiol.* **260**, F240–F430.

Winyard, P.J.D., Nauta, J., Lirenman, D.S. et al (1996a) Deregulation of cell survival in cystic and dysplastic renal development. *Kidney Int.* **49**, 135–146.

Winyard, P.J.D., Risdon, R.A., Sams, V.R., Dressler, G.R. and Woolf, A.S. (1996b) The PAX2 transcription factor is expressed in cystic and hyperproliferative dysplastic epithelia in human kidney malformations. *J. Clin. Invest.* **98**, 451–459.

Woo, D.D.L., Miao, S., Pelayo, J. and Woolf, A.S. (1994) Taxol inhibits congenital polycystic kidney disease progression. *Nature* **368**, 750–753.

Woolf, A.S. (1995) Clinical impact and biological basis of renal malformations. *Seminars Nephrol.* **15**, 361–372.

Woolf, A.S. and Fine, L.G. (1991) Do glomerular hemodynamic adaptations influence the progression of human renal disease? *Pediatr. Nephrol.* **5**, 88–93.

Woolf, A.S. and Winyard, P.J.D. (1995) Unravelling the pathogenesis of cystic kidney diseases. *Arch. Dis. Child.* **72**, 102–105.

Woolf, A.S., Palmer, S.J., Snow, M.J. and Fine, L.G. (1990) Creation of a functioning chimeric mammalian kidney. *Kidney Int.* **38**, 991–997.

Woolf, A.S., Bosch, R.J. and Fine, L.G. (1993) Gene transfer into the mammalian kidney: first steps towards renal gene therapy. *Kidney Int.* **43**, S116–S119.

Woolf, A.S., Neuhaus, T.J., Kolatsi, M., Winyard, P.J.D. and Klein, N.J. (1994) Nephron formation is inhibited by lipopolysaccharide and tumor necrosis factor-α. *J. Am. Soc. Nephrol.* **5**, 641.

Woolf, A.S., Kolatsi, M., Hardman, P. et al (1995) Roles of HGF/SF and the MET receptor in early development of the metanephros. *J. Cell Biol.* **128**, 171–184.

Yeong-Hau, H., Hunt, R., Siskind, M.S. and Zukoski, C. (1993) Association of cyclosporin A with acquired cystic disease of the native kidneys in renal transplant recipients. *Kidney Int.* **44**, 613–616.

Zerres, K., Mucher, G., Bachner, L. et al (1994) Mapping of the gene for autosomal recessive polycystic kidney disease (ARPKD) to chromosome 6p21–cen. *Nature Genetics* **7**, 429–432.

15 The Teeth

IRMA THESLEFF

Institute of Dentistry and Institute of Biotechnology, University of Helsinki, Finland

DEVELOPMENTAL ANATOMY

The early stages of tooth morphogenesis resemble closely those of different derivatives of the skin. The first morphological sign of tooth initiation is the thickening of the surface ectoderm covering the facial processes. Subsequently this epithelium forms a **bud**, which is accompanied by the condensation of the surrounding mesenchymal cells (Figure 15.1). At this stage the appearance of the tooth primordium is similar to that of many other organs which also develop from epithelial and mesenchymal tissue components, such as the hairs, salivary glands, mammary glands, kidneys and lungs.

The bud stage of tooth development is followed by the **cap stage** during which the future cuspal pattern of the tooth is determined. Part of the mesenchymal cells form a **dental papilla** which becomes surrounded by the epithelial **enamel organ**. The rest of the condensed mesenchyme forms the dental sac or **dental follicle**, which surrounds the enamel organ and gives rise to the periodontal tissues connecting the tooth to the alveolar bone.

During the **bell stage**, the tooth germ grows rapidly and undergoes a morphogenesis characteristic for each individual tooth. The terminal differentiation of the tooth-specific secretory cells starts at this stage. The mesenchymal cells underlying the enamel organ epithelium differentiate into **odontoblasts** laying down the organic matrix of dentin, and the juxtaposed epithelial cells differentiate into **ameloblasts** which deposit the enamel matrix. Differentiation and matrix deposition always start at the sites of the tips of the future cusps, and during the entire development of the tooth crown, a gradient of differentiation is seen where the stage of development decreases from the cuspal tip towards the cemento-enamel junction. After completion of crown development, the root starts to form, and the tooth erupts to the oral cavity (Figure 15.1).

Dentin resembles bone in its composition although the histological appearance is different, as the secretory odontoblasts do not get incorporated into the dentin matrix. Instead, each odontoblast leaves behind a cytoplasmic process which becomes embedded in dentin and thereby contributes to the formation of a dentin tubule. Odontoblast cell bodies remain as a confluent cell layer between the dentin and the cells of dental pulp. The **enamel** matrix is composed of unique enamel proteins which direct the mineralization of enamel into the hardest tissue

Embryos, Genes and Birth Defects. Edited by P. Thorogood.
© 1997 John Wiley & Sons Ltd.

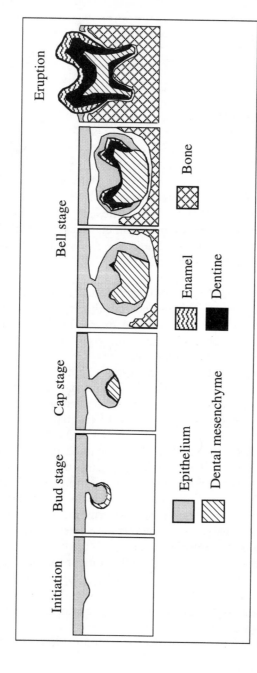

Figure 15.1 Stages in tooth morphogenesis. The thickened ectoderm of the facial processes forms a bud and as a result of interactions with the surrounding neural crest-derived mesenchyme, morphogenesis proceeds into cap and bell stages. Mesenchymal odontoblasts deposit the dentin matrix and epithelial ameloblasts, the enamel. After crown morphogenesis, roots develop and the tooth erupts. Figure provided by Jukka Jernvall

in the body. Mineralization of the dentin and enamel matrices starts when a small amount of dentin matrix has been laid down and the first enamel is deposited. After the end of the secretory phase, the ameloblasts regulate the maturation of enamel, and they degenerate during tooth eruption.

The period during which the human teeth develop spans an extremely long time, starting from the second month of embryonic development until completion during adolescence. The first **deciduous** or **primary teeth** are initiated during the 5th week of gestation, and their mineralization starts during the 14th week. At this time, the first **permanent teeth** have reached the bud stage, and they start to mineralize prior to birth. The first primary teeth normally erupt in children at 6 months of age, and the first permanent teeth at the age of 5–6 years. The last teeth to be formed, the third molars, are initiated post-natally and their crown development is completed between 12 and 16 years of age. Hence, tooth germs are present in fetuses and children of various ages at many different stages of development.

The primary, or deciduous dentition of humans comprises 20 teeth and the secondary, or permanent dentition, 32 teeth. It is important to note that the human teeth are heterodont, i.e. there are different shapes in different groups of teeth (as compared with the homodont dentitions in lower vertebrates, e.g. reptiles, in which all teeth are similar in shape). The human teeth fall into three groups: incisiform, caniniform and molariform teeth. The shapes of individual teeth are remarkably constant, and the variation in tooth shape has been an important tool in studies on the evolution of man as well as of other vertebrates. This is obviously due to the fact that only teeth and bones have usually been preserved from the extinct species. Detailed descriptions of the histology and timing of tooth development can be found in many textbooks (e.g. Ten Cate, 1994).

ABERRATIONS IN TOOTH DEVELOPMENT

For most mammals, a complete and well-functioning dentition is essential for survival. Although dental anomalies do not threaten human lives, they present challenging clinical problems in dentistry, and their aetiology and pathogenesis have always been of interest to those working in the field. The most common dental anomalies are described in many textbooks, and more comprehensive presentations, mainly on genetic aspects of dental anomalies and their association with other congenital defects, can be found in Stewart and Prescott (1976), Sofaer (1990) and Gorlin et al (1990).

ABERRATIONS IN NUMBER, SHAPE AND SIZE OF TEETH

Hypodontia, or missing teeth, is a common anomaly that occurs in many different forms and is often also seen as a trait in certain malformation syndromes. Simple hypodontia affecting one or several permanent teeth in certain tooth groups is most common in third molars, in which it is seen in 25% of the normal population. The frequency of premolar and incisor hypodontia affecting usually maxillary lateral incisors and/or second premolars varies from 5 to 25% according to population. It is probably caused by an autosomal dominant gene with reduced penetrance. It should be noted that hypodontia is extremely rare in the deciduous dentition.

Oligodontia refers to hypodontia of several (usually more than six) teeth and is less common. It may be seen as an isolated trait, but it is more commonly associated with other congenital defects. Such syndromes include **ectodermal dysplasias**, in which deficient development is seen in teeth as well as in sweat glands and hair (see Chapter 12). In the most severe forms of ectodermal dysplasia there is complete anodontia, i.e. all teeth are missing. Hypodontia of varying degrees is frequent in children with clefts of the lip and/or palate (Ranta, 1986). In addition, dozens of other syndromes exist in which hypodontia is associated with anomalies in different organ systems, notably in derivatives of the skin and in the limbs.

Supernumerary teeth, or **hyperodontia**, is less common than hypodontia. Simple hyperodontia is usually seen in the form of 'mesiodens' developing between the upper central incisors or as paramolars. The best known syndrome with hyperodontia is **cleidocranial dysplasia**, an autosomal dominant disorder affecting mainly bone development, where the number of supernumerary teeth varies, and they appear to constitute a partial third dentition (Jensen and Kreiborg, 1990).

Aberrant shape or size of teeth appears most often as a reduction of tooth size, conical teeth or abnormal number of cusps. **Macrodontia** as well as various types of fusions between teeth are rare. Reduction in tooth size, or **microdontia**, has long been known to be associated with congenital absence of teeth. For instance, small and peg-shaped lateral incisors are frequently associated with simple hypodontia, and hence the traits have a common genetic basis. Also, in the different syndromes exhibiting hypodontia, such as ectodermal dysplasias, the remaining teeth are often conical in shape and reduced in size.

DEFECTS IN STRUCTURE OF DENTIN AND ENAMEL

Inherited defects in the structure of dentin or enamel are rare. Especially those affecting the enamel show several modes of inheritance indicating different gene mutations. Heritable dentin defects have been classified into two main types: **dentinogenesis imperfecta** and **dentin dysplasia**. While one type of dentinogenesis imperfecta (DI type I) is associated with osteogenesis imperfecta, the other subtype(s) occur as a single trait (DI type II), as do the two types of dentin dysplasia (Witkop, 1989).

Amelogenesis imperfecta appears in several clinically different forms, and it has been classified according to the primary process of differentiation, matrix deposition or mineralization (Witkop, 1989). Enamel defects appear as traits in several syndromes, mostly in association with skin diseases and metabolic diseases, but these are very rare conditions. Genetic enamel and dentin defects are always manifested in both deciduous and permanent dentitions.

Enamel **hypoplasias**, which appear as localized discolorations or surface defects, are infrequent in deciduous teeth, but quite common in permanent teeth. They are mostly caused by harmful environmental factors, such as high doses of fluorides, dietary factors, diseases or medicines. Enamel develops postnatally in all permanent teeth, and because the development of the tooth crown proceeds in a vertical gradient, as described above, the timing of the insult can be determined according to the level of the hypoplastic lesions.

STUDIES SHEDDING LIGHT ON MECHANISM OF NORMAL DEVELOPMENT

The tooth is an exceptionally good model to study various general mechanisms of organogenesis, including the development of form or morphogenesis, cell differentiation, as well as the production of tissue-specific extracellular matrices (Thesleff et al, 1995). As a consequence, the tooth is one of the organs for which a considerable amount of developmental information has accumulated over many decades, and it is now quite actively studied using contemporary molecular approaches.

DESCRIPTION OF MOLECULAR CHANGES ASSOCIATED WITH ADVANCING TOOTH DEVELOPMENT

The analysis of the expression of individual molecules at the cellular level became possible with immunohistochemical techniques in the 1970s, when antibodies were produced and used for localization of specific molecular epitopes in tissue sections (Figure 15.2). With the progress in molecular biology, in-situ hybridization analysis was developed in the late 1980s. This allows the localization of mRNA in tissue sections by labelled cDNA probes (Figure 15.3). With these two methods, the expression of a large number of molecules has been analysed during branchial arch and tooth development. Based on observed changes in expression patterns, developmental roles for many of these molecules have been suggested.

Homeobox-containing transcription factors appear to specify positional information during embryonic development, and there is both descriptive and experimental evidence that in the branchial arches specific combinations of these genes (called the 'Hox code') regulate the patterning of individual structures (Hunt and Krumlauf, 1991; see also Chapters 7, 10 and 13). Expression of the Hox cluster genes has not been detected anterior to the second branchial arch, but other homeobox-containing genes have been localized which are thought to be important for the development of the head (Chapter 10). Homeobox genes in the Dlx and Msx groups are expressed in the area of tooth initiation in such patterns that they have been suggested to regulate the development of the functional dental pattern (Weiss, 1993; Sharpe, 1995).

Roles for **homeobox-containing genes** as well as for other transcription factors have also been suggested in the regulation of early tooth morphogenesis.

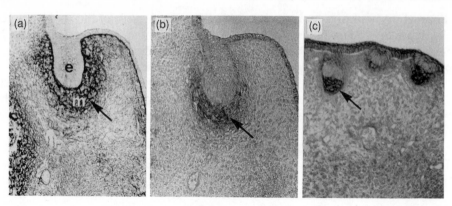

Figure 15.2 Immunohistological localization of two structural molecules during early tooth and hair development. (a) The matrix glycoprotein tenascin and (b) the cell surface proteoglycan syndecan-1 are intensely expressed in dental mesenchyme at bud stage (Thesleff et al, 1990a). (c) Syndecan-1 expression is also intense in the mesenchymal papilla of the developing vibrissae. Syndecan is a multifunctional proteoglycan that regulates cell behaviour by interacting with growth factors and extracellular matrix molecules in the microenvironment of the cell. e, epithelium; m, mesenchyme; arrows, mesenchymal cell condensates

Transcription factors that have been associated with tooth development include *Egr-1*, N-*myc*, c-*fos*, *Dlx-2*, *Msx-1*, *Msx-2* and *Lef-1* (Thesleff et al, 1995). Two of these, *Msx-1* and *Lef-1*, have been shown to be necessary for tooth development (Satokata and Maas, 1994; van Genderen et al, 1995; see below). Interestingly, a mutation in the *MSX1* gene was recently shown to be the cause of missing teeth in a family with oligodontia (Vastardis et al, 1996; see below). The expression of *Msx-1* is restricted to dental mesenchyme (Figure 15.3) (MacKenzie et al, 1991), whereas that of *Lef-1* first appears in the thickened presumptive dental epithelium and subsequently shifts to mesenchyme (Oosterwegel et al, 1993).

Growth factors of most families as well as their receptors are expressed in developing teeth. Localization of receptors for **epidermal growth factor** (EGF) by analysing the binding of ^{125}I-labelled EGF to developing teeth indicated that the expression of EGF receptors is developmentally regulated (Partanen and Thesleff, 1987a). Of particular interest is the restricted expression of **fibroblast growth factor-3** (FGF-3) in dental mesenchyme (Wilkinson et al, 1989) and FGF-4 in dental epithelium (Niswander and Martin, 1992). FGF-4 expression is restricted to the non-dividing cells of the enamel knot, and a role for this growth factor was recently proposed in the initiation of tooth cusp formation and hence in the determination of the shape of the crown (Jernvall et al, 1994).

The expression patterns of growth factors and their receptors are in many cases suggestive of roles in signalling between the epithelial and mesenchymal components of the tooth. In particular, factors in the **transforming growth factor-β** (TGF-β) family, including TGF-β1 and the **bone morphogenetic proteins** BMP-2 and BMP-4, have been proposed to act as signals (Lyons et al, 1990; Pelton et al, 1991; Vaahtokari et al, 1991; Vainio et al, 1993), and there is, in

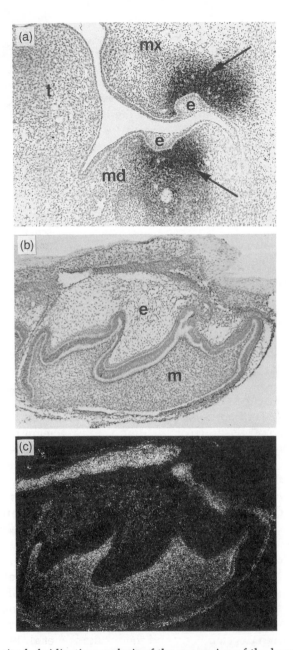

Figure 15.3   In situ hybridization analysis of the expression of the homeobox-containing gene *Msx-1* during (a) the bud stage and (b) late bell stage of tooth development. (c) Dark-field image of (b). Intense expression is restricted to dental mesenchyme (MacKenzie et al, 1991). Inhibition of *Msx-1* gene function in transgenic mice results in cleft palate and missing teeth (Satokata and Maas, 1994). e, epithelium; m, mesenchyme; t, tongue; mx, maxilla; md, mandible; arrows, *Msx-1* mRNA expression

fact, experimental evidence for signalling functions for the BMPs (Vainio et al, 1993; see below).

The molecular changes that are associated with advancing determination and differentiation of those dental mesenchymal cells that end up as odontoblasts have been well characterized, and the possible roles of various molecules at various stages of development have been assessed (Thesleff et al, 1990a). The cell surface proteoglycan **syndecan,** and the extracellular matrix glycoprotein **tenascin,** were the first molecules shown to be up-regulated in condensing dental mesenchyme during the bud stage, suggesting that they could play roles in the aggregation of cells (Figure 15.2) (Thesleff et al, 1990b). It is, however, obvious that although the expression patterns of various molecules correlate with developmental events, the associations alone do not indicate that they have developmental roles. The functions can only be analysed in experimental studies.

EXPERIMENTAL TISSUE RECOMBINATION STUDIES ANALYSING EPITHELIAL–MESENCHYMAL INTERACTIONS

As early as the 1930s experimental embryologists demonstrated that tooth morphogenesis in amphibians depends on interactions between epithelial and mesenchymal tissues (Huggins et al, 1934; Sellman, 1946). They also showed that the mesenchymal component of the tooth, i.e. all tissues except the enamel, is derived from the cranial **neural crest** cells which had migrated to the **branchial arches** (Sellman, 1946; Chibon, 1967). The regulatory roles of **epithelial– mesenchymal interactions** for mammalian tooth morphogenesis and differentia- tion of odontoblasts and ameloblasts were established in the 1960s (Kollar and Baird, 1970). In typical **tissue recombination** studies, the epithelial and mesen- chymal components are separated from tooth rudiments at different stages of development and cultured in vitro or as transplants in various combinations (Figure 15.4). In the first experiments on mouse tooth development, cap- and bell-stage teeth were studied, and it was demonstrated that the mesenchymal dental papilla of the tooth has the capacity to 'instruct' tooth morphogenesis as well as the differentiation of epithelial cells into ameloblasts (Kollar and Baird, 1970). The enamel organ epithelium of incisor teeth was instructed to develop into molariform teeth when cultured with molar dental papilla, and vice versa. Furthermore, the dental papilla mesenchyme of mouse embryos induced the differentiation of ameloblasts in various non-dental epithelia, including chick epithelium (Kollar and Fisher, 1980).

In the 1980s, similar tissue recombination experiments were performed during earlier stages of tooth development, and the results were essentially opposite to the earlier ones. Teeth developed when (non-dental) mesenchyme from the second branchial arch was cultured with (presumptive) dental epithelium, dissected from the first branchial arch prior to the bud stage (E10 or E11 mouse embryos) (Mina and Kollar, 1987). Also, when premigratory neural crest cells from the trunk region were cultured with the presumptive dental epithelium, teeth developed (Lumsden, 1988). Hence, these experiments indicate that the interactions regulating tooth development are sequential and reciprocal. The inductive signals clearly go both ways and start very early, but which tissue is the first expressing odontogenic potential still remains obscure. At the time of the earliest experiments (E9 mouse embryos) the neural crest cells had already migrated into the first branchial arch, and it is possible that they had been programmed earlier, either during patterning of the neural crest or during their migration from the crest, and that they had therefore already exerted inductive effects on the epithelium.

In the above experiments, it was also directly demonstrated that neural crest cells have the potential to participate in mammalian tooth development (Lumsden, 1988). This, together with the finding that teeth did not form if the presumptive dental epithelium was combined with other than neural-crest-derived mesenchyme, supported the earlier assumption, based on experiments with amphibians (Sellman, 1946; Chibon, 1967), that dental mesenchyme in mammals is also derived from neural crest cells. Most of the current knowledge on neural crest cell migration and determination has come from experiments on birds, which, unfortunately, do not have teeth. Recently, **lineage studies** have also been performed in mouse embryos by labelling premigratory crest cells with fluorescent dyes (Osumi-Yamashita and Eto, 1990; Serbedzija et al, 1992). Hence, routes of cell migration to the tooth-bearing areas of the first branchial arch and the frontonasal process are becoming clarified (Bronner-Fraser, 1993; see also Chapter 10).

In-vitro recombination of dental epithelial and mesenchymal tissues has been used for analysing the roles of tissue interactions in the regulation of expression of many molecules (Figure 15.4). Thus, it has been shown that the expression of syndecan and tenascin in the dental mesenchyme is induced by the epithelium (Vainio et al, 1989). Also, *Msx-1* and *Msx-2* expression as well as cell proliferation are regulated by the dental epithelium (Vainio and Thesleff, 1992; Jowett et al, 1993).

The role of growth factors as signals transmitting epithelial–mesenchymal interactions has been studied in tissue recombination cultures by the application of beads that have been incubated first with the growth factor and then placed on dental tissue in organ culture (Figure 15.4). BMP recombinant protein was shown to mimic the effects of early dental epithelium on dental mesenchyme. Most significantly, it induced the expression of *Msx-1* and *Msx-2* (Figure 15.5) (Vainio et al, 1993). In the same model system, FGF-4 stimulates cell proliferation in both the epithelium and mesenchyme (Figure 15.5) (Jernvall et al, 1994).

Effects of epithelial–mesenchymal interactions in the regulation of odontoblast and ameloblast cell differentiation have also been studied in detail by experimental tissue recombination studies. By interposing Nuclepore filters with different pore sizes between epithelium and mesenchyme dissected from bell-stage tooth germs, it was shown that the epithelial basement membrane triggers the differentiation of dental papilla cells into odontoblasts (Thesleff et al, 1977). A series of molecular studies has indicated that the interaction is mediated by cell surface molecules of the preodontoblasts and extracellular matrix components, notably **fibronectin** in the basement membrane (Lesot et al, 1990). Organ culture

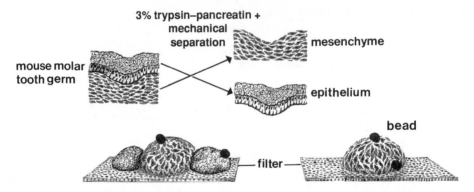

Figure 15.4 Experimental analysis of epithelial–mesenchymal interactions and of the role of growth factors during early odontogenesis. The area of developing lower molars is dissected from a 11- to 12-day-old mouse embryo, and the epithelial and mesenchymal tissues are separated. They are placed in various recombinations in organ culture (e.g. Trowell-type culture as shown in Figure 15.6). Beads that release growth factors or other molecules can be placed in contact with the tissue.

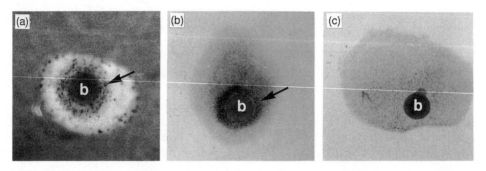

Figure 15.5 Effects of fibroblast growth factor (FGF-4) and bone morphogenetic protein (BMP-2) on dental mesenchyme in experiments as shown in Figure 15.4. The growth factors mimic the effects of dental epithelium on mesenchyme. (a) FGF-4 has stimulated cell proliferation around the bead; dividing cells are labelled with bromodeoxyuridine (arrow) (Jernvall et al, 1994). (b) BMP-2 has induced the expression of *Msx-1*; whole mount in-situ hybridization (Vainio et al, 1993). (c) Control bead, releasing no growth factors, has not induced *Msx-1* expression. b, bead.

experiments where isolated dental papillae from E17 mouse embryonic molars were cultured in the presence of extracellular matrix and growth factors indicate that, in addition to the matrix molecules, TGF-β family growth factors, notably BMP-2, are required for the induction of odontoblast differentiation (Bégue-Kirn et al, 1992). Similar studies analysing factors that regulate the differentiation of ameloblasts from dental epithelium indicate that molecules in the predentin extracellular matrix are involved (Ruch, 1987). These may include both extracellular matrix components, as suggested by experimental studies (Karcher-Djuricic et al, 1985), and growth factors, as suggested by localization studies of growth factor expression (Vaahtokari et al, 1991; Vainio et al, 1993).

FUNCTIONAL STUDIES IN VITRO

Organ culture and transplantation studies have shown that teeth develop quite independently of other tissues. The first branchial arches from 9-day-old mouse embryos will generate teeth when transplanted in the anterior chamber of the eye (Lumsden, 1988). In organ culture, teeth develop into bud or cap stage in lower jaws from 10-day-old mouse embryos (Slavkin, 1988), and when bud-stage teeth are dissected free from surrounding tissues and placed in organ culture, their development proceeds all the way to the bell stage when enamel and dentin mineralize (Figure 15.6) (Partanen et al, 1985). Chemically defined culture media have been designed that support tooth development in culture, and in these conditions the nutritional requirements of tooth morphogenesis can be analysed. An absolute requirement for early morphogenesis is **transferrin**, which is needed for the transport of iron into cells (Partanen and Thesleff, 1987b).

The developmental functions of individual molecules have been analysed in vitro by adding them to the culture medium or by inhibiting their expression in cultured teeth. **Insulin** and **growth hormone** have trophic effects on morphogenesis and dentinogenesis in vitro (Figure 15.7) (Partanen, 1993; Young et al, 1993). EGF affects tooth morphogenesis, and the effects are associated with epithelial-mesenchymal interactions (Partanen et al, 1985). When added to the culture medium, **antisense oligonucleotides** against mRNA for EGF inhibit

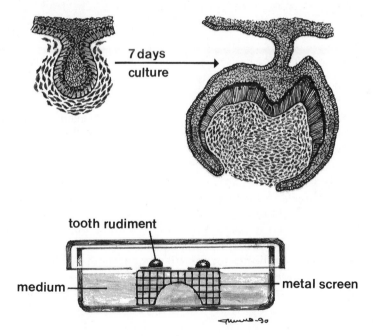

Figure 15.6 Use of the Trowell-type organ culture method for the analysis of tooth morphogenesis. During 1 week of culture a mouse molar tooth germ develops from the bud stage to the bell stage when dentin and enamel matrices start to be deposited

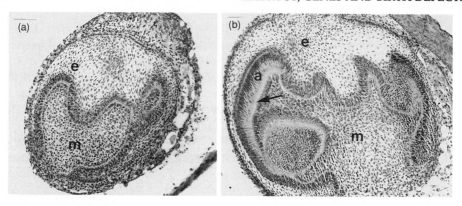

Figure 15.7 Effect of insulin on tooth morphogenesis in an organ culture experiment as shown in Figure 15.6. (a) After 6 days in the control medium the bud-stage tooth germ has reached the early bell stage. (b) In the presence of 1 μg/ml insulin, morphogenesis has been enhanced, and the odontoblasts and ameloblasts have differentiated (Partanen, 1993). e, epithelium; m, mesenchyme; a, ameloblasts; arrow, predentin

tooth morphogenesis in the lower jaw of 9-day-old mouse embryos (Kronmiller et al, 1991). As the sense oligonucleotides had no effect, it was suggested that EGF is a necessary growth factor for tooth initiation. Antisense oligonucleotides against three different TGF-β growth factors were recently added to the culture media of mandibles from 10-day-old mouse embryos. The findings suggested that TGF-β2 is involved in the regulation of tooth size (Chai et al, 1994).

FUNCTIONAL STUDIES IN VIVO BY PRODUCING TRANSGENIC MICE

The generation of **transgenic mice** with targeted null mutations (gene knockout experiments) is the most direct way to test the functions of individual genes (see Chapter 4). Recently two transgenic mouse lines have been generated where tooth development is inhibited, and both involve transcription factors. The mice that are deficient for the homeobox-containing *Msx-1* gene have cleft palate and underdeveloped jaws in addition to lacking teeth (Satokata and Maas, 1994). The other toothless transgenic mice lack a functioning *Lef-1* gene, and the phenotype is quite different. In addition to teeth, development is inhibited in several other ectodermally derived organs, including hair, vibrissae and mammary glands (van Genderen et al, 1995). It is noteworthy that in both *Msx-1* and *Lef-1* deficient mice, tooth development proceeds until the bud stage. The generation of these mice obviously indicates an absolute requirement of *Msx-1* and *Lef-1* for maintained tooth development.

The role of *Lef-1* was recently analysed in detail using recombinations between tissues from *Lef-1* deficient and normal embryos. It was shown that, although *Lef-1* expression shifts between the epithelial and mesenchymal tissues, expression is only needed in dental epithelium during budding, and the effect of *Lef-1* thereafter shifts to mesenchyme (Kratochwil et al, 1996). *Msx-1*, on the other hand, is expressed exclusively in dental mesenchyme.

ANALYSIS OF DENTIN AND ENAMEL FORMATION

Biochemical studies over the last decades have characterized the molecular compositions of dentin and enamel matrices. Dentin, like bone, is mainly composed of **type I collagen** (Linde and Goldberg, 1993). Odontoblasts and osteoblasts have unique regulatory mechanisms controlling type I collagen expression, which has become evident in studies on a mouse mutant in which retroviral insertion in the promoter region of the type I collagen gene inhibited collagen transcription in fibroblasts, but not in odontoblasts and osteoblasts (Kratochwil et al, 1989). The regulation of type I collagen expression in odontoblasts is presently being studied in transgenic mice using engineered promoter constructs, and the location of important regulatory elements in the collagen promoter has been specified (Thomas et al, 1995).

Besides type I collagen, dentin shares several other components with bone, but in addition, dentin contains unique molecules, in particular phosphoproteins (Linde and Goldberg, 1993). Recently, a novel dentin-specific acidic phospho-protein AG1 (also called dentin matrix protein-1, DMP-1) was identified by screening a cDNA library prepared from cells of the rat incisor odontoblast–pulp complex (George et al, 1993). The *AG1* gene has been localized to human chromosome 4q21 (George et al, 1994).

Enamel is composed of several proteins, including **amelogenins** and **enamelins**, which are postulated to play major roles in the mineralization and structural organization of forming enamel (Deutsch et al, 1991; Sasaki and Shimokawa, 1995). The characterization of enamel proteins by biochemical analysis of enamel matrix met with difficulties for a long time as the proteins are degraded very rapidly after secretion. With the aid of cDNA and genomic studies, the complete primary structure of amelogenin, the major component of enamel matrix, has been established in several species including humans (Salido et al, 1992; Catalano-Sherman et al, 1993). The amelogenin gene has been localized in the X and Y chromosomes in humans, but only in the X chromosome in the mouse (Lau et al, 1989; Gibson et al, 1992). The first acidic enamelin protein that was cloned and sequenced was called **tuftelin** (Deutsch et al, 1991), and the gene was subsequently localized to the human chromosome 1 (Deutsch et al, 1995).

The cloning of enamel protein genes has made it possible to study their expression in developing teeth. By using **RT-PCR** (reverse-transcription-polymerase chain reaction) analysis, amelogenin transcripts were localized in developing mouse teeth as early as the cap stage. This indicates that the fate of the ameloblasts is determined very early, in fact long before morphological changes are evident in the epithelial cells (Couwenhoven and Snead, 1994).

HOW DO STUDIES OF NORMAL DEVELOPMENT ELUCIDATE ABNORMAL DEVELOPMENT?

The important conclusion from the tissue recombination experiments is that the interactions between epithelium and mesenchyme that regulate tooth development are reciprocal and sequential. The first interactions regulate tooth initiation and the last direct the deposition and mineralization of dentin and enamel as well as root development. Hence, defective function of either epithelial or mesenchymal cells may result in abnormal development of any dental tissue. For instance, a lack of a signalling molecule may disrupt development, but a defect in its receptor or in the downstream targets in the responding tissue could also lead to inhibited morphogenesis. Therefore, it is not possible to conclude, simply on the basis of the phenotype of a dental anomaly, in which tissue the primary defect has been. This point is particularly well demonstrated in the *Msx-1* and *Lef-1* deficient mice; although *Msx-1* is expressed in mesenchyme and *Lef-1* expression is needed only in epithelium (see above), the tooth phenotype in both knockouts is similar. This obviously also points out that the defective function of many different genes may result in similar phenotypic alteration in tooth development.

All the molecules that have been analysed so far in association with tooth development (excluding enamel and dentine-specific proteins) have been implicated in the development of other organs as well (Thesleff et al, 1995). This includes transcription factors (*Lef-1, Msx-1,* etc.; Figure 15.3), syndecan and tenascin (which are expressed in organ-specific mesenchyme in several epithelio-mesenchymal organs; Figure 15.2), as well as all growth factors and receptors analysed. Hence, all these genes are candidates for causing various syndromes in which dental defects are part of the condition.

Interestingly, the X-chromosomal gene causing anhidrotic ectodermal dysplasia was identified recently. It encodes a transmembrane protein of unknown function (Kere et al, 1996). It is expressed in epithelial cells and presumably is associated with epithelial–mesenchymal interactions regulating the development of teeth, hair and sweat glands. As there exists the mouse counterpart of the ectodermal dysplasia, the *Tabby* mouse, it will serve as a useful model to analyse the developmental function of the gene.

On the other hand, we have learned from transgenic mouse experiments that one has to be cautious in drawing conclusions from the distribution patterns only. All the molecules that are expressed in the developing teeth may not be necessary for dental development. For instance, mice with a non-functional tenascin gene have no apparent malformations in teeth or any organs (Saga et al, 1992), indicating that tenascin, which is intensely expressed in condensed dental mesenchyme and later in dental pulp (Figure 15.2) (Thesleff et al, 1987; Lukinmaa et al, 1991), either is not needed for tooth development or can be compensated for by other molecules. In EGF receptor knockouts, many organs show deficient development but teeth are normal (Miettinen et al, 1995), although EGF receptors are intensely expressed during tooth morphogenesis (Partanen and Thesleff, 1987a). A further example is the *Msx-1* deficient transgenic mouse, which has no detectable limb malformations despite the intense and developmentally regulated expression of the gene in limbs (Satokata and Maas, 1994). It is conceivable that in this case the effect of *Msx-1* is compensated by *Msx-2*.

Interestingly, a missense mutation in the homeodomain of the *MSX1* gene was recently shown to be the cause of oligodontia in one family (Vastardis et al,

1996). As no other organs were affected in the patients, the effect of *MSX1* apparently cannot be compensated by other genes in teeth. In fact, *Msx-2*, which co-expressed with *Msx-1* in most organs studied, is not expressed in the dental mesenchyme during bud stage, i.e. the stage in which development is arrested in the *Msx-1* knockout mice (Satokata and Maas, 1994). It is also possible that the lack of an *MSX1* gene is the cause of hypodontia in some syndromes, such as Wolf–Hirschhorn syndrome, showing deletion of parts of chromosome 4 where the *MSX1* gene is located (Ivens et al, 1990). *MSX1* has, however, been excluded as the gene causing the common premolar and incisor hypodontia (Nieminen et al, 1995). *EGF* and its receptor, as well as *FGF3*, have also been excluded as causative factors in simple hypodontia (Arte et al, 1996).

The characterization of several molecules of the enamel and dentin matrices and the cloning of their genes have made it possible to study their involvement in hereditary dentin and enamel defects by molecular genetic studies. The chromosomal locations of amelogenin and tuftelin are known, and so far mutations in the amelogenin gene have been shown to be the cause of the X-linked form of amelogenesis imperfecta (Lagerström et al, 1991; Aldred et al, 1992; Lench et al, 1994). Mutations in type I collagen genes cause dentinogenesis imperfecta associated with **osteogenesis imperfecta** (Byers et al, 1992), and the gene defect causing a similar dentin defect occurring as a single trait (DI type II) has been mapped to chromosome 4 (Gusella et al, 1986). The locus of the major dentin phosphoprotein is not associated with DI type II (MacDougall et al, 1992), but the location of the *AG1* (DMP-1) dentin phosphoprotein gene maps to the same region. Hence, *AG1* can be considered as a candidate gene for DI type II (George et al, 1994). It is obvious that the defective genes causing dentin and enamel defects may involve structural molecules of the hard-tissue matrices as well as regulatory genes. In the future we can expect the classifications of the various forms of dentin and enamel defects to be based on their specific gene mutations.

AN AGENDA FOR THE FUTURE

Although our understanding of the mechanisms and molecules that regulate tooth development has increased tremendously during recent years, there is still much to be learned. We do not understand how the functional dental pattern is specified; nor do we know when, where and how the neural crest cells and the oral ectodermal cells that participate in tooth development become committed. Obviously, there is a need to continue lineage studies in this area. Also, although the distribution patterns of numerous molecules have been mapped during tooth development, and some have even been shown to be necessary for tooth development, we do not understand how they regulate the shape and size of the tooth. The analysis of the functions of the known molecules should be continued, but it is also important to search for new, perhaps tooth-specific, molecules. One approach is to clone genes from cDNA libraries of dental tissue on the basis of sequence similarity to genes that are known to be important developmental regulators in invertebrate organisms such as *Drosophila*. Also, the **mutation screening** of zebrafish embryos, which is now in progress in some laboratories (Mullins et al, 1994) will conceivably result in identification of genes that affect tooth development.

When a gene has been predicted to be important for tooth development on the basis of its expression pattern, the most direct way to test its developmental function is by production of transgenic mice with altered gene function. This approach should clearly be continued. Not only can the effects of lacking gene function be analysed, as was the case in the *Msx-1* and *Lef-1* knockout mice, but almost any type of mutations can be created in the genes. This ability to manipulate the mouse genome will provide good animal models for studies on tooth development. For instance, the analysis of tissues from various transgenic mice with tissue recombination and other in-vitro techniques can be expected to increase our understanding of the functions of the genes.

Although inhibition of tooth development has so far been detected in two lines of knockout transgenic mice, this approach is not feasible if the gene under study is vital for early embryonic development. Tooth development is a relatively late event during embryogenesis, and hence the embryo may die before reaching the stage of tooth formation. In such cases it will be possible to target the expression of the transgene by regulating the location or timing of expression with specific enhancer or promoter constructs (see Chapter 4). Recently, a 3.5-kb segment of the putative promoter sequence of the amelogenin gene was identified and, when this region was linked to an indicator gene, its expression could be directed to the enamel organ in transgenic mice (Chen et al, 1994). Thus, now it is feasible to target a gene construct to enamel organ cells and, undoubtedly, the cloning of other tooth-specific genes as well as identification of novel segments that direct expression in dental cells will offer new possibilities.

Organ culture techniques continue to be valuable in meeting the challenge to analyse the developmental functions of different molecules. Inhibition of molecular functions by neutralizing antibodies should shed light on their specific roles. Also, by using antisense oligonucleotides it may be possible to inhibit translation specifically. There have, however, been problems in using this approach, as the oligonucleotides penetrate some cells poorly, and they also commonly have toxic effects. In addition to inhibition studies, the 'positive' effects of molecules should be analysed whenever purified proteins are available. For instance, in-vitro studies on the effects of potential signalling molecules such as growth factors are valuable. In general, full proof that a gene has an important developmental role requires demonstration that it is expressed at the right time and in the right place, that it has a meaningful biological function and that inhibition of its function leads to aberrant development.

ACKNOWLEDGEMENT

I thank Dr Pirjo-Liisa Lukinmaa for many helpful comments during the preparation of the manuscript.

REFERENCES

Aldred, M.J., Crawford, P.J.M., Roberts, E. and Thomas, N.S.T. (1992) Identification of a nonsense mutation in the amelogenin gene (AMELX) in a family with X-linked amelogenesis imperfecta (AIH1). *Hum. Genet.* **90**, 413–416.

Arte, S., Nieminen, P., Pirinen, S., Thesleff, I. and Peltonen, L. (1996) Gene defect in hypodontia: exclusion of *EGF*, *EGFR* and *FGF-3* as candidate genes. *J. Dent. Res.* **75**, 1346–1352.

Bégue-Kirn, C., Smith, A.J., Ruch, J.V. et al (1992) Effects of dentin proteins, transforming growth factor β1 (TGFβ1) and bone morphogenetic protein 2 (BMP2) on the differentiation of odontoblast *in vitro*. *Int. J. Dev. Biol.* **36**, 491–503.

Bronner-Fraser, M. (1993) Segregation of cell lineage in the neural crest. *Curr. Opin. Gen. Dev.* **3**, 641–647.

Byers, P.H., Pyeritz, R.E. and Uitto, J. (1992) Research perspectives in heritable disorders of connective tissue. *Matrix* **12**, 333–342.

Catalano-Sherman, J., Palmon, A., Burstein, Y. and Deutsch, D. (1993) Amino acid sequence of a major human amelogenin protein employing Edman degradation and cDNA sequencing. *J. Dent. Res.* **72**, 1566–1572.

Chai, Y., Mah, A., Crohin, C. et al (1994) Specific transforming growth factor-β subtypes regulate embryonic mouse Meckel's cartilage and tooth development. *Dev. Biol.* **162**, 85–103.

Chen, E., Piddington, R., Decker, S. et al (1994) Regulation of *amelogenin* gene expression during tooth development. *Dev. Dyn.* **199**, 189–198.

Chibon, P. (1967) Etude expérimentale par ablations, greffes et autoradiographie, de l'origine des dents chez l'amphibien urodele *Pleurodeles waltlii* Michah. *Arch. Oral Biol.* **12**, 745–753.

Couwenhoven, R.I. and Snead, M.L. (1994) Early determination and permissive expression of amelogenin transcription during mouse mandibular first molar development. *Dev. Biol.* **164**, 290–299.

Deutsch, D., Palmon, A., Fisher, L.W. et al (1991) Sequencing of bovine enamelin ('tuftelin') a novel acidic enamel protein. *J. Biol. Chem.* **266**, 16021–16028.

Deutsch, D., Catalano-Sherman, J., Dafni, L., David, S. and Palmon, A. (1995) Enamel matrix proteins and ameloblast biology. *Conn. Tiss. Res.* **32**, 97–107.

George, A., Sabsay, B., Simonian, P.A. and Veis, A. (1993) Characterization of a novel dentin matrix acidic phosphoprotein: implications for induction of biomineralization. *J. Biol. Chem.* **268**, 12624–12630.

George, A., Gui, J., Jenkins, N.A. et al (1994) In situ localization and chromosomal mapping of the *AG1* (Dmp1) gene. *Int. J. Histochem. Cytochem.* **42**, 1527–1531.

Gibson, C.W., Golub, E.E., Abrams, W.R. et al (1992) Bovine amelogenin message heterogeneity: alternative splicing and Y-chromosomal gene transcription. *Biochemistry* **31**, 8384–8388.

Gorlin, R.J., Cohen, J.M.M. and Levin, L.S. (1990) *Syndromes of the Head and Neck*. 3rd edn. Oxford University Press: New York.

Gusella, J.A., Gilliam, T.C., MacDonald, M.E., Cheng, S.V. and Tanzi, R.E. (1986) Molecular genetics of human chromosome 4. *J. Med. Genet.* **23**, 193–199.

Huggins, C.B., McCarroll, H.R. and Dahlberg, A.A. (1934) Transplantation of tooth germ elements and the experimental heterotopic formation of dentin and enamel. *J. Exp. Med.* **60**, 199–210.

Hunt, P. and Krumlauf, R. (1991) Deciphering the Hox code: clues to patterning branchial regions of the head. *Cell* **66**, 1075–1078.

Ivens, A., Flavin, N., Williamson, R. et al (1990) The human homeobox gene HOX7 maps to chromosome 4p16.1 and may be implicated in Wolf–Hirschhorn syndrome. *Hum. Genet.* **84**, 473–476.

Jensen, B.L. and Kreiborg, S. (1990) Development of the dentition in cleidocranial dysplasia. *J. Oral Pathol. Med.* **19**, 89–93.

Jernvall, J., Kettunen, P., Karavanova, I., Martin, L.B. and Thesleff, I. (1994) Evidence for the role of the enamel knot as a control center in mammalian tooth cusp formation: non-dividing cells express growth stimulating Fgf-4 gene. *Int. J. Dev. Biol.* **38**, 463–469.

Jowett, A.K., Vainio, S., Ferguson, M.W.J., Sharpe, P.T. and Thesleff, I. (1993) Epithelial–mesenchymal interactions are required for *msx 1* and *msx 2* gene expression in the developing murine molar tooth. *Development* **117**, 461–470.

Karcher-Djuricic, V., Staubli, A., Meyer, J.M. and Ruch, J.V. (1985) Acellular dental matrices promote functional differentiation of ameloblast. *Differentiation* **29**, 169–175.

Kere, J., Srivastava, A.K., Montonen, O. et al (1996) X-linked anhidrotic (hypohidrotic) ectodermal dysplasia is caused by mutation in a novel transmembrane protein. *Nature Genetics* **13**, 409–416.

Kollar, E.J. and Baird, G.R. (1970) Tissue interactions in embryonic mouse tooth germs: II. The inductive role of the dental papilla. *J. Embryol. Exp. Morphol.* **24**, 173–186.

Kollar, E.J. and Fisher, C. (1980) Tooth induction in chick epithelium: expression of quiescent avian genes for enamel synthesis. *Science* **207**, 993–995.

Kratochwil, K., von der Mark, K., Kollar, E.J. et al (1989) Retrovirus-induced insertional mutation in *Mov13* mice affects collagen I expression in a tissue-specific manner. *Cell* **57**, 807–816.

Kratochwil, K., Dull, M., Farinas, I., Galceran, J. and Grosschedl, R. (1996) *Lef1* expression is activated by BMP-4 and regulates inductive tissue interactions in tooth and hair development. *Genes Dev.* **10**, 1382–1394.

Kronmiller, J.E., Upholt, W.B. and Kollar, E.J. (1991) EGF antisense oligodeoxynucleotides block murine odontogenesis *in vitro*. *Dev. Biol.* **147**, 485–488.

Lagerström, M., Dahl, N., Nakahori, Y. et al (1991) A deletion in the amelogenin gene (AMG) causes X-linked amelogenesis imperfecta (AIH1). *Genomics* **10**, 971–975.

Lau, E.C., Mohandas, T.K., Shapiro, L.J., Slavkin, H.C. and Snead, M.L. (1989) Human and mouse amelogenin gene loci are on the sex chromosomes. *Genomics* **4**, 162–168.

Lench, N.J., Brook, A.H. and Winter, G.B. (1994) SSCP detection of a nonsense mutation in exon 5 of the amelogenin gene (AMGX) causing X-linked amelogenesis imperfecta (AIH1). *Hum. Mol. Genet.* **3**, 827–828.

Lesot, H., Kubler, M.D., Fausser, J.L. and Ruch, J.V. (1990) A 165 kDa membrane antigen mediating fibronectin–vinculin interaction is involved in murine odontoblast differentiation. *Differentiation* **44**, 25–35.

Linde, A. and Goldberg, M. (1993) Dentinogenesis. *Curr. Rev. Oral Biol. Med.* **4**, 679–728.

Lukinmaa, P.L., Mackie, E.J. and Thesleff, I. (1991) Immunohistochemical localization of the matrix glycoproteins, tenascin and the ED sequence-containing form of cellular fibronectin, in human permanent teeth and periodontal ligament. *J. Dent. Res.* **70**, 19–26.

Lumsden, A.G.S. (1988) Spatial organization of the epithelium and the role of neural crest cell in the initiation of mammalian tooth germ. *Development* Suppl. **103**, 155–169.

Lyons, K.M., Pelton, R.W. and Hogan, B.L.M. (1990) Organogenesis and pattern formation in the mouse: RNA distribution patterns suggest a role for bone morpho-genetic protein-2A (BMP-2A). *Development* **109**, 833–844.

MacDougall, M., Zeichner-David, M., Murray, J. et al (1992) Dentin phosphoprotein gene locus is not associated with dentinogenesis imperfecta types II and III. *Am. J. Hum. Genet.* **50**, 190–194.

MacKenzie, A., Leeming, G., Jowett, A.K., Ferguson, M.W. and Sharpe, P.T. (1991) The homeobox gene 7.1 has specific regional and temporal expression patterns during early murine craniofacial embryogenesis, especially tooth development in vivo and in vitro. *Development* **111**, 269–285.

Miettinen, P.J., Berger, J.E., Menses, J. et al (1995) Epithelial immaturity and multiorgan failure in mice lacking epidermal growth factor receptor. *Nature* **376**, 337–341.

Mina, M. and Kollar, E.J. (1987) The induction of odontogenesis in non-dental mesenchyme combined with early murine mandibular arch epithelium. *Arch. Oral Biol.* **32**, 123–127.

Mullins, M.C., Hammerschmidt, M., Haffter, P. and Nüsslein-Volhard, C. (1994) Large-scale mutagenesis in the zebrafish: in search of genes controlling development in a vertebrate. *Curr. Biol.* **4**, 189–202.

Nieminen, P., Arte, A., Pirinen, S., Peltonen, L. and Thesleff, I (1995) Gene defect in hypodontia: exclusion of *MSX1* and *MSX2* as candidate genes. *Hum. Genet.* **96**, 305–308.

Niswander, L. and Martin, G.R. (1992) Fgf-4 expression during gastrulation, myogenesis, limb and tooth development in the mouse. *Development* **114**, 755–768.

Oosterwegel, M., Wetering van de, M., Timmerman, J. et al (1993) Differential expression of the HMG box factors *TCF-1* and *LEF-1* during murine embryogenesis. *Development* **118**, 439–448.

Osumi-Yamashita, N. and Eto, K. (1990) Mammalian cranial neural crest cells and facial development. *Develop. Growth and Differ.* **32**, 451–459.

Partanen, A. (1993) Transferrin, EGF, and their receptors in the development of tooth and other embryonic epithelial–mesenchymal organs. Doctoral thesis, University of Helsinki.

Partanen, A.M. and Thesleff, I. (1987a) Localization and quantitation of ^{125}I-epidermal growth factor binding in mouse embryonic tooth and other embryonic tissues at different developmental stages. *Dev. Biol.* **120**, 186–197.

Partanen, A.M. and Thesleff, I. (1987b) Transferrin and tooth morphogenesis: retention of transferrin by mouse embryonic teeth in organ culture. *Differentiation* **34**, 25–31.

Partanen, A.M., Ekblom, P. and Thesleff, I. (1985) Epidermal growth factor inhibits tooth morphogenesis and differentiation. *Dev. Biol* **111**, 84–94.

Pelton, R.W., Saxena, B., Jones, M., Moses, H.L. and Gold, L.I. (1991) Immunohistochemical localization of TGFbeta-1, TGFbeta-2, and TGFbeta-3 in the mouse embryo: expression patterns suggest multiple roles during embryonic development. *J. Cell Biol.* **115**, 1091–1105.

Ranta, R. (1986) A review of tooth formation in children with cleft lip/palate. *Am. J. Orthod. Dentofac. Orthop.* **90**, 11–18.

Ruch, J.V. (1987) Determinisms of odontogenesis. *Cell Biol. Rev.* **14**, 1–112.

Saga, Y., Yagi, T., Ikawa, Y., Sakakura, T. and Aizawa, S. (1992) Mice develop normally without tenascin. *Gen. Dev.* **6**, 1821–1831.

Salido, E.C., Yen, P.H., Koprivnikar, K., Yu, L.C. and Shapiro, L.J. (1992) The human enamel protein gene amelogenin is expressed from both the X and the Y chromosomes. *Am. J. Hum. Genet.* **50**, 303–316.

Satokata, I. and Maas, R. (1994) Msx1-deficient mice exhibit cleft palate and abnormalities of craniofacial and tooth development. *Nature Genetics* **6**, 348–356.

Sasaki, S. and Shimokawa, H. (1995) Biochemistry of the developing enamel matrix. In *Dental Enamel, Formation to Destruction* (Eds: C. Robinson, J. Kirkham and R. Shore), pp. 85–104. CRC Press: Florida.

Sellman, S. (1946) Some experiments on the determination of the larval teeth in *Amblystoma mexicanum. Odont. Tidskr.* **54**, 1–128.

Serbedzija, G., Bronner-Fraser, M. and Fraser, S.E. (1992) Vital dye analysis of cranial neural crest cell migration in the mouse embryo. *Development* **116**, 297–307.

Sharpe, P.T. (1995) Homeobox genes and orofacial development. *Conn. Tiss. Res.* **32**, 17–25.

Slavkin, H.C. (1988) Gene regulation in the development of oral tissues. *J. Dent. Res.* **67**, 1142–1149.

Sofaer, J.A. (1990) Single gene disorders. In *Oral Manifestations of Systemic Disease* (Eds: J.H. Jones and D.K. Mason), 2nd edn, pp. 61–111, Baillière Tindall: London.

Stewart, R.E. and Prescott, G.H. (Eds) (1976) *Oral Facial Genetics.* C.V. Mosby: St Louis, MO.

Ten Cate, A.R. (1994) *Oral Histology: Development, Structure and Function.* Mosby-Year Book: St Louis, MO.

Thesleff, I., Lehtonen, E., Wartiovaara, J. and Saxén, L. (1977) Interference of tooth differentiation with interposed filters. *Dev. Biol.* **58**, 197–203.

Thesleff, I., Mackie, E., Vainio, S. and Chiquet-Ehrismann, R. (1987) Changes in the distribution of tenascin during tooth development. *Development* **101**, 289–296.

Thesleff, I., Vaahtokari, A. and Vainio, S. (1990a) Molecular changes during determination and differentiation of the dental mesenchymal cell lineage. *J. Biol. Buccale* **18**, 179–188.

Thesleff, I., Vainio, S., Salmivirta, M. and Jalkanen, M. (1990b) Syndecan and tenascin: induction during early tooth morphogenesis and possible interactions. *Cell Differ. Dev.* **32**, 383–390.

Thesleff, I., Vaahtokari, A. and Partanen, A.-M. (1995) Regulation of organogenesis: common molecular mechanisms regulating the development of teeth and other organs. *Int. J. Dev. Biol.* **39**, 35–50.

Thomas, H.F., Feldman, J.A., Bedalov, A. et al (1995) Identification of regulatory elements necessary for the expression of the COL1A1 promoter in murine odontoblast. *Conn. Tiss. Res.* **33**, 81–85.

Vaahtokari, A., Vainio, S. and Thesleff, I. (1991) Associations between transforming growth factor β1 RNA expression and epithelial–mesenchymal interactions during tooth morphogenesis. *Development* **113**, 985–994.

Vainio, S., Jalkanen, M. and Thesleff, I. (1989) Syndecan and tenascin expression is induced by epithelial–mesenchymal interactions in embryonic tooth mesenchyme. *J. Cell Biol.* **108**, 1945–1954.

Vainio, S. and Thesleff, I. (1992) Coordinated induction of cell proliferation and syndecan expression in dental mesenchyme by epithelium: evidence for diffusible signals. *Dev. Dyn.* **194**, 105–117.

Vainio, S., Karavanova, I., Jowett, A. and Thesleff, I. (1993) Identification of BMP-4 as a signal mediating secondary induction between epithelial and mesenchymal tissues during early tooth development. *Cell* **75**, 45–58.

van Genderen, C., Okamura, R.M., Farinas, I. et al (1995) Development of several organs that require inductive epithelial–mesenchymal interactions is impaired in *LEF-1* deficient mice. *Genes Dev.* **8**, 2691–2703.

Vastardis, H., Karimbux, N., Guthua, S.W., Seidman, J.G. and Seidman, C.E. (1996) A human *MSX1* homeodomain missense mutation causes selective tooth agenesis. *Nature Genetics* **13**, 417–421.

Weiss, K.M. (1993) A tooth, a toe and a vertebra: the genetic dimensions of complex morphological traits. *Evol. Anthr.* **2**, 121–134.

Wilkinson, D.G., Bhatt, S. and McMahon, A.P. (1989) Expression pattern of the FGF-related proto-oncogene *int-2* suggests multiple roles in fetal development. *Development* **105**, 131–136.

Witkop, C.J. (1989) Amelogenesis imperfecta, dentinogenesis imperfecta and dentin dysplasia revisited: problems in classification. *J. Oral Pathol. Med.* **17**, 547–553.

Young, W.G., Zhang, C.Z., Li, H., Lobie, P.E. and Waters, M.J. (1993) A bromodeoxy-uridine immunocytochemical and morphometric study of the influence of growth hormone on cell proliferation in odontogenic mesenchyme of the Lewis dwarf rat. *Arch. Oral Biol.* **38**, 207–214.

Index